T0309121

Respiratory Syncytial Virus: Diagnosis and Treatment

Respiratory Syncytial Virus: Diagnosis and Treatment

Editor: Brock Hewson

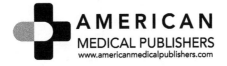

AMERICAN
MEDICAL PUBLISHERS
www.americanmedicalpublishers.com

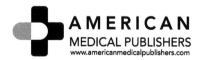

AMERICAN
MEDICAL PUBLISHERS
www.americanmedicalpublishers.com

Cataloging-in-Publication Data

Respiratory syncytial virus : diagnosis and treatment / edited by Brock Hewson.
    p. cm.
Includes bibliographical references and index.
ISBN 978-1-63927-796-4
1. Respiratory syncytial virus. 2. Respiratory syncytial virus--Diagnosis.
3. Respiratory syncytial virus--Treatment. 4. Respiratory organs--Diseases.
I. Hewson, Brock.
RC740 .R473 2023
616.2--dc23

© American Medical Publishers, 2023

American Medical Publishers,
41 Flatbush Avenue,
1st Floor, New York,
NY 11217, USA

ISBN 978-1-63927-796-4 (Hardback)

Contents

Permissions

List of Contributors

Index

Preface

The main aim of this book is to educate learners and enhance their research focus by presenting diverse topics covering this vast field. This is an advanced book which compiles significant studies by distinguished experts in the area of analysis. This book addresses successive solutions to the challenges arising in the area of application, along with it; the book provides scope for future developments.

Respiratory syncytial virus (RSV) is a respiratory virus which results in symptoms similar to cold. This virus spreads through the drops coming from the nose and throat of an infected person, while sneezing and coughing. It can also spread from dried respiratory secretions on the clothes and bed sheets of an infected person. This virus can sustain on hard surfaces for many hours and on skin for a small duration of time. The symptoms of RSV include coughing, fever, sneezing, runny nose, wheezing and loss of appetite. Majority of the people infected from RSV recover within weeks, but it can take a severe form in the case of aged people and infants. There is no treatment for RSV, but its symptoms can be relieved by taking over the counter medicines like ibuprofen and acetaminophen. The symptoms can also be relieved by consuming enough fluids. The topics included in this book on respiratory syncytial virus are of utmost significance and bound to provide incredible insights to readers. Researchers and students in the field engaged in its study will be assisted by it.

It was a great honour to edit this book, though there were challenges, as it involved a lot of communication and networking between me and the editorial team. However, the end result was this all-inclusive book covering diverse themes in the field.

Finally, it is important to acknowledge the efforts of the contributors for their excellent chapters, through which a wide variety of issues have been addressed. I would also like to thank my colleagues for their valuable feedback during the making of this book.

Editor

Diversity and Adaptation of Human Respiratory Syncytial Virus Genotypes Circulating in Two Distinct Communities: Public Hospital and Day Care Center

Luiz Gustavo Araujo Gardinassi [3,†], Paulo Vitor Marques Simas [1,†], Deriane Elias Gomes [2,†], Caroline Measso do Bonfim [1], Felipe Cavassan Nogueira [1], Gustavo Rocha Garcia [3], Claudia Márcia Aparecida Carareto [1], Paula Rahal [1] and Fátima Pereira de Souza [2,*]

[1] Universidade Estadual Paulista, Instituto de Biociências, Letras e Ciências Exatas de São José do Rio Preto, SP. Departamento de Biologia - Rua Cristóvão Colombo, 2265, Jardim Nazareth – Cep: 15054-000, Brazil; E-Mails: simaspvm@yahoo.com.br (P.V.M.S.); carolbonfim@yahoo.com.br (C.M.B.); cavassan@yahoo.com.br (F.C.N.); carareto@ibilce.unesp.br (C.M.A.C.); rahalp@yahoo.com.br (P.R.)
[2] Universidade Estadual Paulista, Instituto de Biociências, Letras e Ciências Exatas de São José do Rio Preto, SP. Departamento de Física - Rua Cristóvão Colombo, 2265, Jardim Nazareth – Cep: 15054-000 Brazil; E-Mail: deribela@yahoo.com.br
[3] Universidade de São Paulo, Faculdade de Medicina de Ribeirão Preto, SP. Departamento de Bioquímica e Imunologia – Av. dos Bandeirantes, 3900 Monte Alegre – Cep: 14049-900 Brazil; E-Mails: gugard@gmail.com (L.G.A.G.); gugarg10@usp.br (G.R.G.)

[†] These authors contributed equally to this work.

[*] Author to whom correspondence should be addressed; E-Mail: fatyssouza@yahoo.com.br

Abstract: HRSV is one of the most important pathogens causing acute respiratory tract diseases as bronchiolitis and pneumonia among infants. HRSV was isolated from two distinct communities, a public day care center and a public hospital in São José do Rio Preto – SP, Brazil. We obtained partial sequences from G gene that were used on phylogenetic and selection pressure analysis. HRSV accounted for 29% of respiratory infections in hospitalized children and 7.7% in day care center children. On phylogenetic analysis of 60 HRSV strains, 48 (80%) clustered within or adjacent to the GA1 genotype; GA5, NA1, NA2, BA-IV and SAB1 were also observed. SJRP GA1 strains presented variations among deduced amino acids composition and lost the potential O-glycosilation site at amino acid position 295, nevertheless this resulted in an insertion of two potential O-glycosilation sites at positions 296 and 297. Furthermore, a potential O-glycosilation site insertion, at position 293, was only observed for hospital strains. Using SLAC and MEME methods, only amino acid 274 was identified to be under positive selection. This is the first report on HRSV circulation and genotypes classification derived from a day care center community in Brazil.

Keywords: respiratory syncytial virus; attachment protein (G); genetic variability; O-glycosilation; selection pressure

---

1. Introduction

Human Respiratory Syncytial Virus (HRSV) is a major viral agent causing serious respiratory tract diseases in the pediatric population worldwide [1]. Of the estimated 2 million children under the age of 5 years who require care for HRSV infections annually, 78% are over the age of 1 year [2], although it has been recognized as a main cause of morbidity in children under 1 year of age [3]. HRSV infection results in several outcomes, ranging from common cold-like symptoms to more severe bronchiolitis and pneumonia in children, immunocompromised and elderly individuals [4,5].

HRSV is classified into the *Pneumovirus* genus of the *Paramyxoviridae* family and is composed of an envelope with a negative-sense single-stranded RNA genome, which encodes for 11 proteins. Based on reactions with monoclonal antibodies against the G and F glycoproteins, beyond molecular differences in several genes [6,7], two major groups, HRSVA and HRSVB, have been described [7–10]. Several HRSVA genotypes were identified in different geographical regions, which include GA1 to GA7 [9,10], SAA1 (South Africa, A1) [11], NA1 and NA2 [12], and most recently ON1 [13]. Thirteen HRSVB genotypes are currently known and designated as GB1 to GB4 [9], SAB1 to SAB3 (South Africa) [11], and BA1 to BA6 (Buenos Aires) [14]. Therefore, the antigenic variability of HRSV strains has been a relevant subject on discussions of the key features contributing to the ability of the virus to re-infect people and cause large-scale yearly outbreaks [15].

The sequence variability of the attachment (G) protein gene, which shows the largest antigenic and genetic differences between the two HRSV groups [16], is commonly used for genotyping HRSVA and HRSVB viruses [13]. The G protein is a type II glycoprotein of 289 to 299 amino acids in length, consisting of the cytoplasmic tail (amino acids [AAs] 1–38), transmembrane domain (AA 38–66), and the ectodomain (AA 66–298) [17]. The C-terminal ectodomain of G protein is comprised of two variable regions, separated by a highly conserved region between amino acids 164 and 176 assumed to represent a receptor-binding site [17]. The two variable regions of the ectodomain contain high serine and threonine residues, which are potential acceptor sites for O-linked sugars affecting the antigenic structure of the G protein as well as impacting on virus infectivity [18,19].

Few studies have evaluated the epidemiology and HRSV genotypes circulating in São Paulo State, Brazil [20–26] and furthermore this is the first report on HRSV genotypes isolated from children attending a day care center in Brazil. Accordingly, we aimed to identify HRSV strains features by analyzing the genetic variability in the second hypervariable region of the attachment (G) gene of viruses isolated from clinical samples collected in a public day care center, and a public hospital in São José do Rio Preto-SP (SJRP), Brazil. Phylogenetic analyses were performed to establish the relation between SJRP′s strains and previously described HRSV genotypes deposited in Genbank and further selection pressure analysis was performed to examine the replacement behavioral patterns of G protein ectodomain encoded amino acids.

2. Results and Discussion

2.1. HRSV Epidemiology and Cohorts Characterization

Brazil is a country of large territorial extension, but few studies have evaluated HRSV circulation patterns and genotypes, which are limited to hospital-based studies performed at Southeast and Northeast regions [20–22,24–26]. Studies including children that attended day care centers have been done mainly in Scandinavia, the United States and England [27], and evidenced that children who attended day care centers from the beginning of infancy present higher risks of respiratory infections comparing to children that did not attend day care centers [28]. Based on these works and due to the lack of informative data, we aimed to understand features, such as the diversity, genotypes and adaptation of HRSV strains circulating in two communities of São José do Rio Preto-SP, Brazil: children that attended a public day care center, and children that were hospitalized due to respiratory infections.

The day care center cohort was composed of 231 children, aged 1 to 78 months (average age of 30.85 months), 44.5% female and 55.5% male, which presented an HRSV frequency of 7.7%. From July 2003 to April 2004, this pathogen was mainly detected and isolated on winter and spring seasons, while in 2005, outbreaks were observed in late autumn and winter seasons. These results contrasts with the previously reported HRSV frequency of 29% [29], detected between May 2004 and September 2005 in clinical samples derived from the hospital, which was composed of 272 children including 57% male and 43% female, whose ages varied between 1 to 68 months. HRSV hospital outbreaks were observed in winter and spring 2004 and autumn 2005 [29].

Such variations on HRSV circulation patterns in both communities may have occurred due to environmental factors such as temperature or relative air humidity, co-circulation and competition with other respiratory pathogens as reported previously in São José do Rio Preto [29] or even due to virulence features as high infectivity and limited antigenic diversity of HRSV strains [30].

Episodes of respiratory infection, on HRSV positive children from the day care center, were characterized by the absence of severe symptoms and were generally limited to upper airways, whit no need of hospitalization during the respiratory infection. The most frequent symptom was runny nose (93.2%), followed by cough (58.2%), nasal obstruction (14.6%), wheezing (3.7%) and fever (2.4%). In contrast, HRSV positive children from the hospital, developed severe diseases such as pneumonia (24.1%), bronchiolitis (64%), and acute wheezing (16.2%) [29]. The most frequent symptoms were cough (93.1%), fever (91%) and coryza (62.1%) and nasal obstruction (50%) [29]. It is evident that strains isolated from the hospital were more pathogenic, accounting for severe symptoms, thus suggesting that multiple lineages co-circulated in São José do Rio Preto.

2.2. Phylogenetic Analysis

In order to understand the diversity and establish the relation between SJRP HRSV strains, we performed phylogenetic analyses of partial sequences obtained from the C-terminal ectodomain of the attachment protein (G) gene (n = 60). Results showed that SJRP's HRSV strains were grouped into three distinct clusters (Supplementary Figure 1) and evidenced the co-circulation of multiple HRSV antigenic groups and genotypes, as reported in several regions of Brazil and São Paulo State [20,21,25,29].

Therefore, we proceeded to an analysis of SJRP's HRSV sequences along with 32 HRSVA and 30 HRSVB reference strains derived from Genbank (Supplementary Table 1), including sequences derived from HRSV isolated in Brazil. The analysis confirmed the co-circulation of both HRSVA and HRSVB antigenic groups, however, most of the sequences (n = 55) were clustered to HRSVA group, while five sequences were associated to HRSVB group (Figure 1). Oliveira and collaborators (2008) also reported a predominance of HRSVA strains over HRSVB in Uberlândia-MG, which agrees with most of the studies performed to identify on antigenic group subtypes, while Cintra and collaborators (2001) have found higher frequencies of both antigenic groups circulating in Ribeirão Preto-SP. Although Ribeirão Preto, Uberlândia and São José do Rio Preto are nearly located (between 200–300 km of distance), different geographical and demographical characteristics must be accounted and also, HRSV antigenic group analysis were performed in different seasons and years, which may contribute for differences on the HRSV subgroups detection.

It has been widely recognized that both subtypes circulate concurrently [31]. Zlateva and collaborators (2004) found the presence of multiple identical sequences among Belgian isolates, which suggested that certain strains predominated in a given epidemic season. Peret and colleagues (2000) also found a dominance of HRSVA over HRSVB, and predominance of 1–2 genotypes in five communities [10]. The predominance of HRSV-A viruses has been attributed to the higher variability among the HRSV-A strains [32]. Usually, the dominant strains shift yearly, suggesting a mechanism for frequent re-infections by evasion of immunity induced by previous strains [33].

Genotype classification through phylogenies demonstrated that SJRP HRSVA isolates, derived from both communities, were more related to GA1 (n = 48), while GA5 (n = 2), NA1 (n = 3), NA2 (n = 2) were detected only in samples from hospitalized children (Figure 1a). These results contrast with previous reports, which showed major prevalence of GA2 genotype during 1999 in Salvador-Ba [21], and during 2004 in Campinas-SP [24]. Interestingly, three Brazilian HRSV reference sequences (RP221/5, BR266-05 and BR292-05), circulating in São Paulo State during 2005 epidemic season, that have been previously described as GA2 genotypes, were clustered together with NA2, a recently identified genotype in Japan, that is genetically close to GA2 [12]. The fact that the three Brazilian strains may be more related to NA2 genotype is supported by the absence of NA2 sequences on phylogenetic analysis performed at the time they were reported, thus contributing to the association with GA2 genotype.

Indeed, inter-continental circulation of HRSV had been reported [14]. Viruses of the BA-I genotype circulated extensively in Buenos Aires from June to August of 1999. In December of the same year, the first BA-I sequence with an exact copy of the duplicated 60 nucleotide segment on the third hypervariable domain of G gene, from a non-Argentinean sample, was found in Belgium. Thus, it is clear that HRSV crossed the Atlantic (in either direction) in a period of few months [14], supporting that NA2 strains may have circulated in Brazil and Japan.

There was a strong phylogenetic association (bootstrapping value of 75%) between sequences obtained from GA1 isolates MMM05C and FAC03C from the day care center with the isolates 7004HB and 27905HB from the hospital. SJRP GA1 isolates were further divided into two major clusters, I and II, which suggested that individual lineages of GA1 genotype could be co-circulating in the period of analysis (Figure 1a), as also proposed by Eshaghi and collaborators (2012), that identified two NA1 lineages circulating in Ontario, Canada.

HRSVB strains were classified as SAB1 (n = 1) (Figure 1b), also reported by Botosso and collaborators (2009) in São Paulo-SP and BA-IV (n = 4). Although, BA genotype had been isolated in Brazil [23], this is the first time HRSVB strains are associated to BA-IV, which was also identified in Buenos Aires, Argentina in 2004 epidemic season, Quebec, Canada through 2001–2003, Kenya in 2003, Belgium in 1999, 2001-2003 [14] and most recently in China through 2006–2009 epidemic seasons [16].

2.3. Molecular Analysis of HRSV GA1 Genotype

By comparing the nucleotide composition and the pattern of mutations among the 60 HRSV isolates, remarkable genetic flexibility could be observed, as previously noted worldwide [31,34–36]. However, two major clusters comprising several groups of identical sequences were identified only among the GA1 genotype strains, thus further analysis were carried out on this group due the lack of sampling of other genotypes. The alignments of nucleotides of the second hypervariable region of HRSV G gene from representative isolates for each GA1 group, compared to the HRSVA reference strain A2 (originally isolated in Australia in 1961), showed possible deletion/insertion sites on nucleotide positions 853, 854, 864, 865, 866 and 879 of the day care center strains, and on nucleotide position 877 of hospital strains (Supplementary Figure 2). Consequently, these variations accounted for changes on the deduced amino acid sequences of SJRP's GA1 isolates, compared to A2 strain amino acid sequence. High variability of day care center sequences was observed mainly from residue 285 to 299, contrasting to hospital sequences which present high variability from residue 293 to the 299 (Figure 2). Such diversification is expected since a high level of genetic variation may be associated with the fact the G protein plays a key role in facilitating re-infections in HRSV—allowing evasion from cross-protective immune responses—and hence in the fluctuating patterns of viral circulation [25].

Since the two variable regions of the ectodomain contain high serine and threonine residues, which are potential acceptor sites for O-linked sugars affecting the antigenic structure of the G protein as well as impacting on virus infectivity [18,19], we performed an O-glycosylation site analysis on deduced aminoacid sequences from SJRP GA1 isolates. Third four sites were potentially O-glycosylated, among GA1 strains isolated from the day care center, while hospital GA1 strains retrieved third five potentially O-glycolsilated sites (G scores of 0.5–0.7) (Figure 2). Several amino acid positions that are likely to have O linked side chains (serine at 267, 270, 275, 283, 287 and threonine at 227, 231, 235, 253, and 282), reported by [37] were conserved in all SJRP GA1 isolates. SJRP GA1 strains lost the potential O-glycosilation site at amino acid position 295, nevertheless this resulted in an insertion of two potential O-glycosilation sites at positions 296 and 297. Furthermore, a potential O-glycosilation site insertion, at position 293, was only observed for hospital strains. It is possible that strains that have lost or changed O glycosylation can escape the immune system by losing recognition of a carbohydrate epitope [38]. We also performed N-glycosylation site analysis, which resulted in potential for N-glycosilation at sites 237 (G score of 0.6340) and 251 (G score of 0.5601). These sites were conserved among all SJRP sequences.

Eshaghi and colleagues (2012) found 21 and 27 potentially O-glycosylation sites in ON/RSV89 and ON/RSV181 (GA5 genotypes isolates) respectively, whereas an average of 33 sites were potentially O-glycosylated in NA1 isolates. By analyzing the same region, four putative N-glycosylation sites (Asn-X-Ser/Thr) were identified among Ontario circulating strains. Zlateva and collaborators (2004) predicted that serine residues at sites 117 and 290 are O glycosylated with a high potential and the positive selected threonine residue at site 225 was also predicted to be O- glycosylated (GA2 and GA5 genotypes).

Figure 1. (a) Phylogenetic tree of José do Rio Preto-SP (SJRP) HRSVA nucleotide sequences of 265–270 in length, from the second variable region of the G gene. Reference strains representing known genotypes are indicated by a solid circle. SW8/60 (subtype B) was used as outgroup, marked by an open square. (b) Phylogenetic tree of SJRP HRSVB nucleotide sequences from the second variable region of the G gene. Reference strains representing known genotypes are indicated by a solid square. Long (subtype A) was used as outgroup, marked by an open circle. Multiple sequences alignment and phylogenetic tree was constructed using Clustal W and Neighbor-joining method running within MEGA 5.05 software. Tree topology was supported by bootstrap analysis with 1000 pseudo replicate datasets. Bootstrap values greater than 50 are shown at the branch nodes. HB refers to strains isolated from the hospital (indicated by a solid lozenge) and C refers to strains isolated in the day care center (indicated by an open triangle).

(a) HRSVA

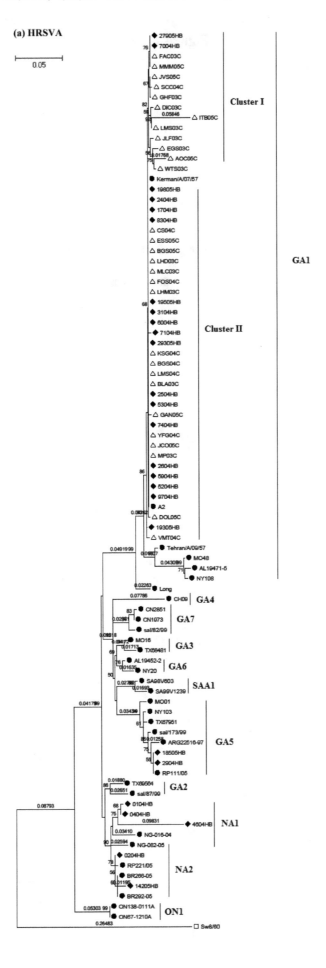

Figure 1. *Cont.*

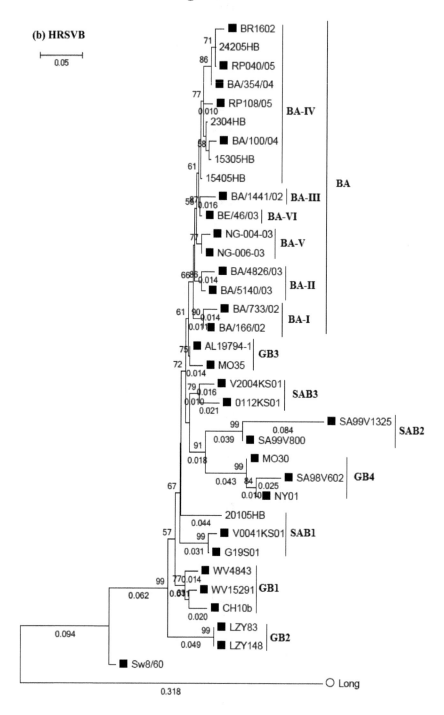

Figure 2. Alignment of deduced amino acid sequence of the G protein of HRSV GA1 genotype strains isolated in São José do Rio Preto-SP. Alignments are shown relative to the sequence of prototype strain A2. The amino acids shown correspond to positions 212 to 298 of the second hypervariable region of HRSVA strain A2 G protein. The alignment was done by the Clustal W algorithm running with BioEdit. Identical residues are represented as dots. Potential O-glycosylation sites conserved between HRSVA strain A2 and SJRP GA1 isolates are shaded in red. Potential O-glycosylation sites present only on SJRP GA1 isolates are shaded in yellow.

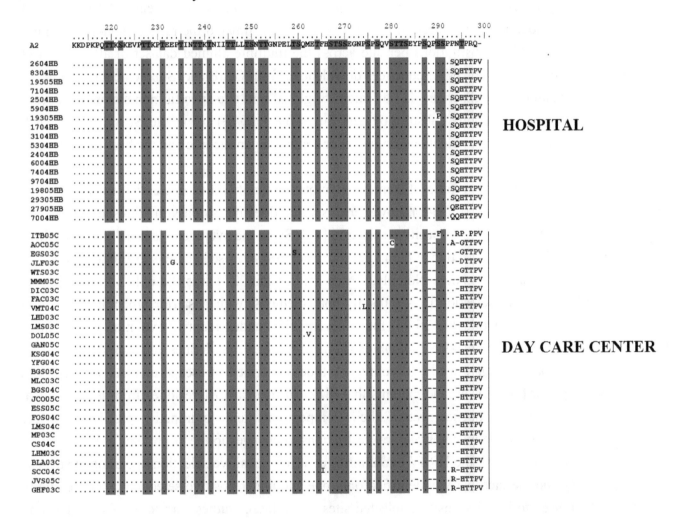

Virus infectivity has been shown to be sensitive to the limited removal of N-linked or O-linked oligosaccharides [19]. Thus, sequence changes may influence the location of carbohydrate side chains, which are important determinants of the G glycoprotein antigenic structure [38]. Modifications observed on nucleotide sequences and consequently on the deduced amino acid residues composing the G protein ectodomain (Supplementary Figure 2 and Figure 2) of SJRP GA1 strains, also accounted for changes on potential O-glycosylation sites, thus suggesting that hospital and day care center strains could have different patterns of replication and virulence.

2.4. Selective Pressure

The second hypervariable region of HRSV G gene has been reported to be an important domain of diversity and adaptation between HRSV strains [17,25,38,39]. Therefore, in order to test neutrality deviations on SJRP GA1 strains and obtain first evidence of selection pressure action on this region of the G gene, we performed the Tajima's Neutrality Test [40], which resulted in D value: $-2,32187$ with a p-value < 0.001 and thus suggested the occurrence of sites under positive/purifying selection on GA1 genotype circulating in São José do Rio Preto (Table 1).

To test the hypothesis that the C-terminal hypervariable region of G proteins of SJRP's GA1 isolates could be under action of selection pressure forces, we estimated the ratio of non-synonymous (dN) to synonymous (dS) substitutions per site across the multiple aligned dataset of all SJRP GA1 sequences, including all 32 HRSVA sequences downloaded from GenBank (Supplementary Table 1). We used the Datamonkey webserver [41] to calculate global and site-specific non-synonymous (d_N) and synonymous (d_S) nucleotide substitution rate ratios ($\omega = d_N/d_S$) using the SLAC and MEME methods, which are based on a neighbor-joining generated phylogenetic tree and the best-fit nucleotide substitution model.

We observed a high average ratio of non-synonymous to synonymous nucleotide substitutions in the G glycoprotein gene ($\omega = 0. 0.645$), however this value does not surpass the threshold of $\omega > 1$, and it is therefore not indicative of positive selection [42]. Since the average ω is usually not sensitive enough to detect Darwinian selection at the molecular level [38], we used codon substitution models to detect sites under positive selection. Notably, amino acid residue 274 was the only site found to be subject of robust positive selection ($p < 0.05$) by both methods, with posterior probability of 1.000 (100%). In fact, previous works [13,25,43] found several sites under adaptive evolution within the G protein, including amino acid residue 274, which is one of the sites that defines genotypes and lineages within genotypes, and correlate well with known epitopes described in escape-mutants selected with specific Mabs [44,45]. HRSV escape mutants that differ in their last 81 residues from the canonical Long prototype protein sequence, retain their compositions and hydropathy profiles, strongly suggesting that there may be indeed structural restrictions to changes in the G protein [25]. According to previous works [13,38,43], the HRSV evolution is driven by positive selection operating at specific codon positions and the fact that we identified only one site under positive selection could be due to the method we used to identify positive selected sites, since these studies carried out the analysis on the PAML program.

Table 1. Nucleotide diversity (π), Tajima D test (D), genetic distances (d) and statistical significance for Tajima D test (p) of identified human respiratory syncytial virus (HRSV) strains and GA1 genotype.

HRSV	N	Π	D	d	p
A	55	0.03465	−2.14299	0.048	p < 0.05
B	5	0.03878	−0.85185	0.040	p > 0.10
GA1	48	0.00924	−2.32187	0.010	p < 0.01

3. Experimental Procedures

3.1. Cohorts and Clinical Specimens

A total of 1,089 respiratory samples were obtained from children aged between 0 and 6 years in the period of July 2003 to September 2005. Two cohorts were included, one composed of children that were hospitalized at São José do Rio Preto Public Hospital (HB) (272 samples), presenting lower respiratory tract diseases (such as bronchiolitis and pneumonia), and another composed of children presenting acute respiratory infections (ARI) (characterized by single or combined occurrence of the following physical signs and symptoms: cough, pharyngitis, rhinorrhea, nasal congestion, headache, low grade fever, facial pressure and sneezing), that attended the Maria Ines Arnal Day Care Center (C) (817 samples) in São José do Rio Preto-SP, Brazil. Nasopharyngeal washes were obtained after instillation of 0.5 mL of sterile PBS (Phosphate Buffered Saline - NaCl, Na2HPO4, NaH2PO4) into each nostril with immediate aspiration through a sterile neonatal canula inserted into the child's nasopharynx. The sample was transferred to a sterile vial and immediately transported to the laboratory, processed and frozen at −80 °C in Trizol LS (Invitrogen, Carlsbad, CA) for later RNA extraction and RT-PCR testing.

3.2. Viral Detection and Nucleotide Sequencing

Total RNA was extracted from nasopharyngeal washes using guanidinium isothiocyanate phenol (Trizol LS, InvitrogenH, Carlsbad, CA, USA) according to the manufacturer's instructions. Reverse transcription was performed with High Capacity cDNA Archive Kit – Applied Biosystems (USA) according to the manufacturer's instructions.

Partial HRSV G gene amplification was performed by a semi-nested PCR procedure. First, cDNA was amplified using the primer FV: 5′- GTTATGACACTGGTATACCAACC-3′ (based on sequences complementary to nucleotides 186 to 163 of the F protein gene [46] – and the forward primer GAB: 5`- YCAYTTTGAAGTGTTCAACTT-3′ (G gene, 504–524 nt). A semi-nested PCR was then performed with primers F1AB 5`- CAACTCCATTGTTATTTGCC-3′ (F gene, 3–22 nt) and GAB [9,10]. PCR assay was carried out in a reaction mixture containing 200 ng of cDNA, 1 mM MgCl2, 0,2 mM dNTPs, 20 pmol of each primer, 2 U of Taq DNA Polimerase (Biotools, ESP) in a final volume of 50 μL. Amplification was performed in a GeneAmp PCR System 9700 thermocycler (Applied Biosystems Inc.) with the following parameters: 95 °C for 5 min, followed by 40 cycles of 1 min at 94 °C, 1 min at 55 °C and 1 min at 72 °C, and finally 7 min of extension at 72 °C.

The semi nested PCR was carried under the same conditions, with 20 pmol of each primer on a final volume of 50 μL. Both cDNA synthesis and PCR followed strict procedures to prevent contamination, including redundant negative controls and segregated environments for pre- and post-amplification procedures. Amplified products of the G gene were purified with a commercial kit (Qiagen PCR Purification Kit (Qiagen – USA)), according to the manufacturer's instructions.

Sanger sequencing, of a 490-bp fragment of the G gene, was carried out with the same primer pair used for semi-nested PCR amplification on the ABI PRISM 3100 and 377 DNA sequencers (Applied Biosystems Inc.) using the BigDye Terminator v3.1 cycle sequencing kit (Applied Biosystems).

3.3. Phylogenetic Analysis

Sequences were assembled with the Sequence Navigator program version 1.0 (Applied Biosystems Inc., EUA) resulting in contigs of 265 nucleotides on average, to isolates from the day care center, and contigs of 270 and 330 nucleotides on average to isolates from the hospital. These contigs were compared to HRSV G gene nucleotides from reference strains representing different HRSVA and HRSVB genotypes identified in other cities or states of Brazil, South America, South Africa as well as HRSV sequences from other countries available at GenBank (Supplementary Table 1). Multiple sequence alignments of the obtained fragments compared to globally sampled reference strains were performed using the Clustal W algorithm [47] and Bioedit sequence alignment-editing software. Phylogenetic associations were determined using Maximum Likelihood (ML) and Neighbor-Joining (NJ) methods running with MEGA 5.05 software [48]. Node support of each clade was evaluated using bootstrap analysis (1000 replicates) and the evolutionary distances were derived using the Kimura-2 parameter method [49].

3.4. O-glycosylation and N-glycosilation Site Analysis

Potential O-glycosylation and N-glycosylation sites were predicted using and NetOGlyc 3.1 [50] and NetNGlyc 1.0. The deduced AA sequences of the second hypervariable region of HRSV GA1 genotypes (encompassing AA 212 to the end of the G protein) were compared to those of HRSV-A2 strain.

3.5. Selection Pressure Analysis

Neutrality Tajima's D test [40] was performed by DnaSP version 5.10.01 software [51] to verify statistically significant deviations among sequences and provide first evidence of selection acting on SJRP HRSV isolates.

To determine the selection pressures acting on the ectodomain of the G gene of GA1 genotype isolates, we estimated the numbers of non-synonymous (dN) to synonymous (dS) nucleotide changes per site; when dN>dS, this was indicative of positive selection. Site-specific (that is, codon-specific) selection pressures were determined using the Single Likelihood Ancestral Counting (SLAC) available in the HyPhy package [52] and Mixed Effects Model of Evolution (MEME) [53] methods, accessed through the Datamonkey webserver [41]. These methods were run using best fit nucleotide model on a neighbor-joining phylogenetic tree. Using this procedure, only codon 274 contained statistically significant evidence for positive selection.

3.6. Ethics Statement

A Written Consent signed by the parents or legal responsible guardians was obtained for each child. This study was approved by Research Ethics Committee from Unesp/IBILCE, Project Number 3777/2001 by opinion n° 062/2001 on 11 June 2001 in São José do Rio Preto, Brazil.

Acknowledgments

The authors have received financial support from FAPESP, process n°. 2010/50444-4.

References

1. Glezen, P.; Denny, F.W. Epidemiology of acute lower respiratory disease in children. *N. Engl. J. Med.* **1973**, *288*, 498–505.
2. Hall, C.B.; Weinberg, G.A.; Iwane, M.K.; Blumkin, A.K.; Edwards, K.M.; Staat, M.A.; Auinger, P.; Griffin, M.R.; Poehling, K.A.; Erdman, D.; *et al.* The burden of respiratory syncytial virus infection in young children. *N. Engl. J. Med.* **2009**, *360*, 588–598.
3. Anderson, L.J.; Parker, R.A.; Strikas, R.L. Association between respiratory syncytial virus outbreaks and lower respiratory tract deaths of infants and young children. *J. Infect. Dis.* **1990**, *161*, 640–646.
4. Falsey, A.R.; Walsh, E.E. Respiratory syncytial virus infection in adults. *Clin. Microbiol. Rev.* **2000**, *13*, 371–384.
5. Widjojoatmodjo, M.N.; Boes, J.; van Bers, M.; van Remmerden, Y.; Roholl, P.J.; Luytjes, W. A highly attenuated recombinant human respiratory syncytial virus lacking the G protein induces long-lasting protection in cotton rats. *Virol. J.* **2010**, *7*, 114.
6. Cane, P.A. Molecular epidemiology of respiratory syncytial virus. *Rev. Med. Virol.* **2001**, *11*, 103–116.
7. Mufson, M.A.; Orvell, C.; Rafnar, B.; Norrby, E. Two distinct subtypes of human respiratory syncytial virus. *J. Gen. Virol.* **1985**, *66 (Pt 10)*, 2111–2124.
8. Anderson, L.J.; Hierholzer, J.C.; Tsou, C.; Hendry, R.M.; Fernie, B.F.; Stone, Y.; McIntosh, K. Antigenic characterization of respiratory syncytial virus strains with monoclonal antibodies. *J. Infect. Dis.* **1985**, *151*, 626–633.
9. Peret, T.C.; Hall, C.B.; Schnabel, K.C.; Golub, J.A.; Anderson, L.J. Circulation patterns of genetically distinct group A and B strains of human respiratory syncytial virus in a community. *J. Gen. Virol.* **1998**, *79 (Pt 9)*, 2221–2229.

10. Peret, T.C.; Hall, C.B.; Hammond, G.W.; Piedra, P.A.; Storch, G.A.; Sullender, W.M.; Tsou, C.; Anderson, L.J. Circulation patterns of group A and B human respiratory syncytial virus genotypes in 5 communities in North America. *J. Infect. Dis.* **2000**, *181*, 1891–1896.

11. Venter, M.; Madhi, S.A.; Tiemessen, C.T.; Schoub, B.D. Genetic diversity and molecular epidemiology of respiratory syncytial virus over four consecutive seasons in South Africa: Identification of new subgroup A and B genotypes. *J. Gen. Virol.* **2001**, *82*, 2117–2124.

12. Shobugawa, Y.; Saito, R.; Sano, Y.; Zaraket, H.; Suzuki, Y.; Kumaki, A.; Dapat, I.; Oguma, T.; Yamaguchi, M.; Suzuki, H. Emerging genotypes of human respiratory syncytial virus subgroup A among patients in Japan. *J. Clin. Microbiol.* **2009**, *47*, 2475–2482.

13. Eshaghi, A.; Duvvuri, V.R.; Lai, R.; Nadarajah, J.T.; Li, A.; Patel, S.N.; Low, D.E.; Gubbay, J.B. Genetic variability of human respiratory syncytial virus a strains circulating in ontario: A novel genotype with a 72 nucleotide G gene duplication. *PLoS One* **2012**, *7*, e32807.

14. Trento, A.; Viegas, M.; Galiano, M.; Videla, C.; Carballal, G.; Mistchenko, A.S.; Melero, J.A. Natural history of human respiratory syncytial virus inferred from phylogenetic analysis of the attachment (G) glycoprotein with a 60-nucleotide duplication. *J. Virol.* **2006**, *80*, 975–984.

15. Sullender, W.M. Respiratory syncytial virus genetic and antigenic diversity. *Clin. Microbiol. Rev.* **2000**, *13*, 1–15.

16. Zhang, R.F.; Jin, Y.; Xie, Z.P.; Liu, N.; Yan, K.L.; Gao, H.C.; Song, J.R.; Yuan, X.H.; Xiao, N.G.; Guo, M.W.; *et al.* Human respiratory syncytial virus in children with acute respiratory tract infections in China. *J. Clin. Microbiol.* **2010**, *48*, 4193–4199.

17. Johnson, P.R.; Spriggs, M.K.; Olmsted, R.A.; Collins, P.L. The G glycoprotein of human respiratory syncytial viruses of subgroups A and B: Extensive sequence divergence between antigenically related proteins. *Proc. Natl. Acad. Sci. USA* **1987**, *84*, 5625–5629.

18. Garcia-Beato, R.; Martinez, I.; Franci, C.; Real, F.X.; Garcia-Barreno, B.; Melero, J.A. Host cell effect upon glycosylation and antigenicity of human respiratory syncytial virus G glycoprotein. *Virology* **1996**, *221*, 301–309.

19. Lambert, D.M. Role of oligosaccharides in the structure and function of respiratory syncytial virus glycoproteins. *Virology* **1988**, *164*, 458–466.

20. Cintra, O.A.; Owa, M.A.; Machado, A.A.; Cervi, M.C.; Figueiredo, L.T.; Rocha, G.M.; Siqueira, M.M.; Arruda, E. Occurrence and severity of infections caused by subgroup A and B respiratory syncytial virus in children in southeast Brazil. *J. Med. Virol.* **2001**, *65*, 408–412.

21. Moura, F.E.; Blanc, A.; Frabasile, S.; Delfraro, A.; de Sierra, M.J.; Tome, L.; Ramos, E.A.; Siqueira, M.M.; Arbiza, J. Genetic diversity of respiratory syncytial virus isolated during an epidemic period from children of northeastern Brazil. *J. Med. Virol.* **2004**, *74*, 156–160.

22. Oliveira, T.F.; Freitas, G.R.; Ribeiro, L.Z.; Yokosawa, J.; Siqueira, M.M.; Portes, S.A.; Silveira, H.L.; Calegari, T.; Costa, L.F.; Mantese, O.C.; *et al.* Prevalence and clinical aspects of respiratory syncytial virus A and B groups in children seen at Hospital de Clinicas of Uberlandia, MG, Brazil. *Mem. Inst. Oswaldo Cruz* **2008**, *103*, 417–422.

23. Da Silva, L.H.; Spilki, F.R.; Riccetto, A.G.; de Almeida, R.S.; Baracat, E.C.; Arns, C.W. Genetic variability in the G protein gene of human respiratory syncytial virus isolated from the Campinas metropolitan region, Brazil. *J. Med. Virol.* **2008**, *80*, 1653–1660.

24. Riccetto, A.G.; Silva, L.H.; Spilki, F.R.; Morcillo, A.M.; Arns, C.W.; Baracat, E.C. Genotypes and clinical data of respiratory syncytial virus and metapneumovirus in brazilian infants: A new perspective. *Braz. J. Infect. Dis.* **2009**, *13*, 35–39.

25. Botosso, V.F.; Zanotto, P.M.; Ueda, M.; Arruda, E.; Gilio, A.E.; Vieira, S.E.; Stewien, K.E.; Peret, T.C.; Jamal, L.F.; Pardini, M.I.; *et al.* Positive selection results in frequent reversible amino acid replacements in the G protein gene of human respiratory syncytial virus. *PLoS Pathog.* **2009**, *5*, e1000254.

26. Lima, H.N.; Botosso, V.F.; Oliveira, D.B.; Campos, A.C.; Leal, A.L.; Silva, T.S.; Bosso, P.A.; Moraes, C.T.; Filho, C.G.; Vieira, S.E.; *et al.* Molecular epidemiology of the SH (small hydrophobic) gene of human respiratory syncytial virus (HRSV), over 2 consecutive years. *Virus Res.* **2012**, *163*, 82–86.

27. McCutcheon, H.; Fitzgerald, M. The public health problem of acute respiratory illness in childcare. *J. Clin. Nurs.* **2001**, *10*, 305–310.

28. Lu, N.; Samuels, M.E.; Shi, L.; Baker, S.L.; Glover, S.H.; Sanders, J.M. Child day care risks of common infectious diseases revisited. *Child Care Health Dev.* **2004**, *30*, 361–368.

29. Gardinassi, L.G.A.; Simas, P.V.M.; Salomão, J.B.; Durigon, E.L.; Trevisan, D.M.Z.; Cordeiro, J.A.; Lacerda, M.N.; Rahal, P.; Souza, F.P. Seasonality of viral respiratory infections in Southeast of Brazil: The influence of temperature and air humidity. *Braz. J. Microbiol.* **2012**, *43*, 98–108.

30. Collins, P.L.; Graham, B.S. Viral and host factors in human respiratory syncytial virus pathogenesis. *J. Virol.* **2008**, *82*, 2040–2055.

31. Hall, C.B.; Walsh, E.E.; Schnabel, K.C.; Long, C.E.; McConnochie, K.M.; Hildreth, S.W.; Anderson, L.J. Occurrence of groups A and B of respiratory syncytial virus over 15 years: Associated epidemiologic and clinical characteristics in hospitalized and ambulatory children. *J. Infect. Dis.* **1990**, *162*, 1283–1290.

32. Mufson, M.A.; Belshe, R.B.; Orvell, C.; Norrby, E. Respiratory syncytial virus epidemics: Variable dominance of subgroups A and B strains among children, 1981–1986. *J. Infect. Dis.* **1988**, *157*, 143–148.

33. Hall, C.B. Respiratory syncytial virus and parainfluenza virus. *N. Engl. J. Med.* **2001**, *344*, 1917–1928.

34. Matthijnssens, J.; Rahman, M.; van Ranst, M. Loop model: Mechanism to explain partial gene duplications in segmented dsRNA viruses. *Biochem. Biophys. Res. Commun.* **2006**, *340*, 140–144.

35. Ballard, A.; McCrae, M.A.; Desselberger, U. Nucleotide sequences of normal and rearranged RNA segments 10 of human rotaviruses. *J. Gen. Virol.* **1992**, *73 (Pt 3)*, 633–638.

36. Kojima, K.; Taniguchi, K.; Kawagishi-Kobayashi, M.; Matsuno, S.; Urasawa, S. Rearrangement generated in double genes, NSP1 and NSP3, of viable progenies from a human rotavirus strain. *Virus Res.* **2000**, *67*, 163–171.

37. Collins, P.L.; Chanock, R.M.; Murphy, B.R. Respiratory syncytial virus. In *Fields Virology*, 4th ed.; Howley, D.M.K.P.M., Ed.; Lippincott Williams & Wilkins: Philadelphia, PA, USA, 2001; pp. 1443–1485.

38. Zlateva, K.T.; Lemey, P.; Vandamme, A.M.; van Ranst, M. Molecular evolution and circulation patterns of human respiratory syncytial virus subgroup a: Positively selected sites in the attachment g glycoprotein. *J. Virol.* **2004**, *78*, 4675–4683.

39. Zlateva, K.T.; Lemey, P.; Moes, E.; Vandamme, A.M.; van Ranst, M. Genetic variability and molecular evolution of the human respiratory syncytial virus subgroup B attachment G protein. *J. Virol.* **2005**, *79*, 9157–9167.

40. Tajima, F. Statistical method for testing the neutral mutation hypothesis by DNA polymorphism. *Genetics* **1989**, *123*, 585–595.

41. Pond, S.L.K.; Frost, S.D.W. Datamonkey: Rapid detection of selective pressure on individual sites of codon alignments. *Bioinformatics* **2005**, *21*, 2531–2533.

42. Yang, Z.; Nielsen, R.; Goldman, N.; Pedersen, A.M. Codon-substitution models for heterogeneous selection pressure at amino acid sites. *Genetics* **2000**, *155*, 431–449.

43. Gaunt, E.R.; Jansen, R.R.; Poovorawan, Y.; Templeton, K.E.; Toms, G.L.; Simmonds, P. Molecular epidemiology and evolution of human respiratory syncytial virus and human metapneumovirus. *PLoS One* **2011**, *6*, e17427.

44. Garcia, O.; Martin, M.; Dopazo, J.; Arbiza, J.; Frabasile, S.; Russi, J.; Hortal, M.; Perez-Brena, P.; Martinez, I.; Garcia-Barreno, B.; *et al.* Evolutionary pattern of human respiratory syncytial virus (subgroup A): Cocirculating lineages and correlation of genetic and antigenic changes in the G glycoprotein. *J. Virol.* **1994**, *68*, 5448–5459.

45. Rueda, P.; Delgado, T.; Portela, A.; Melero, J.A.; Garcia-Barreno, B. Premature stop codons in the G glycoprotein of human respiratory syncytial viruses resistant to neutralization by monoclonal antibodies. *J. Virol.* **1991**, *65*, 3374–3378.

46. Zheng, H.; Peret, T.C.; Randolph, V.B.; Crowley, J.C.; Anderson, L.J. Strain-specific reverse transcriptase PCR assay: Means to distinguish candidate vaccine from wild-type strains of respiratory syncytial virus. *J. Clin. Microbiol.* **1996**, *34*, 334–337.

47. Thompson, J.D.; Higgins, D.G.; Gibson, T.J. CLUSTAL W: Improving the sensitivity of progressive multiple sequence alignment through sequence weighting, position-specific gap penalties and weight matrix choice. *Nucleic Acids Res.* **1994**, *22*, 4673–4680.

48. Tamura, K.; Peterson, D.; Peterson, N.; Stecher, G.; Nei, M.; Kumar, S. MEGA5: Molecular evolutionary genetics analysis using maximum likelihood, evolutionary distance, and maximum parsimony methods. *Mol. Biol. Evol.* **2011**, *28*, 2731–2739.

49. Kimura, M. A simple method for estimating evolutionary rates of base substitutions through comparative studies of nucleotide sequences. *J. Mol. Evol.* **1980**, *16*, 111–120.

50. Julenius, K.; Molgaard, A.; Gupta, R.; Brunak, S. Prediction, conservation analysis, and structural characterization of mammalian mucin-type O-glycosylation sites. *Glycobiology* **2005**, *15*, 153–164.

51. Librado, P.; Rozas, J. DnaSP v5: A software for comprehensive analysis of DNA polymorphism data. *Bioinformatics* **2009**, *25*, 1451–1452.
52. Pond, S.L.; Frost, S.D.; Muse, S.V. HyPhy: Hypothesis testing using phylogenies. *Bioinformatics* **2005**, *21*, 676–679.
53. Murrell, B.; Wertheim, J.O.; Moola, S.; Weighill, T.; Scheffler, K.; Kosakovsky Pond, S.L. Detecting individual sites subject to episodic diversifying selection. *PLoS Genet.* **2012**, *8*, e1002764.

2

Dendritic Cells in Human *Pneumovirus* and *Metapneumovirus* Infections

Antonieta Guerrero-Plata [1,2]

[1] Department of Pathobiological Sciences, Louisiana State University, Baton Rouge, LA 70803, USA; E-Mail: aguerrp@lsu.edu
[2] Center for Experimental Infectious Disease Research, Louisiana State University, Baton Rouge, LA 70803, USA

Abstract: Lung dendritic cells (DC) play a fundamental role in sensing invading pathogens, as well as in the control of tolerogenic responses in the respiratory tract. Their strategic localization at the site of pathogen entry makes them particularly susceptible to initial viral invasion. Human respiratory syncytial virus (hRSV) and human metapneumovirus (hMPV) belong to the *Paramyxoviridae* family, within the *Pneumovirus* and *Metapneumovirus* genera, respectively. hRSV and hMPV are significant human respiratory pathogens that cause similar clinical manifestations and affect many of the same subpopulations. However, they differentially activate the host immune response, including DC, which represents a fundamental link between the innate and adaptive immune response. In this review, the role of DC in the immune response against hRSV and hMPV infections, as well as the inhibitory effects of these paramyxoviruses on the DC immunity will be discussed.

Keywords: dendritic cells; human metapneumovirus; respiratory syncytial virus; lung; paramyxovirus

1. Introduction

Human respiratory syncytial virus (hRSV) and human metapneumovirus (hMPV) are classified within the *Paramyxoviridae* family, *Pneumovirinae* subfamily, which is divided into the *Pneumovirus* and the *Metapneumovirus* genera. Both viruses belong to the order Mononegavirales and contain a nonsegmented, negative-sense RNA with genomic organization, which is similar, but not identical [1–4]. Metapneumoviruses lack the nonstructural proteins NS1 and NS2, and the gene order is different from that of pneumoviruses. hRSV is the type species of the *Pneumovirus* genus, while (based on the biological properties and genomic sequence) hMPV has been assigned to the *Metapneumovirus* genus. hRSV encodes 11 proteins (nonstructural (NS) protein1, NS2, nucleocapsid (N), phosphoprotein (P), matrix (M)1, small hydrophobic (SH), attachment (G), fusion (F), M2-1, M2-2 and polymerase (L), Figure 1), while hMPV encodes nine proteins (N, P, M1, F, M2-1, M2-2, SH, G and L, Figure 1).

Figure 1. Schematic representation of human *Pneumovirus* and *Metapneumovirus*. Gene maps and encoded proteins of members of the subfamily Pneumovirinae: human respiratory syncytial virus (hRSV) and human metapneumovirus (hMPV), which belong to the genera *Pneumovirus* and *Metapneumovirus*, respectively. Genes are represented as boxes with the corresponding encoded protein.

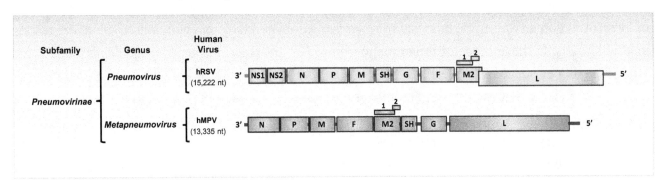

hRSV was first isolated in 1956 from an infected chimpanzee [5] and represents the most important cause of bronchiolitis and pneumonia in infants and young children worldwide. More than 95% of children are infected with hRSV by two years of age [1]. hMPV was first identified in 2001 following its isolation from infants and children with lower respiratory tract infections (LTRI) of unknown etiology [2]. Serologic evidence indicated that hMPV seropositivity is almost universal by the age of five years. The clinical manifestations of hMPV infection in young children are indistinguishable from those of hRSV infection. LRTI associated with hMPV in infants and young children is a frequent cause of hospitalization. Several studies indicate that hMPV likely accounts for 5% to 15% of LRTI hospitalizations in infants and young children and is second only to hRSV as a cause of bronchiolitis in early childhood [6–10]. Both viruses can be transmitted mainly by large droplets from infected individuals [11,12], and the incubation period could last between three and seven days for hRSV and four to six days for hMPV [13]. hRSV and hMPV are present year-round, but their incidence increases in the fall, peaks in the winter and goes down in early spring [1,14,15]. Host risk factors for these infections include premature birth, congenital heart disease, immunodeficiency, elderly individuals, gender and Down's syndrome, among others [16–18]. Adults and older children are commonly reinfected without complications by these paramyxoviruses, because the natural infection does not induce lifelong immunological protection. However, it is in infants, elderly and immunosuppressed individuals that severe disease can result [19–21]. Currently, there are no vaccines available against hRSV or hMPV. However, infected individuals can be treated with ribavirin and immunoglobulins [22].

Knowledge of the critical aspects of the host immune response to these infections has been crucial to understanding the pathology associated with hRSV and hMPV infections. In that regard, dendritic cells (DC) play a pivotal role in shaping antiviral immune response in the respiratory tract, as they represent the perfect link between innate and adaptive immune response [23–25]. Although the mechanisms underlying the activation of these cells by paramyxovirus infections still is largely unknown, substantial progress towards our understanding of the DC response to hRSV has been made, and the role of these cells in hMPV infection has also been explored.

2. Dendritic Cells in the Respiratory Tract

Dendritic cells are professional antigen-presenting cells within the immune system. They arise from both myeloid and lymphoid progenitors within the bone marrow and are widely distributed (as immature DC) into both lymphoid and nonlymphoid tissues [26–28]. Respiratory tract dendritic cells are present within airway epithelium, submucosa and associated lung parenchymal tissue under resting conditions [29]. In the absence of inflammation, lung DC are present at an average density of several hundred cells per square millimeter in the large airways, decreasing to less than a hundred DC per square millimeter within smaller intrapulmonary airways [30]. Pulmonary DC have a rapid turnover, with a half-life of ≤2 days [30,31]. Their strategic localization at the site of pathogen entry makes them particularly susceptible to initial viral invasion. After detection, uptake and degradation of viruses, DC initiate immune responses via the secretion of interferon, chemokines and proinflammatory cytokines, as well as the upregulation of a variety of costimulatory molecules and receptors, a process globally known as cell maturation. After maturation, DC efficiently present antigens and initiate adaptive immune response by migrating into lymph nodes (LN) to activate the virus-specific T-cell response [32].

3. Activation and Inhibition of DC Infected with hRSV and hMPV *in Vitro*

3.1. DC Maturation and Cytokine Production

DC maturation is necessary for the transition from innate to adaptive immunity. In human monocyte-derived DC (moDC), hRSV and hMPV are able to induce cell maturation, indicated by an upregulation of MHC class I and class II molecules, as well as the overexpression of CD80, CD86, CD38 and CD83 [33–37]. Cytokine production by these cells is differentially induced by hRSV and hMPV, hRSV being a more potent inducer of IL-10, TNF-α, IL-1β and IL-12p70, while hMPV induces a more robust response of type I IFN than hRSV. IFN induction is dependent of viral replication, as UV-inactivated virus failed to induce IFN in hRSV- or hMPV-infected cells [34–36,38]. The response of human primary blood myeloid DC to hRSV has also been characterized, and it resembles that of moDC [39]. hRSV also induces maturation in mouse DC. Bone marrow-derived DC (BMDC) exhibited an increased expression of CD40, CD80, CD86, MHC class I and class II and higher production of IL-6, IL-10 and IL-12p70. Consistent with reports in human cells, hRSV replication was required also for DC maturation [40]. However, DC are not highly permissive to hRSV or hMPV infections, regardless of their source (PBMCs, cord-blood or primary DC), as demonstrated by the low percentage (4% to 25%) of antigen positive cells by flow cytometry analysis [33–37,39,41]. This suggests a critical role of the virus-induced cytokines, such as type I IFN, during the maturation process, as reported in BMDC [42]. Infection of plasmacytoid *dendritic cells* (pDC) by hRSV and hMPV induce differential expression of cytokines and chemokines. As in moDC, hRSV is a more potent inducer of IL-6, IL-10, GM-CSF, TNF-α, IL-1β, IL-12p70 and G-CSF than hMPV. However, both viruses induce a similar response of IFN-α release in infected pDC [33].

In understanding the mechanisms of activation and maturation by hRSV, Munir *et al.* [43] have reported that the NS proteins of hRSV suppress the expression of costimulatory molecules, as well as the secretion of cytokines and chemokines in human moDC in a type I IFN-dependent process. The inhibitory effect was mediated mostly by NS1 protein, but was enhanced by the combined deletion of NS2 in the same recombinant hRSV virus. More recently, Johnson *et al.* [44] reported that the interaction of hRSV G protein with the DC/L-SIGN (C-type lectins commonly found in DC) inhibits maturation of primary human DC. They found that when this interaction was neutralized with specific antibodies, RSV-infected myeloid DC and pDC increased both maturation and cytokine/chemokine production [44]. The role of cellular mechanisms critical for DC function has also been explored. Morris *et al.* [45] investigated the role of autophagy, a cellular mechanism that involves cell degradation of unnecessary or dysfunctional cellular components [46]. They found that cytokine production and the expression of surface markers (MHC class II, CD40, CD80 and CD86) was inhibited when autophagy was blocked in hRSV-infected BMDC, indicating that autophagy is a critical cellular process for DC maturation during hRSV infection [45].

3.2. Activation and Inhibition of IFN Responses

Interferons (IFNs) are a heterogeneous family of cytokines with demonstrated antiviral, antitumor and immunomodulatory activities. The IFN family includes type I (IFN-α, -β, -ε, -κ and -ω), type II (IFN-γ) and type III (IFN-λ1, -λ2 and -λ3) IFNs [47,48]. Local production of IFNs plays an important defensive role in many respiratory virus infections by limiting viral replication until virus-specific host defense mechanisms develop [49]. It is known that hRSV and hMPV are able to induce and inhibit the IFN response in human and mouse DC. Moreover, they use different molecular mechanisms depending of the DC subset infected (Table 1). The induction of IFN production by RNA viruses is triggered by the activation by several pattern recognition receptors that recognize different viral components. Among them, the cytosolic RNA helicases, retinoic acid-inducible gene (RIG-I) and melanoma differentiation-associated gene 5 (MDA5) play a role in recognizing short or long dsRNA, respectively [50]. Other receptors include Toll-like receptors (TLR3 and TLR7) found in the endosomal compartment, which recognize dsRNA and ssRNA, respectively [51].

As previously reported, both hRSV and hMPV induce a robust response of IFN-α in human pDC, and this production is dependent on viral replication [33,38,52–54]. Using splenic mouse pDC, it has been further demonstrated that IFN production by hMPV is dependent on TLR7 expression [54].

Unlike in pDC, moDC produce IFN-α mostly after infection with hMPV, not with hRSV [33,38]. Using human moDC, previous results from my laboratory have demonstrated that the cytosolic helicase, MDA5, contributes to the production of type I and type III IFNs after hMPV infection. Those observations were further confirmed in an *in vivo* model of infection using MDA5$^{-/-}$ mice [55]. Activation of TLR4 has also been reported to contribute to the production of IFN-β in moDC after hMPV infection [56].

Although the mechanisms underlying the differential activation of IFN response by hRSV and hMPV in moDC have not been fully elucidated, some experimental evidence indicates the involvement of several viral proteins. Munir *et al*. [43] demonstrated that the hRSV NS1 and, to a lesser extent, NS2 protein suppress the expression of IFN-α/β by using recombinant RSVs bearing deletions of the NS1 and/or NS2 protein [43]. In the case of hMPV, it is the expression of the protein G that is responsible for the reduced production of IFN-α/β in infected moDC [56].

hRSV and hMPV infections are also known to subvert the immune responses by interfering with DC functions. The modulating mechanisms of DC immunity by these viruses have been investigated in several *in vitro* systems, including human DC. It has been shown that hRSV and hMPV inhibit the production of IFN-α in human pDC in response to TLR7 and TL9 agonists [33,52] and in moDC after TLR3 activation [33]. In addition, the soluble form of the G protein of hRSV and hMPV has also been reported to block the IFN response after TLR activation in moDC [56,57].

Overall, these data indicate that hRSV and hMPV activate and inhibit the IFN responses in DC, most possibly through different mechanisms. This critical knowledge contributes to our understanding of the molecular mechanisms of hRSV and hMPV immunopathogenesis and may help to explain the lack of protective immunity after natural infection and the multiple reinfections by these viruses.

Table 1. Activation and inhibition of IFN responses by human respiratory syncytial virus (hRSV) and human metapneumovirus (hMPV) in dendritic cells (DC). pDC, plasmacytoid *dendritic cells*; moDC, monocyte-derived DC.

Virus	Effect	DC Subset	References
hRSV	Induce IFN-α	pDC	[33,38,52,53]
hRSV	Blocks TLR7 and TLR9 activation	pDC	[33,52]
hRSV	Blocks TLR3 activation	moDC	[33]
hRSV NS1 and NS2	Suppress IFN-α/β production	moDC	[43]
hRSV soluble G	Blocks TLR3 and TLR4 activation	moDC	[57]
hMPV	Induce IFN-α	pDC	[33,54]
hMPV	Induce IFN-α, β, λ	moDC	[33,55]
hMPV	Activates MDA5	moDC	[55]
hMPV	Activates TLR4	moDC	[56]
hMPV	Activates TLR7	pDC	[54]
hMPV	Blocks TLR7 activation	pDC	[33]
hMPV	Blocks TLR3 activation	moDC	[33]
hMPV G	Suppresses IFN-α/β production	moDC	[56]

3.3. Regulation of T-Cell Responses

Another aspect of the biology of hRSV and hMPV is that they reinfect throughout life, suggesting incomplete or transient immunity [19,58–60]. Several pieces of evidence indicate that hRSV and hMPV interact with dendritic cells and that the primary T-cell response to these viruses is altered significantly by this interaction. Human DC infected with hRSV have shown a severely impaired capacity to stimulate naive CD4$^+$ T-cell proliferation [33,36,61]. The possible mechanisms of this inhibition has been attributed to soluble factors in the supernatant of hRSV-infected dendritic cells [36], as well as to direct contact with RSV-infected cells to inhibit proliferation of T-cells [52,61]. In fact, *Gonzalez et al.* [40] demonstrated, in bone marrow-derived DC (BMDC), that immunological synapse assembly between hRSV-infected DC and T-cells was impaired, supporting the notion that contact is necessary for the inhibition of T-cell activation by hRSV infection [40]. Inhibition of T-cell proliferation by hMPV-infected DC, however, has also been attributed to soluble factors secreted by hMPV-infected DC, but not by interference with DC-T-cell immunological synapse formation [62]. Others have not observed this inhibitory effect using hRSV-infected cord blood-derived DC or moDC cultured with naive T-cells and superantigens [37,63]. Whether this discrepancy in the activation of the T-cells by hRSV-infected cells is related to the different experimental conditions remains to be determined. Further characterization of the interaction between T-cells and hRSV- and hMPV-infected DC is warranted.

4. Response of Human Dendritic Cells to hRSV Infection *in Vivo*

Current characterization of human lung DC populations includes three types of DC: two myeloid DC (mDC) in the lung parenchyma (mDC1 (BDCA-1$^+$/HLA-DR$^+$) and mDC2 (CD11c$^+$/BDCA-3$^+$)) and one pDC subset (CD11c$^-$/BDCA-2$^+$/CD123$^+$/CD14$^-$/HLA-DR$^+$) [64–66]. Additional reports have confirmed the presence of these lung DC subsets in human bronchoalveolar lavage samples [67,68]. However, further characterization of human lung DC populations, under the steady state and in response to stimulus, is needed in order to define the composition of human DC in the lung.

There have been a limited number of studies focused on the DC response to hRSV or hMPV infections in humans. In fact, the response of pulmonary DC in hMPV-infected individuals has not yet been reported. However, despite the human sample limitations, analyses of nasal washes from young children with acute hRSV infection have revealed that hRSV attracts both mDC and pDC to the site of viral entry. The number of pDC, and, to a lesser extent, that of mDC, positively correlates with the viral load in the infected individuals [69]. However, hRSV recruits DC to a lesser extent relative to other relevant respiratory viruses, such as influenza virus [70]. On the other hand, the numbers of mDC and pDC decreased in peripheral blood, suggesting that the increase of mDC and pDC in nasal mucosa results from their migration from the blood [69,70]. In line with those data, Silver E. *et al.* [71] has found that the lower levels of pDC in peripheral blood have been associated with asthma after severe hRSV bronchiolitis [71]. Overall, these data indicate a relevant role of DC in hRSV infection in humans. However, the better understanding of the response of DC to hRSV or hMPV has been revealed from *in vitro* experiments using human and mouse cells and from experimental animal models, specifically, the mouse model.

5. Response of Pulmonary DC in Experimental Mouse Models after hRSV and hMPV Infection

Because the study of the human DC at multiple stages of respiratory viral infections is technically and ethically difficult, the experimental mouse model has provided an excellent opportunity to investigate the response of DC *in vivo*. To date, there have been at least three major subsets of murine lung DC described. These include plasmacytoid DC (pDC), the myeloid DC (also known as conventional DC (cDC)) and the interferon-producing killer dendritic cells (IKDC) (Figure 2). All three DC populations have been reported to participate in the innate and adaptive immune response to hRSV and hMPV infections, indicating their critical role in the antiviral immunity to these viruses.

Figure 2. Mouse lung DC activated during hRSV and hMPV infection.

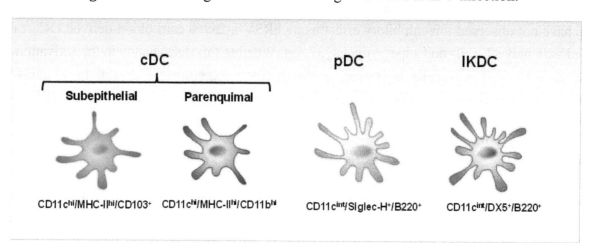

pDC are identified by the expression of $CD11c^{int}/B220^+/Gr-1^+/Siglec-H^+/mPDCA1^+$. They are best known for secreting large amounts of type I interferons (IFN) in response to viral infections [72]. Type I IFN confer resistance to viral infections and promote apoptosis of virally infected cells [73]. Also, type I IFN promote myeloid DC, B-cells, T-cells and natural killer (NK) cell functions [74,75]. Therefore, pDC regulate both innate and adaptive immune response in viral infections. pDC can also present endogenous viral antigens in their activated state to $CD4^+$ T-cells, but they are less efficient antigen-presenting cells, as compared to cDC [76]. Additionally, pDC are able to produce a variety of cytokines and chemokines that are important for the activation and trafficking of $CD4^+$ and $CD8^+$ T-cells to the site of infection [77,78].

cDC are identified as major histocompatibility complex class II $(MHC-II)^{hi}/CD11c^{hi}$. They are considered the main antigen-presenting cells of the immune system [26,79]. In mice, lung cDC comprise two major cDC subpopulations based on the expression of the integrin marker, CD103, and myeloid marker, CD11b, to give place to $MHC-II^{hi}/CD11c^{hi}/CD11b^-/CD103^+$ in the intraepithelial network and the parenchymal $MHC-II^{hi}/CD11c^{hi}/CD11b^+/CD103^-$ DC [79]. These two cDC subsets differ in their relative abilities to prime $CD4^+$ and $CD8^+$ T-cells [80], produce proinflammatory cytokines and generate Foxp3-mediated regulatory function of naive T-cells [81,82]. CD103 (α_E) is the α-chain of the $\alpha_E\beta_7$ integrin that mediates human and mouse T lymphocyte adhesion to epithelial cells through its binding to E-cadherin, which is selectively expressed on the basolateral side of epithelial cells [83]. The MHC-II[hi]/CD11c[hi]/CD11b[-]/CD103[+] DC are also known as migratory DC. CD103[+] DC can migrate to the draining lymph nodes (LN), produce IL-12 and are specialized in cross-presentation [80,82]. MHC-II[hi]/CD11c[hi]/CD11b[+]/CD103[-] DC are more efficient at presenting antigens on MHC II [84].

IKDC are characterized by the expression of CD11c[int]/Gr-1[+]/DX5[+] or NK1.1[+]. They are present in the lung and express cell surface markers of DC, as well as NK cell markers [85,86]. IKDC could be considered as NK-like DC or DC-like NK cells, playing a major role as a distinct population of innate effectors against viral pathogens [85,87,88]. However, their classification [85,86,88–90], origin [91] and physiological roles [85,87,92,93] remain controversial.

More recently, the TNF-α/inducible nitric oxide synthase (iNOS)-producing DC (tipDC) have been identified and found to control viral infections in the lung [94]. However, their role in hRSV or hMPV has not yet been described. TipDC, also known as inflammatory DC or activated macrophages, contribute to the control of the antimicrobial defense and are responsible for severe tissue damage in several models of infection [94–97]. However, based on the overlapping phenotypes of myeloid cells, further characterization of lung tipDC is needed in order to eliminate the possibility that they represent myeloid cells in a transient maturation stage, in response to infection.

5.1. Lung DC Trafficking

Several studies have reported the trafficking and function of respiratory DC in response to hRSV or hMPV infection. Experimental evidence indicates that hRSV induces the recruitment of DC into the lungs and LN of BALB/c [98–100] and C57BL/6 [101] mice. In previous studies, I have observed that IKDC is the smallest DC subset recruited to the airways upon hRSV infection (two-fold) [98], followed by pDC (four-fold) and is the cDC the predominant DC population recruited to the lung after hRSV infection (20-fold) [98]. Some differences in the kinetics of pDC and IKDC into the lung of Hmpv-infected mice have been observed when compared to hRSV, as the recruitment of pDC and IKDC peaked by day eight after hMPV infection *versus* day three in hRSV-infected mice [98]. On the other hand, a similar trafficking pattern of cDC has been observed after hMPV infection when compared to hRSV [98], including a sustained recruitment of this cell population for about 18–21 days beyond the acute phase of infection [98,99]. It has also been found that CD103[+] cDC are substantially decreased after hRSV infection [98,101], and the same effect has been observed in the lungs of hMPV-infected mice in which CD103[+] cDC decreased even after three weeks of infection and returned to basal levels by week eight [98]. By contrast, after either hRSV or hMPV infection, CD11b[hi] cDC increased about four-fold in the lung of infected mice [98,101]. Furthermore, hRSV infection stimulates the mobilization of both populations of cDC, as the numbers of CD103[+] and CD11b[hi] are increased in the lung-draining mediastinal LN [101].

5.2. Lung DC Activation

Upon viral challenge, lung cDC are activated and acquire a mature phenotype [23,26,28,102]. In that regard, previous experimental observations indicate that hRSV or hMPV induce the overexpression of surface molecules, including CD40, CD80, CD86, PD-L1, OX-40L and MHC-II, in pulmonary cDC as early as day one after infection and remained activated until three weeks after infection [98,101,103]. Moreover, the profile of cytokines produced by pulmonary pDC and cDC, infected with hRSV or hMPV, differ substantially. cDC produce IL-10, IL-1α, IL-6, CXCL1 and CCL11, while pulmonary pDC do not. However, both lung cDC and pDC produce IFN-α after hMPV infection *ex vivo*, while infection with hRSV did not stimulate the release of the antiviral cytokine [98]. hRSV also induces maturation of lung pDC, as indicated by the overexpression of CD80, CD86 and MHC class II molecules [104].

5.3. Lung pDC Function in hRSV Infection

It has been demonstrated that the balance between the numbers of pDC and cDC in the lung is important for the regulation of the immune response against hRSV. Smit *et al.* [105] demonstrated that when both pDC and cDC populations were expanded in hRSV-infected mice, that resulted in a decreased Th2 cell response, but an increased Th1 response and lower immunopathology. However, by depleting pDC and expanding cDC, the T-cell response was skewed towards Th2, resulting in an exacerbated inflammatory response.

The specific role of pulmonary pDC in hRSV infection has also been explored by several other groups [100,104,106]. To this end, pDC have also been depleted with the monoclonal antibody (mAb), 120G8, that recognizes the murine surface antigen, CD317 (BST-2; mPDCA1), in several mouse strains [107]. Some studies have reported that the inflammatory response and the airway resistance was substantially exacerbated, and the lung viral titer was increased [100,104], suggesting that pDC play a protective role during hRSV infection. However, it is important to consider that, despite BST-2 antigen being expressed predominantly on pDC in naive mice, it is known that after viral infection or stimulation with type I or type II IFN, BST-2 is induced on most cell types [108]. Therefore, this fact should be taken into consideration for the interpretation of these studies. On the hand, it seems that pDC do not contribute significantly to the production of type I IFN *in vivo* in hRSV infection, as the levels of IFN-α and IFN-β remained unchanged in hRSV-infected mice after successful depletion of pDC [106]. In fact, it has been reported that alveolar macrophages are the primary IFN-α producer in lung infections by RNA viruses [109]. In support to that, Pribul *et al.* [110] has demonstrated that alveolar macrophages significantly contribute to the production of IFN-α in hRSV infection. As for the role of DC subsets in hMPV infection, there are no reports exploring the contribution of these cells in the hMPV-induced immune response. Therefore, future experiments aimed to determine the role of DC subpopulations in hMPV-infected mice are needed to understand the contribution of these cells in hMPV-induced immune response.

5.4. Impairment of Mouse Lung DC Response in hRSV and hMPV

Infection by hRSV and hMPV is characterized by short-lasting virus specific immunity and, often, long-term airway morbidity. Previous studies have revealed that hRSV or hMPV impair the capacity of human DC to present antigens to T-cells *in vitro* [33,101,111]. That detrimental effect has also been observed in experiments *in vivo* using the mouse model [98]. In that system, I have previously observed that, when compared with cDC from mock-infected mice, lung cDC from mice infected with hRSV or hMPV have an impaired capacity to present antigens to CD4$^+$ T-cells that lasted beyond the acute phase of infection, suggesting that acute pneumovirus and metapneumovirus infections can alter the long-term immune function of pulmonary DC. Moreover, that inhibitory effect seems to be selective for lung cells, since that inhibitory effect was not observed when spleen cDC from the same infected mice were used [98]. The mechanisms by which hRSV and hMPV impair cDC function are largely unknown. However, one of the surface molecules that was upregulated after viral infection in lung cDC was programmed death-1 ligand (PD-L1) [98], which is known to inhibit some T-cell functions, including T-cell proliferation [112–114], suggesting that this molecule may play a role in the impaired capacity of cDC to present antigens to T-cells after hRSV and hMPV infection.

The production of type I IFN and other cytokines by lung DC is also altered by hRSV and hMPV infection *in vivo* [98]. I have previously observed that lung pDC isolated from infected mice produced significantly lower levels of IFN-α, IL-6, TNF-α, CCL3, CCL4 and CCL5 in response to CpG ODN [98], indicating that both viruses are able to interfere with the capacity of pulmonary pDC to mount an antiviral response in response to a secondary stimulus. Age is also a factor that negatively impacts DC response in the lung. The recruitment of DC after hRSV infection can be impaired by the age of the infected individuals, as shown by Zhao *et al.* in aged mice (6–22 months-old) where the ability of lung DC to migrate to LN was compromised in hRSV-infected aged mice, with a decline in migration occurring as early as six months of age [115].

5.5. Contribution Lung DC in Vaccine Development

Data *in vivo* using the C57BL/6 mouse model of hRSV infection have indicated that after hRSV intranasal challenge to formalin-inactivated RSV (FI-RSV)-immunized mice, the numbers of CD11b$^+$ and CD103$^+$ cDC recruited into the lung are increased [116]. Considering that differences between these DC populations in priming the T-cell responses exist [80] and that the balance between the numbers of DC subsets influences the CD4$^+$ Th1/Th2 responses in the lung [105], the development of hRSV and hMPV vaccines should consider the characterization of the lung DC subsets response and their contribution to prime an immune response against these viral infections, which will contribute toward the better design of an effective vaccine against these respiratory viral infections.

6. Conclusions

Lung DC participate in the innate and adaptive immune response to hRSV and hMPV infections, indicating their critical role in the antiviral immunity to these paramyxoviruses. hRSV and hMPV can induce similar DC responses, as DC can be activated by both hRSV and hMPV infections *in vivo*. In addition, both viruses can induce the maturation and trafficking of the different DC populations from lung to LN. Moreover, they interfere with the T-cell response, as the antigen-presenting capacity of pulmonary DC to T-cells is impaired after hRSV or hMPV infection, which may contribute to the lack of protection and multiple reinfections by these viruses. On the other hand, hRSV and hMPV differentially induce the production of type I IFN in lung DC, as hMPV is a more potent inducer of the antiviral cytokine.

Although many aspects of the immune mechanisms involving DC in hRSV infection have not been elucidated, considerable progress has been made with respect to our understanding of the role of pulmonary DC in hRSV infection. However, less is known regarding the interaction of hMPV with the lung DC, and in general, the mechanisms that regulate the host immune response to hMPV infection remain largely unknown. Additional studies are necessary to better understand the mechanisms that regulate the DC response in hRSV and hMPV infections.

Acknowledgments

This work was supported by Grants from the National Institute of Allergy and Infectious Diseases AI081171, the National Center for Research Resources 5P20RR020159-09 and the National Institute of General Medical Sciences 8P20GM103458-09 from the National Institutes of Health and the Flight Attendant Medical Research Institute YCSA grant. The author thanks Dawn Simms for critical reading of the manuscript.

References

1.   Collins PL; Crowe, J. Respiratory Syncytial Virus and Metapneumovirus. In *Fileds Virology*, 5th ed.; Knipe, D.M., Howley, P.M., Eds.; Wolters Kluwer: Philadelphia, PA, USA, 2007; Volume 2, pp. 1601–1646.

2.   Van den Hoogen, B.G.; de Jong, J.C.; Groen, J.; Kuiken, T.; de Groot, R.; Fouchier, R.A.; Osterhaus, A.D. A newly discovered human pneumovirus isolated from young children with respiratory tract disease. *Nat. Med.* **2001**, *7*, 719–724.

3.   Domachowske, J.B.; Rosenberg, H.F. Respiratory syncytial virus infection: Immune response, immunopathogenesis, and treatment. *Clin. Microbiol. Rev.* **1999**, *12*, 298–309.

4.   Easton, A.J.; Domachowske, J.B.; Rosenberg, H.F. Animal pneumoviruses: Molecular genetics and pathogenesis. *Clin. Microbiol. Rev.* **2004**, *17*, 390–412.

5.   Blount, R.E., Jr.; Morris, J.A.; Savage, R.E. Recovery of cytopathogenic agent from chimpanzees with coryza. *Proc. Soc. Exp. Biol. Med.* **1956**, *92*, 544–549.

6. Boivin, G.; de Serres, G.; Cote, S.; Gilca, R.; Abed, Y.; Rochette, L.; Bergeron, M.G.; Dery, P. Human metapneumovirus infections in hospitalized children. *Emerg. Infect. Dis.* **2003**, *9*, 634–640.

7. Mullins, J.A.; Erdman, D.D.; Weinberg, G.A.; Edwards, K.; Hall, C.B.; Walker, F.J.; Iwane, M.; Anderson, L.J. Human metapneumovirus infection among children hospitalized with acute respiratory illness. *Emerg. Infect. Dis.* **2004**, *10*, 700–705.

8. Van den Hoogen, B.G.; van Doornum, G.J.; Fockens, J.C.; Cornelissen, J.J.; Beyer, W.E.; de Groot, R.; Osterhaus, A.D.; Fouchier, R.A. Prevalence and clinical symptoms of human metapneumovirus infection in hospitalized patients. *J. Infect. Dis.* **2003**, *188*, 1571–1577.

9. Williams, J.V.; Harris, P.A.; Tollefson, S.J.; Halburnt-Rush, L.L.; Pingsterhaus, J.M.; Edwards, K.M.; Wright, P.F.; Crowe, J.E., Jr. Human metapneumovirus and lower respiratory tract disease in otherwise healthy infants and children. *N. Engl. J. Med.* **2004**, *350*, 443–450.

10. Kahn, J.S. Epidemiology of human metapneumovirus. *Clin. Microbiol. Rev.* **2006**, *19*, 546–557.

11. Hall, C.B.; McCarthy, C.A. Respiratory Syncytial Virus. In *Principles and Practice of Infectious Diseases*; Mandel, G.L., Bennett, J.E., Dolin, R., Eds.; Churchill Livingston: New York, NY, USA, 1995; Volume 4, p. 1501.

12. Hall, C.B.; Douglas, R.G., Jr. Modes of transmission of respiratory syncytial virus. *J. Pediatr.* **1981**, *99*, 100–103.

13. Lessler, J.; Reich, N.G.; Brookmeyer, R.; Perl, T.M.; Nelson, K.E.; Cummings, D.A. Incubation periods of acute respiratory viral infections: A systematic review. *Lancet Infect. Dis.* **2009**, *9*, 291–300.

14. Welliver, R.C. Respiratory syncytial virus and other respiratory viruses. *Pediatr. Infect. Dis. J.* **2003**, *22*, S6–S10; discussion S10–S12.

15. Hermos, C.R.; Vargas, S.O.; McAdam, A.J. Human metapneumovirus. *Clin. Lab. Med.* **2010**, *30*, 131–148.

16. Papenburg, J.; Hamelin, M.E.; Ouhoummane, N.; Carbonneau, J.; Ouakki, M.; Raymond, F.; Robitaille, L.; Corbeil, J.; Caouette, G.; Frenette, L.; *et al.* Comparison of risk factors for human metapneumovirus and respiratory syncytial virus disease severity in young children. *J. Infect. Dis.* **2012**, *206*, 178–189.

17. Papenburg, J.; Boivin, G. The distinguishing features of human metapneumovirus and respiratory syncytial virus. *Rev. Med. Virol.* **2010**, *20*, 245–260.

18. Van Drunen Littel-van den Hurk, S.; Watkiss, E.R. Pathogenesis of respiratory syncytial virus. *Curr. Opin. Virol.* **2012**, *2*, 300–305.

19. Pavlin, J.A.; Hickey, A.C.; Ulbrandt, N.; Chan, Y.P.; Endy, T.P.; Boukhvalova, M.S.; Chunsuttiwat, S.; Nisalak, A.; Libraty, D.H.; Green, S.; *et al.* Human metapneumovirus reinfection among children in Thailand determined by ELISA using purified soluble fusion protein. *J. Infect. Dis.* **2008**, *198*, 836–842.

20. Ebihara, T.; Endo, R.; Ishiguro, N.; Nakayama, T.; Sawada, H.; Kikuta, H. Early reinfection with human metapneumovirus in an infant. *J. Clin. Microbiol.* **2004**, *42*, 5944–5946.

21. Ohuma, E.O.; Okiro, E.A.; Ochola, R.; Sande, C.J.; Cane, P.A.; Medley, G.F.; Bottomley, C.; Nokes, D.J. The natural history of respiratory syncytial virus in a birth cohort: The influence of age and previous infection on reinfection and disease. *Am. J. Epidemiol.* **2012**, *176*, 794–802.

22. Graham, B.S. Biological challenges and technological opportunities for respiratory syncytial virus vaccine development. *Immunol. Rev.* **2011**, *239*, 149–166.

23. Steinman, R.M. Decisions about dendritic cells: Past, present, and future. *Annu. Rev. Immunol.* **2012**, *30*, 1–22.

24. Grayson, M.H.; Holtzman, M.J. Emerging role of dendritic cells in respiratory viral infection. *J. Mol. Med.* **2007**, *85*, 1057–1068.

25. Reis e Sousa, C. Activation of dendritic cells: Translating innate into adaptive immunity. *Curr. Opin. Immunol.* **2004**, *16*, 21–25.

26. Banchereau, J.; Briere, F.; Caux, C.; Davoust, J.; Lebecque, S.; Liu, Y.T.; Pulendran, B.; Palucka, K. Immunobiology of dendritic cells. *Ann. Rev. Immunol.* **2000**, *18*, 767–811.

27. Pulendran, B.; Palucka, K.; Banchereau, J. Sensing pathogens and tuning immune responses. *Science* **2001**, *293*, 253–256.

28. Steinman, R.M.; Cohn, Z.A. Identification of a novel cell type in peripheral lymphoid organs of mice. I. Morphology, quantitation, tissue distribution. *J. Exp. Med.* **1973**, *137*, 1142–1162.

29. Stumbles, P.A.; Upham, J.W.; Holt, P.G. Airway dendritic cells: Co-ordinators of immunological homeostasis and immunity in the respiratory tract. *APMIS* **2003**, *111*, 741–755.

30. Schon-Hegrad, M.A.; Oliver, J.; McMenamin, P.G.; Holt, P.G. Studies on the density, distribution, and surface phenotype of intraepithelial class II major histocompatibility complex antigen (Ia)-bearing dendritic cells (DC) in the conducting airways. *J. Exp. Med.* **1991**, *173*, 1345–1356.

31. McWilliam, A.S.; Napoli, S.; Marsh, A.M.; Pemper, F.L.; Nelson, D.J.; Pimm, C.L.; Stumbles, P.A.; Wells, T.N.; Holt, P.G. Dendritic cells are recruited into the airway epithelium during the inflammatory response to a broad spectrum of stimuli. *J. Exp. Med.* **1996**, *184*, 2429–2432.

32. Manicassamy, S.; Pulendran, B. Dendritic cell control of tolerogenic responses. *Immunol. Rev.* **2011**, *241*, 206–227.

33. Guerrero-Plata, A.; Casola, A.; Suarez, G.; Yu, X.; Spetch, L.; Peeples, M.E.; Garofalo, R.P. Differential response of dendritic cells to human metapneumovirus and respiratory syncytial virus. *Am. J. Respir. Cell Mol. Biol.* **2006**, *34*, 320–329.

34. Le Nouen, C.; Munir, S.; Losq, S.; Winter, C.C.; McCarty, T.; Stephany, D.A.; Holmes, K.L.; Bukreyev, A.; Rabin, R.L.; Collins, P.L.; *et al.* Infection and maturation of monocyte-derived human dendritic cells by human respiratory syncytial virus, human metapneumovirus, and human parainfluenza virus type 3. *Virology* **2009**, *385*, 169–182.

35. Jones, A.; Morton, I.; Hobson, L.; Evans, G.S.; Everard, M.L. Differentiation and immune function of human dendritic cells following infection by respiratory syncytial virus. *Clin. Exp. Immunol.* **2006**, *143*, 513–522.

36. De Graaff, P.M.; de Jong, E.C.; van Capel, T.M.; van Dijk, M.E.; Roholl, P.J.; Boes, J.; Luytjes, W.; Kimpen, J.L.; van Bleek, G.M. Respiratory syncytial virus infection of monocyte-derived dendritic cells decreases their capacity to activate CD4 T cells. *J. Immunol.* **2005**, *175*, 5904–5911.

37. Bartz, H.; Turkel, O.; Hoffjan, S.; Rothoeft, T.; Gonschorek, A.; Schauer, U. Respiratory syncytial virus decreases the capacity of myeloid dendritic cells to induce interferon-gamma in naive T cells. *Immunology* **2003**, *109*, 49–57.

38. Hornung, V.; Schlender, J.; Guenthner-Biller, M.; Rothenfusser, S.; Endres, S.; Conzelmann, K.K.; Hartmann, G. Replication-dependent potent IFN-alpha induction in human plasmacytoid dendritic cells by a single-stranded RNA virus. *J. Immunol.* **2004**, *173*, 5935–5943.

39. Johnson, T.R.; Johnson, C.N.; Corbett, K.S.; Edwards, G.C.; Graham, B.S. Primary human mDC1, mDC2, and pDC dendritic cells are differentially infected and activated by respiratory syncytial virus. *PLoS One* **2011**, *6*, e16458.

40. Gonzalez, P.A.; Prado, C.E.; Leiva, E.D.; Carreno, L.J.; Bueno, S.M.; Riedel, C.A.; Kalergis, A.M. Respiratory syncytial virus impairs T cell activation by preventing synapse assembly with dendritic cells. *Proc. Natl. Acad. Sci. USA* **2008**, *105*, 14999–15004.

41. Bartz, H.; Buning-Pfaue, F.; Turkel, O.; Schauer, U. Respiratory syncytial virus induces prostaglandin E2, IL-10 and IL-11 generation in antigen presenting cells. *Clin. Exp. Immunol.* **2002**, *129*, 438–445.

42. Rudd, B.D.; Luker, G.D.; Luker, K.E.; Peebles, R.S.; Lukacs, N.W. Type I interferon regulates respiratory virus infected dendritic cell maturation and cytokine production. *Viral Immunol.* **2007**, *20*, 531–540.

43. Munir, S.; Le, N.C.; Luongo, C.; Buchholz, U.J.; Collins, P.L.; Bukreyev, A. Nonstructural proteins 1 and 2 of respiratory syncytial virus suppress maturation of human dendritic cells. *J. Virol.* **2008**, *82*, 8780–8796.

44. Johnson, T.R.; McLellan, J.S.; Graham, B.S. Respiratory syncytial virus glycoprotein G interacts with DC-SIGN and L-SIGN to activate ERK1 and ERK2. *J. Virol.* **2012**, *86*, 1339–1347.

45. Morris, S.; Swanson, M.S.; Lieberman, A.; Reed, M.; Yue, Z.; Lindell, D.M.; Lukacs, N.W. Autophagy-mediated dendritic cell activation is essential for innate cytokine production and APC function with respiratory syncytial virus responses. *J. Immunol.* **2011**, *187*, 3953–3961.

46. Kundu, M.; Thompson, C.B. Autophagy: Basic principles and relevance to disease. *Ann. Rev. Pathol.* **2008**, *3*, 427–455.

47. Ank, N.; Paludan, S.R. Type III IFNs: New layers of complexity in innate antiviral immunity. *Biofactors* **2009**, *35*, 82–87.

48. Piehler, J.; Thomas, C.; Garcia, K.C.; Schreiber, G. Structural and dynamic determinants of type I interferon receptor assembly and their functional interpretation. *Immunol. Rev.* **2012**, *250*, 317–334.

49. Garcia-Sastre, A.; Biron, C.A. Type 1 interferons and the virus-host relationship: A lesson in detente. *Science* **2006**, *312*, 879–882.

50. Takeuchi, O.; Akira, S. MDA5/RIG-I and virus recognition. *Curr. Opin. Immunol.* **2008**, *20*, 17–22.

51. Baum, A.; Garcia-Sastre, A. Induction of type I interferon by RNA viruses: Cellular receptors and their substrates. *Amino Acids* **2009**, *38*, 1283–1299.

52. Schlender, J.; Hornung, V.; Finke, S.; Gunthner-Biller, M.; Marozin, S.; Brzozka, K.; Moghim, S.; Endres, S.; Hartmann, G.; Conzelmann, K.K. Inhibition of toll-like receptor 7- and 9-mediated alpha/beta interferon production in human plasmacytoid dendritic cells by respiratory syncytial virus and measles virus. *J. Virol.* **2005**, *79*, 5507–5515.

53. Castro, S.M.; Chakraborty, K.; Guerrero-Plata, A. Cigarette smoke suppresses TLR-7 stimulation in response to virus infection in plasmacytoid dendritic cells. *Toxicol. Vitro* **2011**, *25*, 1106–1113.

54. Goutagny, N.; Jiang, Z.; Tian, J.; Parroche, P.; Schickli, J.; Monks, B.G.; Ulbrandt, N.; Ji, H.; Kiener, P.A.; Coyle, A.J.; *et al.* Cell type-specific recognition of human metapneumoviruses (HMPVs) by retinoic acid-inducible gene I (RIG-I) and TLR7 and viral interference of RIG-I ligand recognition by HMPV-B1 phosphoprotein. *J. Immunol.* **2010**, *184*, 1168–1179.

55. Banos-Lara Mdel, R.; Ghosh, A.; Guerrero-Plata, A. Critical role of MDA5 in the interferon response induced by human metapneumovirus infection in dendritic cells and *in vivo*. *J. Virol.* **2013**, *87*, 1242–1251.

56. Kolli, D.; Bao, X.; Liu, T.; Hong, C.; Wang, T.; Garofalo, R.P.; Casola, A. Human metapneumovirus glycoprotein G inhibits TLR4-dependent signaling in monocyte-derived dendritic cells. *J. Immunol.* **2011**, *187*, 47–54.

57. Shingai, M.; Azuma, M.; Ebihara, T.; Sasai, M.; Funami, K.; Ayata, M.; Ogura, H.; Tsutsumi, H.; Matsumoto, M.; Seya, T. Soluble G protein of respiratory syncytial virus inhibits Toll-like receptor 3/4-mediated IFN-beta induction. *Int. Immunol.* **2008**, *20*, 1169–1180.

58. Henderson, F.W.; Collier, A.M.; Clyde, W.A., Jr.; Denny, F.W. Respiratory-syncytial-virus infections, reinfections and immunity. A prospective, longitudinal study in young children. *N. Engl. J. Med.* **1979**, *300*, 530–534.

59. Falsey, A.R.; Walsh, E.E. Viral pneumonia in older adults. *Clin. Infect. Dis.* **2006**, *42*, 518–524.

60. Hall, C.B.; Walsh, E.E.; Long, C.E.; Schnabel, K.C. Immunity to and frequency of reinfection with respiratory syncytial virus. *J. Infect. Dis.* **1991**, *163*, 693–698.

61. Rothoeft, T.; Fischer, K.; Zawatzki, S.; Schulz, V.; Schauer, U.; Korner Rettberg, C. Differential response of human naive and memory/effector T cells to dendritic cells infected by respiratory syncytial virus. *Clin. Exp. Immunol.* **2007**, *150*, 263–273.

62. Cespedes, P.F.; Gonzalez, P.A.; Kalergis, A.M. Human metapneumovirus keeps dendritic cells from priming antigen-specific naive T cells. *Immunology* **2013**, *139*, 366–376.

63. Le Nouen, C.; Hillyer, P.; Munir, S.; Winter, C.C.; McCarty, T.; Bukreyev, A.; Collins, P.L.; Rabin, R.L.; Buchholz, U.J. Effects of human respiratory syncytial virus, metapneumovirus, parainfluenza virus 3 and influenza virus on CD4+ T cell activation by dendritic cells. *PLoS One* **2010**, *5*, e15017.

64. Demedts, I.K.; Brusselle, G.G.; Vermaelen, K.Y.; Pauwels, R.A. Identification and characterization of human pulmonary dendritic cells. *Am. J. Respir. Cell Mol. Biol.* **2005**, *32*, 177–184.

65. Masten, B.J.; Olson, G.K.; Tarleton, C.A.; Rund, C.; Schuyler, M.; Mehran, R.; Archibeque, T.; Lipscomb, M.F. Characterization of myeloid and plasmacytoid dendritic cells in human lung. *J. Immunol.* **2006**, *177*, 7784–7793.

66. Condon, T.V.; Sawyer, R.T.; Fenton, M.J.; Riches, D.W. Lung dendritic cells at the innate-adaptive immune interface. *J. Leukoc. Biol.* **2011**, *90*, 883–895.

67. Bratke, K.; Lommatzsch, M.; Julius, P.; Kuepper, M.; Kleine, H.D.; Luttmann, W.; Christian Virchow, J. Dendritic cell subsets in human bronchoalveolar lavage fluid after segmental allergen challenge. *Thorax* **2007**, *62*, 168–175.

68. Lommatzsch, M.; Bratke, K.; Bier, A.; Julius, P.; Kuepper, M.; Luttmann, W.; Virchow, J.C. Airway dendritic cell phenotypes in inflammatory diseases of the human lung. *Eur. Respir. J.* **2007**, *30*, 878–886.

69. Gill, M.A.; Palucka, A.K.; Barton, T.; Ghaffar, F.; Jafri, H.; Banchereau, J.; Ramilo, O. Mobilization of plasmacytoid and myeloid dendritic cells to mucosal sites in children with respiratory syncytial virus and other viral respiratory infections. *J. Infect. Dis.* **2005**, *191*, 1105–1115.

70. Gill, M.A.; Long, K.; Kwon, T.; Muniz, L.; Mejias, A.; Connolly, J.; Roy, L.; Banchereau, J.; Ramilo, O. Differential recruitment of dendritic cells and monocytes to respiratory mucosal sites in children with influenza virus or respiratory syncytial virus infection. *J. Infect. Dis.* **2008**, *198*, 1667–1676.

71. Silver, E.; Yin-DeClue, H.; Schechtman, K.B.; Grayson, M.H.; Bacharier, L.B.; Castro, M. Lower levels of plasmacytoid dendritic cells in peripheral blood are associated with a diagnosis of asthma 6 yr after severe respiratory syncytial virus bronchiolitis. *Pediatr. Allergy Immunol.* **2009**, *20*, 471–476.

72. Gilliet, M.; Cao, W.; Liu, Y.J. Plasmacytoid dendritic cells: Sensing nucleic acids in viral infection and autoimmune diseases. *Nat. Rev. Immunol.* **2008**, *8*, 594–606.

73. Honda, K.; Yanai, H.; Takaoka, A.; Taniguchi, T. Regulation of the type I IFN induction: A current view. *Int. Immunol.* **2005**, *17*, 1367–1378.

74. Colonna, M.; Trinchieri, G.; Liu, Y.J. Plasmacytoid dendritic cells in immunity. *Nat. Immunol.* **2004**, *5*, 1219–1226.

75. Swiecki, M.; Colonna, M. Unraveling the functions of plasmacytoid dendritic cells during viral infections, autoimmunity, and tolerance. *Immunol. Rev.* **2010**, *234*, 142–162.

76. Young, L.J.; Wilson, N.S.; Schnorrer, P.; Proietto, A.; ten Broeke, T.; Matsuki, Y.; Mount, A.M.; Belz, G.T.; O'Keeffe, M.; Ohmura-Hoshino, M.; *et al.* Differential MHC class II synthesis and ubiquitination confers distinct antigen-presenting properties on conventional and plasmacytoid dendritic cells. *Nat. Immunol.* **2008**, *9*, 1244–1252.

77. Sozzani, S.; Vermi, W.; Del Prete, A.; Facchetti, F. Trafficking properties of plasmacytoid dendritic cells in health and disease. *Trends Immunol.* **2010**, *31*, 270–277.

78. Villadangos, J.A.; Young, L. Antigen-presentation properties of plasmacytoid dendritic cells. *Immunity* **2008**, *29*, 352–361.

79. Lambrecht, B.N.; Hammad, H. Biology of lung dendritic cells at the origin of asthma. *Immunity* **2009**, *31*, 412–424.

80. Del Rio, M.L.; Rodriguez-Barbosa, J.I.; Kremmer, E.; Forster, R. CD103- and CD103+ bronchial lymph node dendritic cells are specialized in presenting and cross-presenting innocuous antigen to CD4+ and CD8+ T cells. *J. Immunol.* **2007**, *178*, 6861–6866.

81. Coombes, J.L.; Siddiqui, K.R.; Arancibia-Carcamo, C.V.; Hall, J.; Sun, C.M.; Belkaid, Y.; Powrie, F. A functionally specialized population of mucosal CD103+ DCs induces Foxp3+ regulatory T cells via a TGF-beta and retinoic acid-dependent mechanism. *J. Exp. Med.* **2007**, *204*, 1757–1764.

82. Del Rio, M.L.; Bernhardt, G.; Rodriguez-Barbosa, J.I.; Forster, R. Development and functional specialization of CD103+ dendritic cells. *Immunol. Rev.* **2010**, *234*, 268–281.

83. Cepek, K.L.; Shaw, S.K.; Parker, C.M.; Russell, G.J.; Morrow, J.S.; Rimm, D.L.; Brenner, M.B. Adhesion between epithelial cells and T lymphocytes mediated by E-cadherin and the alpha E beta 7 integrin. *Nature* **1994**, *372*, 190–193.

84. Dudziak, D.; Kamphorst, A.O.; Heidkamp, G.F.; Buchholz, V.R.; Trumpfheller, C.; Yamazaki, S.; Cheong, C.; Liu, K.; Lee, H.W.; Park, C.G.; *et al.* Differential antigen processing by dendritic cell subsets *in vivo*. *Science* **2007**, *315*, 107–111.

85. Chan, C.W.; Crafton, E.; Fan, H.N.; Flook, J.; Yoshimura, K.; Skarica, M.; Brockstedt, D.; Dubensky, T.W.; Stins, M.F.; Lanier, L.L.; *et al.* Interferon-producing killer dendritic cells provide a link between innate and adaptive immunity. *Nat. Med.* **2006**, *12*, 207–213.

86. Taieb, J.; Chaput, N.; Menard, C.; Apetoh, L.; Ullrich, E.; Bonmort, M.; Pequignot, M.; Casares, N.; Terme, M.; Flament, C.; *et al.* A novel dendritic cell subset involved in tumor immunosurveillance. *Nat. Med.* **2006**, *12*, 214–219.

87. Bonmort, M.; Dalod, M.; Mignot, G.; Ullrich, E.; Chaput, N.; Zitvogel, L. Killer dendritic cells: IKDC and the others. *Curr. Opin. Immunol.* **2008**, *20*, 558–565.

88. Chauvin, C.; Josien, R. Dendritic cells as killers: Mechanistic aspects and potential roles. *J. Immunol.* **2008**, *181*, 11–16.

89. Blasius, A.L.; Barchet, W.; Cella, M.; Colonna, M. Development and function of murine B220+CD11c+NK1.1+ cells identify them as a subset of NK cells. *J. Exp. Med.* **2007**, *204*, 2561–2568.

90. Vosshenrich, C.A.; Lesjean-Pottier, S.; Hasan, M.; Richard-Le Goff, O.; Corcuff, E.; Mandelboim, O.; di Santo, J.P. CD11cloB220+ interferon-producing killer dendritic cells are activated natural killer cells. *J. Exp. Med.* **2007**, *204*, 2569–2578.

91. Welner, R.S.; Pelayo, R.; Garrett, K.P.; Chen, X.; Perry, S.S.; Sun, X.H.; Kee, B.L.; Kincade, P.W. Interferon-producing killer dendritic cells (IKDCs) arise via a unique differentiation pathway from primitive c-kitHiCD62L+ lymphoid progenitors. *Blood* **2007**, *109*, 4825–4931.

92. Caminschi, I.; Ahmet, F.; Heger, K.; Brady, J.; Nutt, S.L.; Vremec, D.; Pietersz, S.; Lahoud, M.H.; Schofield, L.; Hansen, D.S.; *et al.* Putative IKDCs are functionally and developmentally similar to natural killer cells, but not to dendritic cells. *J. Exp. Med.* **2007**, *204*, 2579–2590.

93. Spits, H.; Lanier, L.L. Natural killer or dendritic: What's in a name? *Immunity* **2007**, *26*, 11–16.

94. Aldridge, J.R., Jr.; Moseley, C.E.; Boltz, D.A.; Negovetich, N.J.; Reynolds, C.; Franks, J.; Brown, S.A.; Doherty, P.C.; Webster, R.G.; Thomas, P.G. TNF/iNOS-producing dendritic cells are the necessary evil of lethal influenza virus infection. *Proc. Natl. Acad. Sci. USA* **2009**, *106*, 5306–5311.

95. Serbina, N.V.; Salazar-Mather, T.P.; Biron, C.A.; Kuziel, W.A.; Pamer, E.G. TNF/iNOS-producing dendritic cells mediate innate immune defense against bacterial infection. *Immunity* **2003**, *19*, 59–70.

96. Bosschaerts, T.; Guilliams, M.; Stijlemans, B.; Morias, Y.; Engel, D.; Tacke, F.; Herin, M.; de Baetselier, P.; Beschin, A. Tip-DC development during parasitic infection is regulated by IL-10 and requires CCL2/CCR2, IFN-gamma and MyD88 signaling. *PLoS Pathog.* **2010**, *6*, e1001045.

97. Hespel, C.; Moser, M. Role of inflammatory dendritic cells in innate and adaptive immunity. *Eur. J. Immunol.* **2012**, *42*, 2535–2543.

98. Guerrero-Plata, A.; Kolli, D.; Hong, C.; Casola, A.; Garofalo, R.P. Subversion of pulmonary dendritic cell function by paramyxovirus infections. *J. Immunol.* **2009**, *182*, 3072–3083.

99. Beyer, M.; Bartz, H.; Horner, K.; Doths, S.; Koerner-Rettberg, C.; Schwarze, J. Sustained increases in numbers of pulmonary dendritic cells after respiratory syncytial virus infection. *J. Allergy Clin. Immunol.* **2004**, *113*, 127–133.

100. Smit, J.J.; Rudd, B.D.; Lukacs, N.W. Plasmacytoid dendritic cells inhibit pulmonary immunopathology and promote clearance of respiratory syncytial virus. *J. Exp. Med.* **2006**, *203*, 1153–1159.

101. Lukens, M.V.; Kruijsen, D.; Coenjaerts, F.E.; Kimpen, J.L.; van Bleek, G.M. Respiratory syncytial virus-induced activation and migration of respiratory dendritic cells and subsequent antigen presentation in the lung-draining lymph node. *J. Virol.* **2009**, *83*, 7235–7243.

102. Mellman, I.; Steinman, R.M. Dendritic cells: Specialized and regulated antigen processing machines. *Cell* **2001**, *106*, 255–258.

103. Wythe, S.E.; Dodd, J.S.; Openshaw, P.J.; Schwarze, J. OX40 ligand and programmed cell death 1 ligand 2 expression on inflammatory dendritic cells regulates CD4 T cell cytokine production in the lung during viral disease. *J. Immunol.* **2012**, *188*, 1647–1655.

104. Wang, H.; Peters, N.; Schwarze, J. Plasmacytoid dendritic cells limit viral replication, pulmonary inflammation, and airway hyperresponsiveness in respiratory syncytial virus infection. *J. Immunol.* **2006**, *177*, 6263–6270.

105. Smit, J.J.; Lindell, D.M.; Boon, L.; Kool, M.; Lambrecht, B.N.; Lukacs, N.W. The balance between plasmacytoid DC *versus* conventional DC determines pulmonary immunity to virus infections. *PLoS One* **2008**, *3*, e1720.

106. Jewell, N.A.; Vaghefi, N.; Mertz, S.E.; Akter, P.; Peebles, R.S., Jr.; Bakaletz, L.O.; Durbin, R.K.; Flano, E.; Durbin, J.E. Differential type I interferon induction by respiratory syncytial virus and influenza a virus *in vivo*. *J. Virol.* **2007**, *81*, 9790–9800.

107. Asselin-Paturel, C.; Brizard, G.; Pin, J.J.; Briere, F.; Trinchieri, G. Mouse strain differences in plasmacytoid dendritic cell frequency and function revealed by a novel monoclonal antibody. *J. Immunol.* **2003**, *171*, 6466–6477.

108. Blasius, A.L.; Giurisato, E.; Cella, M.; Schreiber, R.D.; Shaw, A.S.; Colonna, M. Bone marrow stromal cell antigen 2 is a specific marker of type I IFN-producing cells in the naive mouse, but a promiscuous cell surface antigen following IFN stimulation. *J. Immunol.* **2006**, *177*, 3260–3265.

109. Kumagai, Y.; Takeuchi, O.; Kato, H.; Kumar, H.; Matsui, K.; Morii, E.; Aozasa, K.; Kawai, T.; Akira, S. Alveolar macrophages are the primary interferon-alpha producer in pulmonary infection with RNA viruses. *Immunity* **2007**, *27*, 240–252.

110. Pribul, P.K.; Harker, J.; Wang, B.; Wang, H.; Tregoning, J.S.; Schwarze, J.; Openshaw, P.J. Alveolar macrophages are a major determinant of early responses to viral lung infection but do not influence subsequent disease development. *J. Virol.* **2008**, *82*, 4441–4448.

111. Biacchesi, S.; Skiadopoulos, M.H.; Boivin, G.; Hanson, C.T.; Murphy, B.R.; Collins, P.L.; Buchholz, U.J. Genetic diversity between human metapneumovirus subgroups. *Virology* **2003**, *315*, 1–9.

112. Erickson, J.J.; Gilchuk, P.; Hastings, A.K.; Tollefson, S.J.; Johnson, M.; Downing, M.B.; Boyd, K.L.; Johnson, J.E.; Kim, A.S.; Joyce, S.; *et al.* Viral acute lower respiratory infections impair CD8+ T cells through PD-1. *J. Clin. Investig.* **2012**, *122*, 2967–2982.

113. Carter, L.; Fouser, L.A.; Jussif, J.; Fitz, L.; Deng, B.; Wood, C.R.; Collins, M.; Honjo, T.; Freeman, G.J.; Carreno, B.M. PD-1:PD-L inhibitory pathway affects both CD4(+) and CD8(+) T cells and is overcome by IL-2. *Eur. J. Immunol.* **2002**, *32*, 634–643.

114. Freeman, G.J.; Long, A.J.; Iwai, Y.; Bourque, K.; Chernova, T.; Nishimura, H.; Fitz, L.J.; Malenkovich, N.; Okazaki, T.; Byrne, M.C.; *et al.* Engagement of the PD-1 immunoinhibitory receptor by a novel B7 family member leads to negative regulation of lymphocyte activation. *J. Exp. Med.* **2000**, *192*, 1027–1034.

115. Zhao, J.; Legge, K.; Perlman, S. Age-related increases in PGD(2) expression impair respiratory DC migration, resulting in diminished T cell responses upon respiratory virus infection in mice. *J. Clin. Investig.* **2011**, *121*, 4921–4930.

116. Kruijsen, D.; Schijf, M.A.; Lukens, M.V.; van Uden, N.O.; Kimpen, J.L.; Coenjaerts, F.E.; van Bleek, G.M. Local innate and adaptive immune responses regulate inflammatory cell influx into the lungs after vaccination with formalin inactivated RSV. *Vaccine* **2011**, *29*, 2730–2741.

3

Apoptosis in Pneumovirus Infection

Elske van den Berg, Job B.M. van Woensel and Reinout A. Bem *

Pediatric Intensive Care Unit, Emma Children's Hospital, Academic Medical Center,
Meibergdreef 9, Amsterdam 1105 AZ, The Netherlands;
E-Mails: elske.vandenberg@amc.nl (E.B.); j.b.vanwoensel@amc.nl (J.B.M.W.)

* Author to whom correspondence should be addressed; E-Mail: r.a.bem@amc.nl

Abstract: Pneumovirus infections cause a wide spectrum of respiratory disease in humans and animals. The airway epithelium is the major site of pneumovirus replication. Apoptosis or regulated cell death, may contribute to the host anti-viral response by limiting viral replication. However, apoptosis of lung epithelial cells may also exacerbate lung injury, depending on the extent, the timing and specific location in the lungs. Differential apoptotic responses of epithelial cells *versus* innate immune cells (e.g., neutrophils, macrophages) during pneumovirus infection can further contribute to the complex and delicate balance between host defense and disease pathogenesis. The purpose of this manuscript is to give an overview of the role of apoptosis in pneumovirus infection. We will examine clinical and experimental data concerning the various pro-apoptotic stimuli and the roles of apoptotic epithelial and innate immune cells during pneumovirus disease. Finally, we will discuss potential therapeutic interventions targeting apoptosis in the lungs.

Keywords: respiratory syncytial virus; cell death; host defense; acute lung injury

1. Introduction

Pneumoviruses are single-stranded, negative-sense, enveloped RNA viruses belonging to the family *Paramyxoviridae*, subfamily *Pneumovirinae*, and include several closely related, but species-limited, members (reviewed by Easton *et al.* [1]). The human pneumovirus respiratory syncytial virus (hRSV) is a leading respiratory pathogen in young children and the elderly worldwide and is associated with considerable morbidity and mortality and high health care costs [2,3]. Likewise, bovine RSV (bRSV) causes outbreaks of respiratory disease in young beef and dairy cattle. Both bRSV infection in cattle and infection of mice by the rodent-specific pneumovirus pneumonia virus of mice (PVM) have been studied extensively as a model for hRSV disease in humans [4]. Pneumovirus infections in humans and animals cause a wide spectrum of respiratory disease symptoms, ranging from mild upper airway illness, such as coryza and cough, to lower respiratory tract disease (e.g., bronchiolitis and bronchopneumonia), which may eventually lead to impaired gas-exchange and life threatening respiratory failure. Human infants with hRSV infection are prone to develop acute respiratory distress syndrome (ARDS), an acute-onset life threatening inflammatory lung condition associated with widespread lung injury [5,6]. Currently, as no specific treatment options for severe hRSV disease in humans exist, there is an ongoing research effort focusing on pneumovirus biology and host-interaction, ultimately to find novel therapies.

Apoptosis, a highly regulated energy-dependent type of cell death with distinct morphological and biochemical characteristics [7], is a basic biological response of cells to virus entry and replication [8]. While apoptosis of virus-infected cells may be an important first line host defense mechanism to limit pathogen replication and spread, many viruses have evolved strategies to evade and modulate intracellular pro-apoptotic signaling in the early replication phase [9,10]. Conversely, it has become clear that viruses may also *exploit* the cellular pro-apoptotic machinery in the formation and spread of infectious progeny virions in the late phase or in the elimination of immune cells, thereby evading host defense [10,11]. At the same time, from the host's perspective, extensive pro-apoptotic signaling may be beneficial in attacking a virus, but may become devastating upon the occurrence of an overshoot in apoptosis, leading to widespread loss of infected and/or uninfected bystander structural cells. Such an unbalanced extensive apoptotic response is implicated in the pathogenesis of a wide variety of diseases, including the development of diffuse lung epithelial injury in ARDS [12]. Taken together, the outcome of apoptosis during viral infection for the host may depend on its extent, timing and cell-specificity.

The occurrence and potential role of apoptosis in pneumovirus infections have been investigated in both *in vivo* (human and animal) and *in vitro* studies. The main goal of this manuscript is to provide an overview of the existing literature on pro- and anti-apoptotic signaling in pneumovirus infections with a focus on lung (airway and alveolar) epithelial cells, neutrophils and macrophages as first line cellular responders to acute pneumovirus infection. Furthermore, we will speculate on future apoptosis-based pharmacological therapies in hRSV disease.

2. Apoptotic Signaling Pathways

Cell death in multicellular organisms occurs either by necrosis or apoptosis, however their strict distinction is somewhat artificial, because overlap of their characteristics and cellular pathways may occur [13–15]. Apoptosis is associated with membrane blebbing, cell breakdown into apoptotic bodies and fragmentation of DNA. "Classical" apoptosis refers to the activation of the caspase cascade, a family of intracellular substrate specific proteases of which the final executioner, caspase-3, is a commonly used marker for apoptosis. Non-classical apoptosis occurs independent of caspase activation and involves release of the flavoprotein apoptosis-inducing factor (AIF) from mitochondria. Galluzzi *el al.* have provided an extensive and detailed review on the use and interpretation of caspase-(in)dependent apoptosis assays in laboratory research [16].

Figure 1. Schematic overview of three pathways of caspase-dependent apoptosis. First, the death receptor (extrinsic) pathway is activated upon tumor necrosis factor (TNF) death receptor family ligation by membrane-bound or soluble ligands, such as Fas ligand (FasL) and TNF-related apoptosis-inducing ligand (TRAIL), presented or secreted by local immune cells, including effector lymphocytes, neutrophils (PMN) and/or macrophages. Intracellular adaptor protein interactions through death domain modules follow the death receptor ligation and subsequently lead to activation of initiator caspase-8 and the downstream caspase cascade resulting in apoptosis. The inhibitor of apoptosis proteins (IAPs) can block several caspases, thereby inhibiting cell death. Second, granzymes delivered into the cytosol by effector lymphocytes can interact with several caspases and Bid to induce apoptosis. Third, members of the Bcl-2 family, including Bcl-2, Bax and Bcl-XL and p53, regulate cytochrome c release from the mitochondria (intrinsic pathway) in response to stimuli, such as DNA damage, infection and formation of reactive oxygen species (ROS). Cytochrome c in the cytosol assembles with apoptotic peptidase activating factor 1 (Apaf 1) to activate initiator caspase-9 with subsequent activation of the caspase-cascade and apoptosis. The mitochondrial and death receptor pathway can interact through BH3-interacting domain death agonist (Bid).

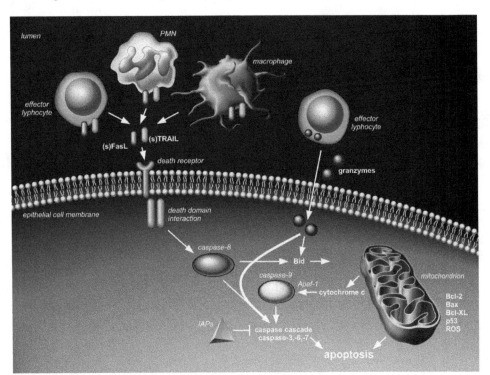

Figure 1 shows the conceptual framework of the major (caspase-dependent) apoptotic pathways, which are relevant to discuss in the context of pneumovirus infection. The intrinsic or mitochondrial pathway involves the release of cytochrome c from mitochondria into the cytoplasm and is regulated by Bcl-2 protein family members. The extrinsic or death receptor pathway is triggered by ligation of transmembrane death receptors that belong to the tumor necrosis factor (TNF) death receptor family, which include TNF receptor (TNFR), Fas (CD95) and TNF-related apoptosis-inducing ligand (TRAIL) death receptors (TRAIL-R1 and -R2). Expression and activation of proteins in both these pathways can be modulated by p53, a major cell stress sensor protein. Finally, the granule-mediated cytotoxic pathway is exploited by effector lymphocytes, which can release serine proteases, known as granzymes, into the cytosol of target cells, which subsequently results in caspase-(in)dependent apoptosis. Activation and modulation of these three apoptotic pathways is associated with pneumovirus infection in humans and animals, as will be discussed below.

3. Lung (Airway and Alveolar) Epithelial Cell Apoptosis

In the lower airways, the bronchiolar epithelium is the primary site of human and animal pneumovirus infection [17–20]. In addition, viral antigen can be detected in alveolar epithelial cells in severe hRSV-, bRSV- and PVM-induced bronchopneumonia [18–21]. An interesting and consistently reported feature of severe pneumovirus disease is the sloughing of dead airway epithelial cells, which form dense plugs with mucus, fibrin and leukocytes, resulting in air trapping and ventilatory failure [18,20–23]. The loss of these epithelial cells has always been thought to occur primarily through necrosis, however Welliver et al. observed marked active caspase-3 immunostaining in bronchiolar epithelium of children with fatal hRSV disease, suggesting that apoptosis is an important mechanism of cell death as well (Figure 2A) [20,24]. Likewise, lung epithelial cells show enhanced DNA fragmentation as detected by terminal dUTP nick-end labeling (TUNEL) in bRSV infected calves and increased caspase-3 activation in PVM infected mice [19,25] (Figure 2B). The relative importance of apoptosis in cell decay in pneumovirus infected lungs is further supported by the finding of a strong correlation between caspase-3 and -7 activity and LDH concentration in the airways in children with hRSV-induced bronchiolitis; however, from this study, the exact cellular source of these markers is not clear [26].

The occurrence of apoptosis in the lung epithelium during the course of pneumovirus infection may serve to limit viral replication. However, the widespread and extensive scale on which this takes place, involving the whole pulmonary system, including the alveoli, may also suggests an overshoot and/or inefficiency of pro-apoptotic signaling during the late and severe phase of pneumovirus infection. This may lead to enhanced respiratory disease, e.g., diffuse alveolar epithelial injury, as seen in human ARDS [12] and influenza virus animal models [27]. We believe three scenarios regarding lung epithelial cell apoptosis during pneumovirus infection may co-exist as described below (Figure 3), and the balance between them is likely to be critical for the development and outcome of host disease.

Figure 2. (**A**) Positive immunohistochemical staining for the apoptosis marker caspase-3 (brown) in bronchiolar epithelial cells in lung tissue from a child with fatal human pneumovirus respiratory syncytial virus (hRSV) disease. From Welliver *et al.* [24], by permission of Oxford University Press. (**B**) Positive immunohistochemical staining for caspase-3 (brown, arrows) in alveolar epithelial cells in lung tissue from a mouse (C57Bl/6 background) with severe pneumonia virus of mice (PVM) disease. From Bem *et al.* [25], Copyright 2010, The American Association of Immunologists, Inc.

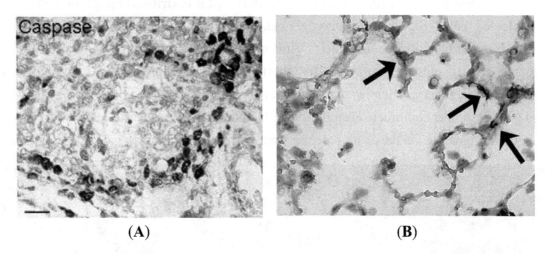

(**A**)   (**B**)

3.1. Pneumovirus Infected Cells May Undergo Apoptosis as a Result of Direct Activation of Intrinsic Pathways.

Based on the results of a number of *in vitro* studies in cultured primary airway epithelial cells and A549 cells (an adenocarcinomic human alveolar basal epithelial cell line) it appears that, although in the early phase of hRSV infection apoptosis does not occur, this type of cell death becomes an important response in the later phase of viral replication [28–39]. It should be noted however that several of these studies show some conflicting results with regard to the time point at which apoptosis is detected, possibly related to the use of different cell lines/cultures, multiplicity of infection, hRSV strains, early versus late apoptosis markers and assays used.

The relative paucity of apoptosis during the early phase of hRSV infection may be explained by viral-induced anti-apoptotic intrinsic pathway signaling, which ensures more time for viral replication and assembly of virions. Mechanisms of early hRSV-induced alteration of the intrinsic pathway towards an anti-apoptotic balance in Bcl-2 family proteins include post-transcriptional regulation of p53 [32], microRNA modulation [40] and three important basic cell survival/proliferation pathways involving nerve growth factor/tyrosine kinase receptor (NGF/Trk) [36], epidermal growth factor receptor (EGFR) [35] and phosphoinositide 3-kinase(PI3K)/Akt signaling [38]. Interestingly, by using recombinant and RNA silencing techniques, it was shown that both the hRSV-encoded small hydrophobic (SH) protein and nonstructural (NS) proteins are critical regulators of the early anti-apoptotic effects [29,31]. The NS proteins have been found to interfere with interferon (IFN) signaling [41], which may affect apoptotic pathways in hRSV infected cells. However, Bitko *et al.* [29] suggested that the early NS protein associated anti-apoptotic effect was mediated through NF-κB and PI3K/Akt signaling, independent of the IFN pathway.

Figure 3. Three theoretical scenarios regarding lung epithelial cell apoptosis during pneumovirus infection, which may co-exist. First (**A**), viral infection triggers the mitochondrial (intrinsic) apoptotic pathway via interaction with Bcl-2 family proteins. Second (**B**), death receptor ligands (either membrane-bound or soluble) presented or secreted by local immune cells activate the death receptor (extrinsic) apoptotic pathway in viral-infected cells. Similarly, granzymes released from effector lymphocytes into the cytosol of target cells induce apoptosis. Viral infection may modulate the susceptibility to death receptor ligands or granzymes by altering the expression of and interaction with the protein machinery, such as surface death receptors, involved in these pathways. Third (**C**), bystander (uninfected) epithelial cells undergo apoptosis as a result of extensive, non-specific signaling via the death receptor (extrinsic) and/or granzyme apoptotic pathway.

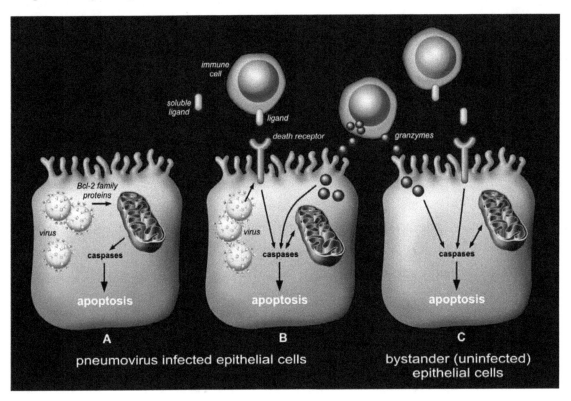

Pro-apoptotic signaling appears to predominate at a later phase of hRSV infection [29,30,34,39]. The hRSV-encoded fusion (F) protein, which is expressed at a later time point as compared to the NS proteins [29], has been found to be critical in the activation of apoptosis by p53-mediated activation of pro-apoptotic Bcl-2 family proteins [30]. Apoptosis markers in hRSV-infected A549 and human primary airway epithelial cells further include caspase activation, detection of phosphatidylserine exposition by Annexin V and TUNEL staining. However, the susceptibility of epithelial cells to pneumovirus-associated apoptosis may vary depending on the specific localization (proximal *versus* distal) in the lungs [34]. Importantly, in the recent study by Villenave *et al.* well-differentiated primary bronchial epithelial cells of children cultured in air-liquid interface showed TUNEL-positive staining in detached cells six days after hRSV infection [39]. This supports the hypothesis that apoptosis contributes to the characteristic sloughing of epithelial cells in the airways of children during the late phase of pneumovirus infection.

3.2. Pneumovirus Infected Cells May Undergo Apoptosis by Activation of Extrinsic and Granule-Mediated Pathways

First, death receptor ligands may trigger apoptosis of virus infected epithelial cells. Several studies have shown enhanced local production of TNFα, FasL and TRAIL by recruited immune cells or neighbor epithelial cells upon pneumovirus infection [4,28,34,39,42,43]. Interestingly, *in vitro* studies have shown that, whereas hRSV infection results in decreased susceptibility to TNFα-induced apoptosis [44], it sensitizes lung epithelial cells to the pro-apoptotic effects of TRAIL [34], which likely occurs as a result of increased expression of death receptors TRAIL-R1 and -R2 [34,42]. Similarly, enhanced epithelial surface expression of Fas in hRSV infection has been found in both *in vitro* and human histopathology studies [20,28,45]. Interestingly, mice with a non-functional FasL (*gld* strain) have been reported to have delayed hRSV clearance [46], but van den Berg *et al.* [47] did not detect differences in lung viral loads in PVM-infected mice with a defective Fas (*lpr* strain) as compared to wild type mice. This differential effect of a dysfunctional Fas/FasL system on viral clearance in these different pneumovirus models may be explained by specific pneumovirus-host interactions, although may potentially also be related to a leaky, incomplete Fas defect in *lpr* mice.

Second, granzymes released from the granules of natural killer cells and cytotoxic T-lymphocytes into virus infected target cells may induce apoptosis. In children with severe hRSV disease, we have found strong release of granzymes in the lungs [48]. Similarly, PVM infected mice show enhanced granzyme expression, however this appears not to affect local viral titers [25], suggesting that the granule-mediated apoptotic pathway does not have an important role in clearance of pneumovirus infected epithelial cells.

3.3. Uninfected Bystander Epithelial Cells May Undergo Apoptosis as a Result of Extensive and Non-Specific Activation of Extrinsic and Granule-Mediated Pathways

Although pneumovirus antigen can be detected in alveolar epithelium in the late and severe phase of human and animal pneumovirus disease, the primary site of replication are (small) airway epithelial cells [17–21]. Interestingly, histopathology studies in humans with fatal hRSV disease and animal models show epithelial cell apoptosis may occur in the entire pulmonary system, including the alveolar compartment [4,19,24,25]. In fact, we have previously detected active caspase-3 immunostaining primarily in alveolar epithelial cells in mice with severe PVM disease, while this apoptosis marker was scarce in bronchial epithelium [25]. Such a potential disparity in the localization between pneumovirus presence and apoptosis may suggest uninfected bystander cells in the lungs are victim of an overshoot and/or inefficiency in pro-apoptotic signaling, and this may lead to enhanced pneumovirus disease.

The bystander injury hypothesis is supported by two *in vivo* studies in mice: Rutigliano *et al.* [46] showed that while a dysfunctional FasL results in delayed hRSV clearance, at the same time it significantly diminishes clinical illness; and, our own group showed that while a deficiency in granzymes did not affect PVM clearance, it resulted in delayed clinical disease in association with a marked decrease in lung caspase-3 activity [25]. In addition, we have previously shown that soluble TRAIL is present in increased levels in bronchoalveolar lavage fluid of children with severe hRSV disease, and this death receptor ligand induced cell death in uninfected primary pediatric airway epithelial cells *in vitro* [42]. Interestingly, similar findings for soluble FasL were found in relation to epithelial injury in human ARDS [49]. When considering the bystander epithelial injury hypothesis, soluble death receptor ligands present in the lung microenvironment during pneumovirus disease are of particular interest due to the potential increased likelihood of non-specific signaling. They may be released into the extracellular space from recruited immune cells, such as macrophages [42] and neutrophils [50] or from (infected) neighbor epithelial cells (paracrine pathway) [51], although *in vitro* studies by Bitko *et al.* [28] suggested a minor role for the latter mechanism.

4. Neutrophil Apoptosis

Neutrophils, recruited by local production of chemoattractants, are the predominant inflammatory cells in the pulmonary compartment during acute pneumovirus infection [4,52–54]. They possess a wide arsenal of defensive strategies against invading microorganisms, including phagocytosis, production of toxic reactive oxygen species and release of immune defense proteins. Although the role of neutrophils in anti-*viral* immunity remains relatively unclarified, several studies have shown a protective effect of neutrophils against influenza virus [55,56]. Both animal and human studies demonstrated that during pneumovirus infection, recruited neutrophils contain virus, suggesting a contributive role to viral clearance [19,57]. This is further supported by *in vitro* studies that showed neutrophil-mediated injury and detachment of hRSV infected lung epithelial cells [58]. On the other hand, it is well recognized that uncontrolled or prolonged neutrophil activity may cause collateral tissue injury [59], such as diffuse alveolar damage in human ARDS [60–62]. Although direct evidence of neutrophil-mediated respiratory disease in pneumovirus infection is lacking, the acute and strong neutrophil influx in the lungs coincides with peak disease severity in animal models [19,25].

To prevent their potential inadvertent harmful effect, the life span of neutrophils is limited by apoptosis. Interestingly, incubation of human neutrophils with hRSV *in vitro* results in activation of anti-apoptotic signaling through the Bcl-2 family proteins [63]. Although this inhibition of neutrophil cell death by hRSV does not require live virus, it does require cellular uptake. Lindemans *et al.* [63] further suggested this effect depends on auto- or paracrine-signaling via the release of IL-6. Others, however, have suggested that the anti-apoptotic effect of hRSV on human neutrophils is primarily mediated by soluble factors via monocyte interaction and, thus, is a secondary response [64]. Regardless of the precise mechanism involved, these *in vitro* studies suggest prolonged neutrophil survival in the setting of hRSV infection and, as such, this may be an important event in the development of lung injury during pneumovirus disease. In contrast, Wang *et al.* [65] reported an increased number of Annexin V positive neutrophils in nasopharyngeal aspirates and the peripheral blood of infants with hRSV disease, as compared to peripheral blood neutrophils of healthy children. This would imply that despite the pro-survival effect of hRSV on neutrophils as observed *in vitro*, pro-apoptotic signaling by mediators (e.g., cytokines) in the lung microenvironment during hRSV disease prevails. Whether this truly would protect against harmful prolonged neutrophil survival remains speculative. In particular, it is possible that different neutrophil apoptotic responses in functionally heterogeneous neutrophil subsets co-exist and change over time [66,67]. As such, it is clear that further research on the precise role of neutrophil apoptosis during pneumovirus infections is highly needed.

5. Macrophage Apoptosis

Macrophages are observed in high numbers in the airways and lungs of humans and animals with pneumovirus disease [4,18–20,22,23,52,54]. Macrophages are key innate immune cells acting in pathogen surveillance and initiation and resolution of inflammation through mechanisms involving antigen processing/presentation, phagocytosis and cytokine production. Macrophage depletion in wild-type mice infected by hRSV or PVM results in increased lung viral titers and greatly affects the local cytokine production [23,68,69]. However, paradoxically in PVM-infected mice, this results in prolonged survival, whereas in hRSV challenged mice, this is associated with enhanced airway occlusion on histopathological examination [23,69], suggesting that the role of macrophages may depend on specific host-pneumovirus interactions. Nevertheless, these findings underline the importance of macrophage biology in pneumovirus infection. As such, dysregulation of (apoptotic) cell death pathways in resident and migrated macrophages in the lungs may have profound consequences for the outcome of pneumovirus infection.

Unfortunately, very few studies have focused on macrophage apoptosis in pneumovirus disease. In the histopathological studies from Welliver *et al.*, fatal hRSV disease in children was associated with relatively low numbers of caspase-3 immunoreactive inflammatory cells in the lungs, as compared to children with fatal influenza virus disease [24]. In mice challenged with PVM, we observed cleaved caspase-3 positive macrophages in the alveolar spaces (unpublished observations, [70]); however, the exact magnitude and role of apoptosis of these cells in this model is not yet clear.

Ex vivo and autopsy studies have shown that virus antigen is detected in macrophages in the airways and lungs of hRSV infected patients [18,71]. In addition, isolated peripheral and cord blood monocytes, as well as alveolar macrophages, are susceptible to hRSV infection *in vitro* [72,73], and PVM was recently shown to replicate in primary mouse macrophage culture [69]. Interestingly, hRSV presence in human monocytes and mouse macrophages results in decreased (susceptibility of) apoptosis, associated with decreased caspase-3 activity and enhanced expression of anti-apoptotic members of the Bcl-2 protein family and inhibitor of apoptosis protein (IAP) family [74,75]. These observations suggest pneumoviruses exploit strategies to escape apoptosis in macrophages and could explain the apparent paucity of evidence for macrophage apoptosis in the aforementioned histopathology studies.

6. Apoptosis-Based Pharmacological Intervention

During the last decades, much progress has been made in the development of apoptosis-based therapeutic agents, including antisense oligodeoxynucleotides, small interfering (si)RNA, peptides/proteins and antibodies (reviewed by Fischer *et al.* [76]). Much attention in this field has been directed towards cancer treatment, however inflammatory and infectious diseases are of emerging focus. The increasing knowledge in the regulation and molecular machinery of apoptotic cell death pathways involving many different target genes and proteins has set the stage for highly promising research in pharmacological intervention. Death receptors, caspases and IAP and Bcl-2 protein family members all belong to prominent targets in current drug development [76]. However, despite the ongoing success of pre-clinical and even clinical studies exploiting the use of apoptosis-based drugs in a wide variety of diseases, many obstacles still have to be overcome, including cell-specificity and permeability, timing of intervention and potential toxicity or interference with other biological processes, such as inflammation.

To our knowledge, up to date, no published studies have directly examined the effects of apoptosis-based pharmacological treatments in pneumovirus disease *in vivo*. Although originally designed to study macrophage depletion rather than directly focusing on apoptosis intervention, Rigaux *et al.* [69] found that intratracheal treatment with clodronate-liposomes, which induces apoptosis upon specific uptake by macrophages [77], prolongs the survival of PVM-infected mice. This suggests that enhancing macrophage apoptosis in pneumovirus disease is of clinical interest. Currently, our own group is studying the use of the irreversible pan-caspase inhibitor, z-VAD-fmk, administered by a systemic route in mice challenged with PVM (study in progress). In addition, we have shown that treatment with DR5-Fc fusion protein, which inhibits TRAIL death receptor signaling, partly attenuates cell death of primary pediatric bronchial airway cells exposed to bronchoalveolar lavage fluid from hRSV-infected children *in vitro* [42]. However the effects of this compound *in vivo* are yet unclear. Given the strong evidence of activation of pro- and anti-apoptotic pathways during pneumovirus infection as described in the above paragraphs, more attention towards this field is highly needed.

Several critical points need to be considered in potential apoptosis-based interventions in pneumovirus disease. First is the cell-specificity. From the present overview, it becomes clear that different cell types in the lungs may show differential apoptotic responses during pneumovirus disease. Interestingly, even within a lung cell population (e.g., epithelial cells), differential responses to a single apoptotic mediator may exist [78,79], including in the setting of pneumovirus infection [34], which further increases the complexity of intervention. This stresses the need for insight in cell-specific pro- and anti-apoptotic targets and for development of small molecule compounds and vehicles for specific local intervention. On the other hand, even without specific target cell delivery systems, animal studies modeling ARDS have shown promising beneficial effects on survival and histopathological changes by using a number of systemic or intratracheal apoptosis-based treatments, including blockade of FasL by decoy receptor-3 [80], Fas:Ig fusion protein [81] or Fas-siRNA [82] and pan-caspase inhibition by z-VAD-fmk [83]. These studies successfully aimed to inhibit lung epithelial cell apoptosis during the process of lung injury. However, it remains to be elucidated whether such strategies also effectively reduce lung epithelial cell death in pneumovirus disease and, subsequently, to what extent this affects viral replication and, most importantly, clinical outcome. Second, given the dynamic course of anti- and pro-apoptotic signaling in lung epithelial cells, timing of apoptotic interventions may be critical, as, for example, inhibitory strategies may be beneficial in the late severe phase of disease, but detrimental in the early stages of viral replication. Third, concurrent iatrogenic treatments with pro-apoptotic effects, such as mechanical ventilation and/or oxygen therapy [70,84], may interact with apoptosis-based interventions in the lungs. Fourth and finally, the effect of modulating apoptosis in the lungs needs to be considered with special focus on age, as apoptosis is an important event in lung development and maturation [85].

7. Conclusion

Pneumovirus infection is associated with both pro- and anti-apoptotic signaling in the lungs, depending on the cell-type, involvement of specific cell death pathway and timing during the course of infection. The balance between these events is likely to be critical for the development and outcome of pneumovirus disease. However, more research is needed to fully understand the dynamic character of apoptosis during this important respiratory illness. In particular, we need to address which factors favor the viral propagation *versus* host defense. Here, we have reviewed the existing literature on this topic and have speculated on future apoptosis-based pharmacological treatments.

Acknowledgments

The authors thank Inge Kos-Oosterling from the AMC Medical Illustration Service for help with the figure drawings. No specific financial support or grants are reported.

References

1. Easton, A.J.; Domachowske, J.B.; Rosenberg, H.F. Animal pneumoviruses: Molecular genetics and pathogenesis. *Clin. Microbiol. Rev.* **2004**, *17*, 390–412.
2. Falsey, A.R.; Hennessey, P.A.; Formica, M.A.; Cox, C.; Walsh, E.E. Respiratory syncytial virus infection in elderly and high-risk adults. *N. Engl. J. Med.* **2005**, *352*, 1749–1759.
3. Nair, H.; Nokes, D.J.; Gessner, B.D.; Dherani, M.; Madhi, S.A.; Singleton, R.J.; O'Brien, K.L.; Roca, A.; Wright, P.F.; Bruce, N.; *et al.* Global burden of acute lower respiratory infections due to respiratory syncytial virus in young children: A systematic review and meta-analysis. *Lancet* **2010**, *375*, 1545–1555.
4. Bem, R.A.; Domachowske, J.B.; Rosenberg, H.F. Animal models of human respiratory syncytial virus disease. *Am. J. Physiol. Lung Cell. Mol. Physiol.* **2011**, *301*, 148–156.

5.   ARDS definition task force Acute respiratory distress syndrome—The Berlin definition. *JAMA* **2012**, *307*, 256–2533.

6.   Dahlem, P.; van Aalderen, W.M.; Hamaker, M.E.; Dijkgraaf, M.G.; Bos, A.P. Incidence and short-term outcome of acute lung injury in mechanically ventilated children. *Eur. Respir. J.* **2003**, *22*, 980–985.

7.   Kerr, J.F.; Wyllie, A.H.; Currie, A.R. Apoptosis: A basic biological phenomenon with wide-ranging implications in tissue kinetics. *Br. J. Cancer* **1972**, *26*, 239–257.

8.   Barber, G.N. Host defense, viruses and apoptosis. *Cell Death Differ.* **2001**, *8*, 113–126.

9.   Benedict, C.A.; Norris, P.S.; Ware, C.F. To kill or be killed: Viral evasion of apoptosis. *Nat. Immunol.* **2002**, *3*, 1013–1018.

10. Galluzzi, L.; Brenner, C.; Morselli, E.; Touat, Z.; Kroemer, G. Viral control of mitochondrial apoptosis. *PLoS Pathog.* **2008**, *4*, e1000018.

11. Herold, S.; Ludwig, S.; Pleschka, S.; Wolff, T. Apoptosis signaling in influenza virus propagation, innate host defense and lung injury. *J. Leukoc. Biol.* **2012**, *92*, 75–82.

12. Martin, T.R.; Hagimoto, N.; Nakamura, M.; Matute-Bello, G. Apoptosis and epithelial injury in the lungs. *Proc. Am. Thorac. Soc.* **2005**, *2*, 214–220.

13. Denecker, G.; Vercammen, D.; Declercq, W.; Vandenabeele, P. Apoptotic and necrotic cell death induced by death domain receptors. *Cell Mol. Life Sci.* **2001**, *58*, 356–370.

14. Leist, M.; Jaattela, M. Four deaths and a funeral: From caspases to alternative mechanisms. *Nat. Rev. Mol. Cell Biol.* **2001**, *2*, 589–598.

15. Wang, X.; Ryter, S.W.; Dai, C.; Tang, Z.L.; Watkins, S.C.; Yin, X.M.; Song, R.; Choi, A.M. Necrotic cell death in response to oxidant stress involves the activation of the apoptogenic caspase-8/bid pathway. *J. Biol. Chem.* **2003**, *278*, 29184–29191.

16. Galluzzi, L.; Aaronson, S.A.; Abrams, J.; Alnemri, E.S.; Andrews, D.W.; Baehrecke, E.H.; Bazan, N.G.; Blagosklonny, M.V.; Blomgren, K.; Borner, C.; *et al.* Guidelines for the use and interpretation of assays for monitoring cell death in higher eukaryotes. *Cell Death Differ.* **2009**, *16*, 1093–1107.

17. Bonville, C.A.; Bennett, N.J.; Koehnlein, M.; Haines, D.M.; Ellis, J.A.; DelVecchio, A.M.; Rosenberg, H.F.; Domachowske, J.B. Respiratory dysfunction and proinflammatory chemokines in the pneumonia virus of mice (PVM) model of viral bronchiolitis. *Virology* **2006**, *349*, 87–95.

18. Johnson, J.E.; Gonzales, R.A.; Olson, S.J.; Wright, P.F.; Graham, B.S. The histopathology of fatal untreated human respiratory syncytial virus infection. *Mod. Pathol.* **2007**, *20*, 108–119.

19. Viuff, B.; Tjornehoj, K.; Larsen, L.E.; Rontved, C.M.; Uttenthal, A.; Ronsholt, L.; Alexandersen, S. Replication and clearance of respiratory syncytial virus: Apoptosis is an important pathway of virus clearance after experimental infection with bovine respiratory syncytial virus. *Am. J. Pathol.* **2002**, *161*, 2195–2207.

20. Welliver, T.P.; Reed, J.L.; Welliver, R.C., Sr. Respiratory syncytial virus and influenza virus infections: Observations from tissues of fatal infant cases. *Pediatr. Infect. Dis. J.* **2008**, *27*, 92–96.

21. Cook, P.M.; Eglin, R.P.; Easton, A.J. Pathogenesis of pneumovirus infections in mice: Detection of pneumonia virus of mice and human respiratory syncytial virus mRNA in lungs of infected mice by *in situ* hybridization. *J. Gen. Virol.* **1998**, *79*, 2411–2417.

22. Aherne, W.; Bird, T.; Court SD; Gardner, P.S.; McQuillin, J. Pathological changes in virus infections of the lower respiratory tract in children. *J. Clin. Pathol.* **1970**, *23*, 7–18.

23. Reed, J.L.; Brewah, Y.A.; Delaney, T.; Welliver, T.; Burwell, T.; Benjamin, E.; Kuta, E.; Kozhich, A.; McKinney, L.; Suzich, J.; *et al.* Macrophage impairment underlies airway occlusion in primary respiratory syncytial virus bronchiolitis. *J. Infect. Dis.* **2008**, *198*, 1783–1793.

24. Welliver, T.P.; Garofalo, R.P.; Hosakote, Y.; Hintz, K.H.; Avendano, L.; Sanchez, K.; Velozo, L.; Jafri, H.; Chavez-Bueno, S.; Ogra, P.L.; *et al.* Severe human lower respiratory tract illness caused by respiratory syncytial virus and influenza virus is characterized by the absence of pulmonary cytotoxic lymphocyte responses. *J. Infect. Dis.* **2007**, *195*, 1126–1136.

25. Bem, R.A.; van Woensel, J.B.; Lutter, R.; Domachowske, J.B.; Medema, J.P.; Rosenberg, H.F.; Bos, A.P. Granzyme A- and B-cluster deficiency delays acute lung injury in pneumovirus-infected mice. *J. Immunol.* **2010**, *184*, 931–938.

26. Laham, F.R.; Trott, A.A.; Bennett, B.L.; Kozinetz, C.A.; Jewell, A.M.; Garofalo, R.P.; Piedra, P.A. LDH concentration in nasal-wash fluid as a biochemical predictor of bronchiolitis severity. *Pediatrics* **2010**, *125*, 225–233.

27. Herold, S.; Steinmueller, M.; von, W.W.; Cakarova, L.; Pinto, R.; Pleschka, S.; Mack, M.; Kuziel, W.A.; Corazza, N.; Brunner, T.; *et al.* Lung epithelial apoptosis in influenza virus pneumonia: The role of macrophage-expressed TNF-related apoptosis-inducing ligand. *J. Exp. Med.* **2008**, *205*, 3065–3077.

28. Bitko, V.; Barik, S. An endoplasmic reticulum-specific stress-activated caspase (caspase-12) is implicated in the apoptosis of A549 epithelial cells by respiratory syncytial virus. *J. Cell Biochem.* **2001**, *80*, 441–454.

29. Bitko, V.; Shulyayeva, O.; Mazumder, B.; Musiyenko, A.; Ramaswamy, M.; Look, D.C.; Barik, S. Nonstructural proteins of respiratory syncytial virus suppress premature apoptosis by an NF-kappaB-dependent, interferon-independent mechanism and facilitate virus growth. *J. Virol.* **2007**, *81*, 1786–1795.

30. Eckardt-Michel, J.; Lorek, M.; Baxmann, D.; Grunwald, T.; Keil, G.M.; Zimmer, G. The fusion protein of respiratory syncytial virus triggers p53-dependent apoptosis. *J. Virol.* **2008**, *82*, 3236–3249.

31. Fuentes, S.; Tran, K.C.; Luthra, P.; Teng, M.N.; He, B. Function of the respiratory syncytial virus small hydrophobic protein. *J. Virol.* **2007**, *81*, 8361–8366.

32. Groskreutz, D.J.; Monick, M.M.; Yarovinsky, T.O.; Powers, L.S.; Quelle, D.E.; Varga, S.M.; Look, D.C.; Hunninghake, G.W. Respiratory syncytial virus decreases p53 protein to prolong survival of airway epithelial cells. *J. Immunol.* **2007**, *179*, 2741–2747.

33. Groskreutz, D.J.; Monick, M.M.; Babor, E.C.; Nyunoya, T.; Varga, S.M.; Look, D.C.; Hunninghake, G.W. Cigarette smoke alters respiratory syncytial virus-induced apoptosis and replication. *Am. J. Respir. Cell Mol. Biol.* **2009**, *41*, 189–198.

34. Kotelkin, A.; Prikhod'ko, E.A.; Cohen, J.I.; Collins, P.L.; Bukreyev, A. Respiratory syncytial virus infection sensitizes cells to apoptosis mediated by tumor necrosis factor-related apoptosis-inducing ligand. *J. Virol.* **2003**, *77*, 9156–9172.

35. Monick, M.M.; Cameron, K.; Staber, J.; Powers, L.S.; Yarovinsky, T.O.; Koland, J.G.; Hunninghake, G.W. Activation of the epidermal growth factor receptor by respiratory syncytial virus results in increased inflammation and delayed apoptosis. *J. Biol. Chem.* **2005**, *280*, 2147–2158.

36. Othumpangat, S.; Gibson, L.F.; Samsell, L.; Piedimonte, G. NGF is an essential survival factor for bronchial epithelial cells during respiratory syncytial virus infection. *PLoS One* **2009**, *4*, e6444.

37. Takeuchi, R.; Tsutsumi, H.; Osaki, M.; Haseyama, K.; Mizue, N.; Chiba, S. Respiratory syncytial virus infection of human alveolar epithelial cells enhances interferon regulatory factor 1 and interleukin-1beta-converting enzyme gene expression, but does not cause apoptosis. *J. Virol.* **1998**, *72*, 4498–4502.

38. Thomas, K.W.; Monick, M.M.; Staber, J.M.; Yarovinsky, T.; Carter, A.B.; Hunninghake, G.W. Respiratory syncytial virus inhibits apoptosis and induces NF-kappa B activity through a phosphatidylinositol 3-kinase-dependent pathway. *J. Biol. Chem.* **2002**, *277*, 492–501.

39. Villenave, R.; Thavagnanam, S.; Sarlang, S.; Parker, J.; Douglas, I.; Skibinski, G.; Heaney, L.G.; McKaigue, J.P.; Coyle, P.V.; Shields, M.D.; *et al. In vitro* modeling of respiratory syncytial virus infection of pediatric bronchial epithelium, the primary target of infection *in vivo*. *Proc. Natl. Acad. Sci. USA* **2012**, *109*, 5040–5045.

40. Othumpangat, S.; Walton, C.; Piedimonte, G. MicroRNA-221 modulates RSV replication in human bronchial epithelium by targeting NGF expression. *PLoS One* **2012**, *7*, e30030.

41. Spann, K.M.; Tran, K.C.; Chi, B.; Rabin, R.L.; Collins, P.L. Suppression of the induction of alpha, beta and lambda interferons by the NS1 and NS2 proteins of human respiratory syncytial virus in human epithelial cells and macrophages. *J. Virol.* **2004**, *78*, 4363–4369.

42. Bem, R.A.; Bos, A.P.; Wosten-van Asperen, R.M.; Bruijn, M.; Lutter, R.; Sprick, M.R.; van Woensel, J.B. Potential Role of Soluble TRAIL in Epithelial Injury in Children with Severe RSV Infection. *Am. J. Respir. Cell Mol. Biol.* **2009**, *42*, 697-705.

43. Aung, S.; Rutigliano, J.A.; Graham, B.S. Alternative mechanisms of respiratory syncytial virus clearance in perforin knockout mice lead to enhanced disease. *J. Virol.* **2001**, *75*, 9918–9924.

44. Domachowske, J.B.; Bonville, C.A.; Mortelliti, A.J.; Colella, C.B.; Kim, U.; Rosenberg, H.F. Respiratory syncytial virus infection induces expression of the anti-apoptosis gene IEX-1L in human respiratory epithelial cells. *J. Infect. Dis.* **2000**, *181*, 824–830.

45. O'donnell, D.R.; Milligan, L.; Stark, J.M. Induction of CD95 (Fas) and apoptosis in respiratory epithelial cell cultures following respiratory syncytial virus infection. *Virology* **1999**, *257*, 198–207.

46. Rutigliano, J.A.; Graham, B.S. Prolonged production of TNF-alpha exacerbates illness during respiratory syncytial virus infection. *J. Immunol.* **2004**, *173*, 3408–3417.

47. Van den Berg E.; van Woensel, J.B.; Bos, A.P.; Bem, R.A.; Altemeier, W.A.; Gill, S.E.; Martin, T.R.; Matute-Bello, G. Role of the Fas/FasL system in a model of RSV infection in mechanically ventilated mice. *Am. J. Physiol. Lung Cell Mol. Physiol.* **2011**, *301*, 451–460.

48. Bem, R.A.; Bos, A.P.; Bots, M.; Wolbink, A.M.; van Ham, S.M.; Medema, J.P.; Lutter, R.; van Woensel, J.B. Activation of the granzyme pathway in children with severe respiratory syncytial virus infection. *Pediatr. Res.* **2008**, *63*, 650–655.

49. Matute-Bello, G.; Liles, W.C.; Steinberg, K.P.; Kiener, P.A.; Mongovin, S.; Chi, E.Y.; Jonas, M.; Martin, T.R. Soluble Fas ligand induces epithelial cell apoptosis in humans with acute lung injury (ARDS). *J. Immunol.* **1999**, *163*, 2217–2225.

50. Serrao, K.L.; Fortenberry, J.D.; Owens, M.L.; Harris, F.L.; Brown, L.A. Neutrophils induce apoptosis of lung epithelial cells via release of soluble Fas ligand. *Am. J. Physiol. Lung Cell Mol. Physiol.* **2001**, *280*, 298–305.

51. Powell, W.C.; Fingleton, B.; Wilson, C.L.; Boothby, M.; Matrisian, L.M. The metalloproteinase matrilysin proteolytically generates active soluble Fas ligand and potentiates epithelial cell apoptosis. *Curr. Biol.* **1999**, *9*, 1441–1447.

52. Everard, M.L.; Swarbrick, A.; Wrightham, M.; McIntyre, J.; Dunkley, C.; James, P.D.; Sewell, H.F.; Milner, A.D. Analysis of cells obtained by bronchial lavage of infants with respiratory syncytial virus infection. *Arch. Dis. Child.* **1994**, *71*, 428–432.

53. Van Woensel, J.B.; Lutter, R.; Biezeveld, M.H.; Dekker, T.; Nijhuis, M.; van Aalderen, W.M.; Kuijpers, T.W. Effect of dexamethasone on tracheal viral load and interleukin-8 tracheal concentration in children with respiratory syncytial virus infection. *Pediatr. Infect. Dis. J.* **2003**, *22*, 721–726.

54. McNamara, P.S.; Ritson, P.; Selby, A.; Hart, C.A.; Smyth, R.L. Bronchoalveolar lavage cellularity in infants with severe respiratory syncytial virus bronchiolitis. *Arch. Dis. Child.* **2003**, *88*, 922–926.

55. Tate, M.D.; Deng, Y.M.; Jones, J.E.; Anderson, G.P.; Brooks, A.G.; Reading, P.C. Neutrophils ameliorate lung injury and the development of severe disease during influenza infection. *J. Immunol.* **2009**, *183*, 7441–7450.

56. Tumpey, T.M.; Garcia-Sastre, A.; Taubenberger, J.K.; Palese, P.; Swayne, D.E.; Pantin-Jackwood, M.J.; Schultz-Cherry, S.; Solorzano, A.; van, R.N.; Katz, J.M.; *et al.* Pathogenicity of influenza viruses with genes from the 1918 pandemic virus: Functional roles of alveolar macrophages and neutrophils in limiting virus replication and mortality in mice. *J. Virol.* **2005**, *79*, 14933–14944.

57. Halfhide, C.P.; Flanagan, B.F.; Brearey, S.P.; Hunt, J.A.; Fonceca, A.M.; McNamara, P.S.; Howarth, D.; Edwards, S.; Smyth, R.L. Respiratory syncytial virus binds and undergoes transcription in neutrophils from the blood and airways of infants with severe bronchiolitis. *J. Infect. Dis.* **2011**, *204*, 451–458.

58. Wang, S.Z.; Forsyth, K.D. The interaction of neutrophils with respiratory epithelial cells in viral infection. *Respirology* **2000**, *5*, 1–10.

59. Segel, G.B.; Halterman, M.W.; Lichtman, M.A. The paradox of the neutrophil's role in tissue injury. *J. Leukoc. Biol.* **2011**, *89*, 359–372.

60. Martin, T.R. Neutrophils and lung injury: Getting it right. *J. Clin. Investig.* **2002**, *110*, 1603–1605.

61. Perl, M.; Lomas-Neira, J.; Chung, C.S.; Ayala, A. Epithelial cell apoptosis and neutrophil recruitment in acute lung injury-a unifying hypothesis? What we have learned from small interfering RNAs. *Mol. Med.* **2008**, *14*, 465–475.

62. Ware, L.B.; Matthay, M.A. The acute respiratory distress syndrome. *N. Engl. J. Med.* **2000**, *342*, 1334–1349.

63. Lindemans, C.A.; Coffer, P.J.; Schellens, I.M.; de Graaff, P.M.; Kimpen, J.L.; Koenderman, L. Respiratory syncytial virus inhibits granulocyte apoptosis through a phosphatidylinositol 3-kinase and NF-kappaB-dependent mechanism. *J. Immunol.* **2006**, *176*, 5529–5537.

64. Coleman, C.M.; Plant, K.; Newton, S.; Hobson, L.; Whyte, M.K.; Everard, M.L. The anti-apoptotic effect of respiratory syncytial virus on human peripheral blood neutrophils is mediated by a monocyte derived soluble factor. *Open Virol. J.* **2011**, *5*, 114–123.

65. Wang, S.Z.; Smith, P.K.; Lovejoy, M.; Bowden, J.J.; Alpers, J.H.; Forsyth, K.D. The apoptosis of neutrophils is accelerated in respiratory syncytial virus (RSV)-induced bronchiolitis. *Clin. Exp. Immunol.* **1998**, *114*, 49–54.

66. Pillay, J.; Ramakers, B.P.; Kamp, V.M.; Loi, A.L.; Lam, S.W.; Hietbrink, F.; Leenen, L.P.; Tool, A.T.; Pickkers, P.; Koenderman, L. Functional heterogeneity and differential priming of circulating neutrophils in human experimental endotoxemia. *J. Leukoc. Biol.* **2010**, *88*, 211–220.

67. Simon, H.U. Neutrophil apoptosis pathways and their modifications in inflammation. *Immunol. Rev.* **2003**, *193*, 101–110.

68. Pribul, P.K.; Harker, J.; Wang, B.; Wang, H.; Tregoning, J.S.; Schwarze, J.; Openshaw, P.J. Alveolar macrophages are a major determinant of early responses to viral lung infection, but do not influence subsequent disease development. *J. Virol.* **2008**, *82*, 4441–4448.

69. Rigaux, P.; Killoran, K.E.; Qiu, Z.; Rosenberg, H.F. Depletion of alveolar macrophages prolongs survival in response to acute pneumovirus infection. *Virology* **2012**, *422*, 338–345.

70. Bem, R.A.; van Woensel, J.B.; Bos, A.P.; Koski, A.; Farnand, A.W.; Domachowske, J.B.; Rosenberg, H.F.; Martin, T.R.; Matute-Bello, G. Mechanical ventilation enhances lung inflammation and caspase activity in a model of mouse pneumovirus infection. *Am. J. Physiol. Lung Cell Mol. Physiol.* **2009**, *296*, 46–56.

71. Midulla, F.; Villani, A.; Panuska, J.R.; Dab, I.; Kolls, J.K.; Merolla, R.; Ronchetti, R. Respiratory syncytial virus lung infection in infants: Immunoregulatory role of infected alveolar macrophages. *J. Infect. Dis.* **1993**, *168*, 1515–1519.

72. Midulla, F.; Huang, Y.T.; Gilbert, I.A.; Cirino, N.M.; McFadden, E.R., Jr.; Panuska, J.R. Respiratory syncytial virus infection of human cord and adult blood monocytes and alveolar macrophages. *Am. Rev. Respir. Dis.* **1989**, *140*, 771–777.

73. Panuska, J.R.; Cirino, N.M.; Midulla, F.; Despot, J.E.; McFadden, E.R., Jr.; Huang, Y.T. Productive infection of isolated human alveolar macrophages by respiratory syncytial virus. *J. Clin. Investig.* **1990**, *86*, 113–119.

74. Krilov, L.R.; McCloskey, T.W.; Harkness, S.H.; Pontrelli, L.; Pahwa, S. Alterations in apoptosis of cord and adult peripheral blood mononuclear cells induced by *in vitro* infection with respiratory syncytial virus. *J. Infect. Dis.* **2000**, *181*, 349–353.

75. Nakamura-Lopez, Y.; Villegas-Sepulveda, N.; Sarmiento-Silva, R.E.; Gomez, B. Intrinsic apoptotic pathway is subverted in mouse macrophages persistently infected by RSV. *Virus Res.* **2011**, *158*, 98–107.

76. Fischer, U.; Schulze-Osthoff, K. Apoptosis-based therapies and drug targets. *Cell Death Differ.* **2005**, *12*, 942–961.

77. Van Rooijen N.; Sanders, A. Liposome mediated depletion of macrophages: Mechanism of action, preparation of liposomes and applications. *J. Immunol. Methods* **1994**, *174*, 83–93.

78. Janssen, W.J.; Barthel, L.; Muldrow, A.; Oberley-Deegan, R.E.; Kearns, M.T.; Jakubzick, C.; Henson, P.M. Fas determines differential fates of resident and recruited macrophages during resolution of acute lung injury. *Am. J. Respir. Crit. Care Med.* **2011**, *184*, 547–560.

79. Nakamura, M.; Matute-Bello, G.; Liles, W.C.; Hayashi, S.; Kajikawa, O.; Lin, S.M.; Frevert, C.W.; Martin, T.R. Differential response of human lung epithelial cells to fas-induced apoptosis. *Am. J. Pathol.* **2004**, *164*, 1949–1958.

80. Matute-Bello, G.; Liles, W.C.; Frevert, C.W.; Dhanireddy, S.; Ballman, K.; Wong, V.; Green, R.R.; Song, H.Y.; Witcher, D.R.; Jakubowski, J.A.; *et al.* Blockade of the Fas/FasL system improves pneumococcal clearance from the lungs without preventing dissemination of bacteria to the spleen. *J. Infect. Dis.* **2005**, *191*, 596–606.

81. Matute-Bello, G.; Liles, W.C.; Frevert, C.W.; Nakamura, M.; Ballman, K.; Vathanaprida, C.; Kiener, P.A.; Martin, T.R. Recombinant human Fas ligand induces alveolar epithelial cell apoptosis and lung injury in rabbits. *Am. J. Physiol. Lung Cell Mol. Physiol.* **2001**, *281*, 328–335.

82. Perl, M.; Chung, C.S.; Lomas-Neira, J.; Rachel, T.M.; Biffl, W.L.; Cioffi, W.G.; Ayala, A. Silencing of Fas, but not caspase-8, in lung epithelial cells ameliorates pulmonary apoptosis, inflammation and neutrophil influx after hemorrhagic shock and sepsis. *Am. J. Pathol.* **2005**, *167*, 1545–1559.

83. Kawasaki, M.; Kuwano, K.; Hagimoto, N.; Matsuba, T.; Kunitake, R.; Tanaka, T.; Maeyama, T.; Hara, N. Protection from lethal apoptosis in lipopolysaccharide-induced acute lung injury in mice by a caspase inhibitor. *Am. J. Pathol.* **2000**, *157*, 597–603.

84. Altemeier, W.A.; Sinclair, S.E. Hyperoxia in the intensive care unit: Why more is not always better. *Curr. Opin. Crit. Care* **2007**, *13*, 73–78.

85. Bem, R.A.; Bos, A.P.; Matute-Bello, G.; van, T.M.; van Woensel, J.B. Lung epithelial cell apoptosis during acute lung injury in infancy. *Pediatr. Crit. Care Med.* **2007**, *8*, 132–137.

4

Use of an Innovative Web-Based Laboratory Surveillance Platform to Analyze Mixed Infections Between Human Metapneumovirus (hMPV) and Other Respiratory Viruses Circulating in Alberta (AB), Canada (2009–2012)

Sumana Fathima [1], Bonita E. Lee [2], Jennifer May-Hadford [3], Shamir Mukhi [4] and Steven J. Drews [1,5,*]

[1] Provincial Laboratory for Public Health (ProvLab), 3030 Hospital Dr. NW, Calgary, AB T2N 4W4, Canada; E-Mail: sumana.fathima@albertahealthservices.ca

[2] University of Alberta, Room 3-588B, ECHA, 11405 – 87 Avenue, Edmonton, AB T6G 1C9, Canada; E-Mail: bonita.lee@albertahealthservices.ca

[3] Public Health Agency of Canada, 130 Colonnade Road A.L. 6501H Ottawa, ON K1A 0K9, Canada; E-Mail: jennifer.may-hadford@phac-aspc.gc.ca

[4] Canadian Network for Public Health Intelligence, Public Health Agency of Canada, 1015 Arlington St, Winnipeg, MB R3E 3R2, Canada; E-Mail: shamir.nizar.mukhi@phac-aspc.gc.ca

[5] University of Calgary, 2500 University Drive Northwest, Calgary, AB T2N 1N4, Canada; E-Mail: steven.drews@albertahealthservices.ca

* Author to whom correspondence should be addressed; E-Mail: steven.drews@albertahealthservices.ca

Abstract: We investigated the proportions of mono *vs.* mixed infections for human metapneumovirus (hMPV) as compared to adenovirus (ADV), four types of coronavirus (CRV), parainfluenza virus (PIV), RSV, and enterovirus/rhinovirus (ERV) in Alberta, Canada. Using the Data Integration for Alberta Laboratories (DIAL) platform, 26,226 respiratory specimens at ProvLab between 1 July 2009 and 30 June 2012 were selected and included in the study. Using the Respiratory Virus Panel these specimens tested positive for one or more respiratory virus and negative for influenza A and B. From our subset hMPV was the fourth most common virus (n = 2,561) with 373 (15%) identified as mixed infection using DIAL. Mixed infection with hMPV was most commonly found in infants less than 6 months old and ERV was most commonly found in mixed infection with hMPV (230/373, 56%) across all age groups. The proportion of mixed-infection *vs.* mono-infection was highest for ADV (46%), followed by CRV 229E (32%), CRV HKU1 (31%), CRV NL63 (28%), CRV OC43 (23%), PIV (20%), RSV (17%), hMPV (15%) and ERV (13%). hMPV was significantly more likely to be identified in mono infection as compared with ADV, CRV, PIV, and RSV with the exception of ERV [$p<0.05$].

Keywords: hMPV; co-infection; testing; epidemiology; respiratory

---

1. Introduction

Respiratory tract infections are a global public health concern and in Canada is the eighth leading cause of death in 2009 [1]. Human metapneumovirus (hMPV) is an RNA virus belonging to *Paramyxoviridae* family. The virus was identified by researchers in the Netherlands in 2001 as an important cause of respiratory infections that affect all age groups [2]. A study from Saskatchewan, Canada by Liu *et al.* [3], using ELISA showed that seroprevalence for hMPV approaches 99% by young adulthood. This virus can affect any age group but several studies have shown that hMPV is a leading cause in lower respiratory tract infections in children [4–6] but it also affects the elderly [7]. Clinical manifestations are similar to Respiratory Syncytial Virus (RSV) primarily leading to pneumonia and bronchiolitis [8]. In Canada, outbreaks associated with hMPV have been reported in Alberta, British Columbia and Quebec mainly in long term and senior care facilities [9–11]. Other common respiratory viruses in these settings include influenza A (FLUA), influenza B (FLUB), parainfluenza virus (PIV), enterovirus/rhinovirus (ERV), adenovirus (ADV), and coronavirus (CRV), which all can cause lower respiratory tract infections [12,13].

Provincial Laboratory for Public Health (ProvLab) in Alberta provides testing for all respiratory virus pathogens for the province of Alberta and surrounding Northern Territories (excluding Yukon) of Canada. The diagnostic testing algorithm for respiratory virus at ProvLab changed during the 2009 H1N1 pandemic. From April 2009, respiratory specimens arriving at ProvLab were screened by an in-house real-time reverse-transcriptase (RT)-PCR for influenza A [14]. Specimens that were positive for influenza A were also subtyped for seasonal H3, seasonal H1 and pandemic H1N1 (2009) genes by RT-PCR. A cost effective approach was adopted in June 2009, to only test specimens negative for both influenza A and B by either singleplex or multiplex real time PCR assays using the Respiratory Virus Panel (RVP) classic assay, a multiplexed assay which detects multiple respiratory viral pathogens including FLUA, FLUB, PIV, ERV, ADV, 4 types of CRV, RSV, and hMPV [15]. Exceptions to this testing policy include samples submitted from a provincial influenza-like-illness surveillance program

(Tarrant Viral Watch) and some samples from patients with severe illness and admission to the intensive care units.

In Alberta, a unique platform was developed for laboratory-based surveillance called Data Integration of Alberta Laboratories (DIAL). DIAL is a secure web based platform, which is used to extract, interpret, collate and analyze respiratory virus testing data from ProvLab, Laboratory Information System (LIS) in real time [16]. DIAL has an automatic engine that extracts raw specimen-based laboratory data from ProvLab LIS, including patient demographics, information of physician and submitting agencies, and test data for specific targets. The second and most important component of DIAL is a built-in Automated Interpretation Engine (AIE) which provides clinically relevant interpretation and final target-specific classifications for each specimen. Finally, DIAL also has an analytical engine which allows users to select and create specific data sets for various targets by different factors, e.g., patient demographics, geographic distribution, time periods, testing methods and perform different types of analysis including graphical presentations, tables, maps, rate calculation and trending analysis. In the case of respiratory specimens from ProvLab, DIAL's AIE was designed to assign positive and negative classifications for each respiratory virus as well as a summary classification that classifies each specimen as: (1) only positive for one specific virus, (2) mixed infection with more than one respiratory virus or (3) negative for all respiratory viruses. Using these final classifications, positive and negative specimens for each virus can easily be selected in DIAL for further analysis.

In this study we used DIAL to select specimen-based data and investigated the proportions of mono vs. mixed infections for hMPV as compared to ADV, CRV, ERV, PIV and RSV for a period of three years, 1 July 2009 to 30 June 2012. In order to create a uniform dataset for this study, we excluded all samples that tested positive for influenza A or B by the in-house real-time PCR assays and included only samples that had undergone RVP testing.

2. Results and Discussion

Using DIAL, 36,824 specimens were identified as positive for one or more respiratory virus during the study period. A total of 10,598 were excluded from this study with 9,340 tested positive for influenza A, 1,065 for influenza B, 7 for both influenza A and B and 185 specimens not tested by RVP even though they were negative for influenza. For the 26,226 RVP positive specimens included in the study, 10,042 (38%) were received between July 2009 and June 2010, 8,450 (32%) between July 2010 and June 2011 and 7,734 (30%) between July 2011 and June 2012. Mixed infection (having more than one virus identified) was found in 2,330 (9%) specimens and 23,896 (91%) had mono-infection (having only one virus identified). The majority of the specimens were collected from the upper respiratory tract as nasopharyngeal/nasal/throat swabs or nasopharyngeal aspirates 84% (n = 22,013), 12% (n = 3076) as respiratory samples with unspecified source, 4% (n = 917) were from the lower respiratory tract e.g., endotracheal aspirates or bronchaveolar lavage, and remaining as unknown sample types and a few tissues and sterile body fluid.

The age distribution of specimens submitted and tested positive for hMPV is summarized in Table 1. The highest number of specimens received was from patients less than 6 months old and the proportion of specimens tested positive for hMPV ranged from 4%–19% among the different age groups ($p < 0.001$, Chi Square test). Overall, mixed infection was detected in 15% of specimens tested positive for hMPV. Using specimens from the youngest age group (less than six months old) as the reference age group, there was significant difference for the proportion of mixed hMPV infection among the various age groups ($p < 0.05$, Binary Logistic Regression) (Table 1). Mixed infection with hMPV was most commonly found in specimens from patients younger than six months and rarely in specimens submitted from older than 70 years old.

Among the 373 specimens with mixed infections with hMPV, the three most commonly found virus was ERV, RSV and PIV, which also were the three most common viruses detected in all the specimens (Table 2). In comparison with ADV, four types of CRV, PIV, and RSV, hMPV had a significantly lower proportion of mixed infection specimens [χ^2 with Bonferroni's correction, $p =< 0.05$] and there was no significant difference of mixed infection comparing hMPV and ERV [χ^2 with Bonferroni's correction, $p = 0.06$].

The age distribution of virus found in mixed infection with hMPV is summarized in Table 3. ERV was the most commonly found virus in hMPV mixed infection across all age groups.

Table 1. Age distribution of specimens tested positive for metapneumovirus (hMPV) using Respiratory Virus Panel (RVP) and the number and % of mixed infection with hMPV.

Age groups	Number of specimens tested (n = 26,226)	Number of specimens tested positive for hMPV (%) (n = 2,561)	Number of specimens with mixed hMPV infection (n = 373)	% with Mixed infection
Unknown	83	13 (16)	5 *	38 *
Less than 6 months	5636	389 (7)	90	23 †
6 months to 1 year	3398	350 (10)	75	21
1 year	4282	467 (11)	75	16 †
2 years	1808	203 (11)	34	17
3 years	1066	141 (13)	19	14 †
4 years	671	88 (13)	8	9 †
5 to 9 years	1386	153 (11)	19	12 †
10 to 19 years	1167	58 (5)	8	14
20 to 29 years	1026	43 (4)	4	9
30 to 39 years	1091	82 (8)	5	6 †
40 to 49 years	999	105 (11)	8	8 †
50 to 59 years	1224	116 (10)	8	7 †
60 to 69 years	996	110 (11)	13	12 †
70 to 79 years	595	102 (17)	0	0 †
80 to 89 years	562	104 (19)	2	2 †
90 to 105 years	236	37 (16)	0	0 †

* 13 specimens with unknown age group, of which five had mixed hMPV infection, were excluded from the binary logistic regression analysis. † Using less than six months old as the reference age group, $p < 0.05$ comparing mono *versus* mixed infection for hMPV among the age groups (Binary Logistics Regression).

Table 2. Number and proportion of positive and mixed infection for the nine respiratory viruses and the frequency of the eight viruses identified in specimens with mixed infection with hMPV.

Virus	Number of specimens tested positive by virus (Total number of specimens tested = 26,226 *)	Number of specimens with mixed infection by virus (%)	Number of specimens found in mixed infections with hMPV (n = 373)	% of virus found in mixed infections with hMPV (n = 373)
Enterovirus/Rhinovirus	14322	1811 (13)	230 †	56
Respiratory Syncytial virus	5959	1020 (17)	48 †	12
Parainfluenza virus	3296	656 (20)	47 †	11
Human Metapneumovirus	2561	373 (15)	Not applicable	Not applicable
Adenovirus	1317	606 (46)	35 †	9
Coronavirus NL63	381	105 (28)	29 †	7
Coronavirus 229E	349	110 (32)	15 †	4
Coronavirus OC43	293	67 (23)	7 †	2
Coronavirus HKU1	263	82 (31)	2 †	1

* Influenza A and B positive samples and samples not tested by RVP were excluded from the analysis. † Some specimens in these subsets had more than one virus identified as co-existing with hMPV.

Table 3. Age distribution of respiratory virus found in mixed virus infection with hMPV.

Age groups	Number of specimens with mixed infection with hMPV (n = 368 *)	Distribution of virus found in specimens with mixed hMPV infections							
		ERV	RSV	PIV	ADV	CRV HKU1	CRV 229E	CRV OC43	CRV NL63
Less than 6 month	90 †	60	16	6	8	9	2	0	0
6 month to 1 year	75 †	46	7	6	9	10	2	1	0
1 year	75 †	52	10	9	8	4	1	1	1
2 years	34 †	16	5	6	7	1	2	0	0
3 years	19 †	13	3	3	0	1	0	0	0
4 years	8 †	6	0	2	1	0	0	0	1
5 to 9 years	19 †	9	0	8	0	1	1	1	0
10 to 19 years	8 †	3	2	1	0	1	2	0	0
20 to 29 years	4	4	0	0	0	0	0	0	0
30 to 39 years	5	2	0	2	1	0	0	0	0
40 to 49 years	8	3	2	1	0	1	1	0	0
50 to 59 years	8	2	1	1	0	1	3	0	0
60 to 69 years	13 †	9	1	1	0	0	1	4	0
70 to 79 years	0	NA	NA	NA	NA	NA	NA	NA	NA
80 to 89 years	2	1	0	1	0	0	0	0	0
90 to 105 years	0	NA	NA	NA	NA	NA	NA	NA	NA

* Five specimens with unknown age group were not tabulated. † Some specimens in these subsets had more than one virus identified as co-existing with hMPV.

Peak hMPV activity was observed in February 2010, June 2011 and November 2011, whereas peak ERV activity was found in the month of September in three consecutive years (2009, 2010 and 2011) (Figure 1). Specimens with mixed infection with these two viruses followed the trend and circulatory pattern of hMPV.

Figure 1. Monthly distribution of hMPV and ERV along with mixed infection with these two viruses.

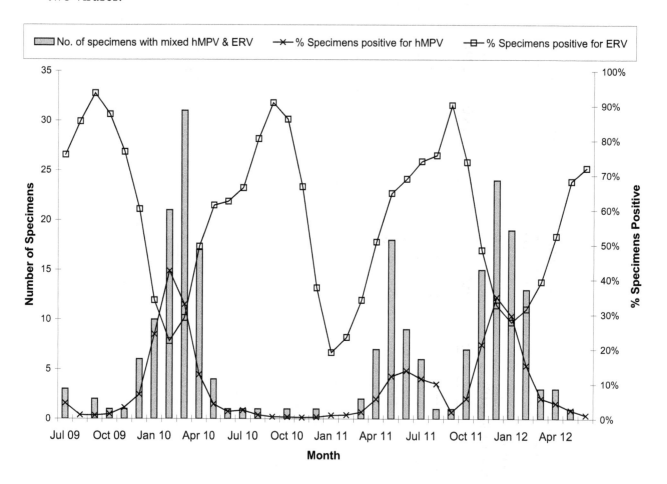

The objective of this study was to describe mono and mixed infections of hMPV in our jurisdiction for a three year period. All specimen data was acquired using ProvLab's DIAL application and we were able to identify that hMPV was more likely to occur in mono infection (85%) than mixed (15%). The results in this study were similar to a previous pilot study in Alberta which identified hMPV mixing with other pathogens in 15% of specimens (118/778) [17]. In other populations, namely hospitalized patients, mixed hMPV infections were in the minority.

Our study also determined that in hMPV mixed infections, the pathogen most likely to co-exist with hMPV is ERV (56%). In contrast, other studies have identified RSV as the leading cause of mixed infection with hMPV [18–20]. There may be several reasons for the difference in findings including the type of diagnostic assays used and the detection of various respiratory targets, clinical setting, patient age, and timing of specimen collection. Many studies have focused on populations mostly consisting of hospitalized pediatric patients and these studies have shown that RSV was the leading pathogen identified in these young children who were between 16 months to 14 years old [21–23]. In contrast, our study examined all age groups, including community-based and hospital-based specimens. ERV and hMPV remained closely linked across all age groups. Mixed infection with hMPV was most commonly found in the age group less than 6 months old. Moreover, ERV was still the dominant virus found to be mixed with hMPV. Our data set included specimens collected during the second phase of 2009 H1N1 pandemic in Alberta and Northern Territories, which made up of more than one third of the specimens included in this study. We found 62% of the samples between July 2009 and June 2010 tested positive for ERV, significantly higher than that found in the other two time periods, July 2010 to June 2011 (49%) and July 2011 to June 2012 (51%) (p < 0.001, Binary Logistic Regression). Other studies have also shown that during the pandemic ERV was a very common circulating virus followed by CRV [22,24,25]. Moreover, this linkage between ERV and hMPV could also be due to the inclusion of a very large group of viruses identified as ERV since RVP could not distinguish between various strains of rhinovirus and enterovirus. There might also be factors related to host immune responses and viral infection kinetics [26–29]. We have only examined the seasonality of hMPV and ERV and the mixed infection between these two viruses because of the relatively lower number of hMPV mixed infections for the other six viruses. Annual variations in peak hMPV activity was observed in our study with one of the peak months occurring in the summer of 2011, which was different from other studies in various Canadian provinces showing peaks of hMPV in the winter (January to April) [30–32]. As expected, the mixed infection of hMPV and ERV followed the circulatory pattern of hMPV but differed from ERV.

Although our findings have shown some trends with hMPV and its ability to exist as mono *versus* mixed infection, there are some important limitations in this study. Firstly, influenza A and B positive samples were excluded mainly because ProvLab does not routinely test influenza positive specimens for hMPV since the pandemic 2009. Excluding influenza viruses from our database may have impacted viral co-infection rates identified in our study. On the other hand, a recent study in England showed a lower prevalence of influenza A (H1N1) in patients positive for hMPV, ADV, RSV, PIV and rhinovirus with statistical significance for this relationship with hMPV and rhinovirus [32]. Another limitation was that the analysis by age group was based on specimen-based data only with duplicate samples from some individuals. Moreover, only limited information is usually provided on the requisition submitted with the specimens so we were not able to study clinical manifestations of mono-infection *versus* mixed infections and explore different settings

Despite the limitations stated, this study has considerable public health implications. This study helps us better understand the frequency of hMPV mono *versus* mixed infection over a period of three years. Better understanding of what mechanisms or conditions support mono *versus* mixed infections and the difference in clinical presentations and prognosis is needed. The prevalence of this virus supports research efforts to develop vaccine strategies which may become available in the future [33]. This also brings us to question whether testing algorithms at ProvLab need to be changed to better understand the interaction between hMPV and influenza A and B. Since hMPV has been shown to be an important pathogen, it should be included in ongoing surveillance and public health strategies.

Enhanced surveillance programs will help us better understand hMPV-associated diseases and maintain our awareness of trends in mono and mixed infections.

3. Experimental Section

ProvLab provides respiratory virus testing for the province of Alberta and surrounding Northern Territories (excluding Yukon) of Canada. Since June 2009, all respiratory specimens arriving at ProvLab was screened by an in-house (RT)-PCR for influenza A [14]. Specimens tested positive for influenza A were also subtyped for seasonal H3, seasonal H1 and pandemic H1N1 (2009) genes by RT-PCR. A multiplex assay to detect both influenza A and B was implemented in February 2010. Only specimens tested negative for both influenza A and B were tested using the RVP classic assay, a multiplexed assay which detects multiple respiratory viral pathogens including FLUA, FLUB, PIV, ERV, ADV, four types of CRV, RSV, and hMPV [14]. Exceptions to this testing policy included samples submitted from a provincial influenza-like-illness surveillance program (Tarrant Viral Watch) and some samples from patients with severe illness and admitted to the intensive care units. Specimens tested by RVP and tested positive for one or more respiratory virus excluding influenza A and B between July 2009 and June 2012 identified using the DIAL application was included in this study. DIAL provided classification of the specimens by each respiratory virus target as well as mono *versus* mixed infection. DIAL also allowed a user to select specimens based on the type of testing and over various geographic and time periods and age groups.

Statistical analysis of the proportion of mono *versus* mixed infections for the different virus was performed using Pearson Chi-squared (χ^2) test with Bonferroni's adjustment for multiple analyses. The proportion of hMPV as mixed infection by age group and ERV positive specimens by analysis of age group and time periods was analyzed using binary logistic regression. The SPSS software version 20.0 (IBM® SPSS® Statistics, IBM Corp., USA) was used for statistical analysis with the level of significance set at $p < 0.05$.

4. Conclusions

In this study we used DIAL to provide user-defined data sets of respiratory virus testing data and found that over a period of 3 years, July 2009 to June 2012, hMPV is significantly more likely to be identified in mono infection (86%) as compared with ADV, four types of CRV, PIV, and RSV with the exception of ERV. The three viruses most likely to be found in mixed infection with hMPV in this study were ERV, PIV and RSV with a higher proportion of mixed infection found in young infants.

Acknowledgments

The authors would like to acknowledge the staff of the Provincial Laboratory of Public Health who performed all laboratory testing and the Canadian Network for Public Health Intelligence program for their development work on the DIAL platform.

References

1. Statistics Canada. Leading causes of death in Canada 2009. Available online: http://www.statcan.gc.ca/pub/84-215-x/2012001/tbl/T001-eng.pdf (accessed 31 October 2012).

2. Van den Hoogen, B.G.; de Jong, J.C.; Groen, J.; Kuiken, T.; Fouchier, R.A.; Osterhaus, A.D. A newly discovered human pneumovirus isolated from young children with respiratory tract disease. *Nat. Med.* **2001**, *7*, 719–724.

3. Liu, L.; Bastien, N.; Sidaway, F.; Chan, E.; Li, Y. Seroprevalence of human metapneumovirus (hMPV) in the Canadian province of Saskatchewan analyzed by a recombinant nucleocapsid protein-based enzyme-linked immunosorbent assay. *J. Med. Virol.* **2007**, *79*, 308–313.

4. Manoha, C.; Espinosa, S.; Aho, S.L.; Huet, F.; Pothier, P. Epidemiological and clinical features of hMPV, RSV and RVs infections in young children. *J. Clin. Virol.* **2007**, *38*, 221–226.

5. Mullins, J.A.; Erdman, D.D.; Weinberg, G.A.; Edwards, K.; Hall, C.B.; Walker, F.J.; Iwane, M.; Anderson, L.J. Human metapneumovirus infection among children hospitalized with acute respiratory illness. *Emerg. Infect. Dis.* **2004**, *10*, 700–705.

6. Kaida, A.; Iritani, N.; Kubo, H.; Shiomi, M.; Kohdera, U.; Murakami, T. Seasonal distribution and phylogenetic analysis of human metapneumovirus among children in Osaka City, Japan. *J. Clin. Virol.* **2006**, *35*, 394–399.

7. Falsey, A.R.; Erdman, D.; Anderson, L.J.; Walsh, E.E. Human metapneumovirus infections in young and elderly adults. *J. Infect. Dis.* **2003**, *187*, 785–790.

8. Boivin, G.; Abed, Y.; Pelletier, G.; Ruel, L.; Moisan, D.; Cote, S.; Peret, T.C.; Erdman, D.D.; Anderson, L.J. Virological features and clinical manifestations associated with human metapneumovirus: A new paramyxovirus responsible for acute respiratory-tract infections in all age groups. *J. Infect. Dis.* **2002**, *186*, 1330–1334.

9. Boivin, G.; De, S.G.; Hamelin, M.E.; Cote, S.; Argouin, M.; Tremblay, G.; Maranda-Aubut, R.; Sauvageau, C.; Ouakki, M.; Boulianne, N.; Couture, C. An outbreak of severe respiratory tract infection due to human metapneumovirus in a long-term care facility. *Clin. Infect. Dis.* **2007**, *44*, 1152–1158.

10. Louie, J.K.; Schnurr, D.P.; Pan, C.Y.; Kiang, D.; Carter, C.; Tougaw, S.; Ventura, J.; Norman, A.; Belmusto, V.; Rosenberg, J.; Trochet, G. A summer outbreak of human metapneumovirus infection in a long-term-care facility. *J. Infect. Dis.* **2007**, *196*, 705–708.

11. Towgood, L.; Miller, M.; McKay, D.; Parker, R. Human metapneumovirus outbreak in a senior's care facility, British Columbia. *Canada Communicable Disease Report (CCDR) Weekly* **2008**.

12. Van Asten, L.; van den Wijngaard, C.; van Pelt, W.; van de Kassteele, J.; Meijer, A.; van der Hoek, W.; Kretzschmar, M.; Koopmans, M. Mortality attributable to 9 common infections: Significant effect of influenza a, respiratory syncytial virus, influenza B, norovirus, and parainfluenza in elderly persons. *J. Infect. Dis.* **2012**, *206*, 628–639.

13. Xie, Z.D.; Xiao, Y.; Liu, C.Y.; Hu, Y.H.; Yao, Y.; Yang, Y.; Qian, S.Y.; Geng, R.; Wang, J.W.; Shen, K.L. Three years surveillance of viral etiology of acute lower respiratory tract infection in children from 2007 to 2010. *Zhonghua Er. Ke. Za Zhi.* **2011**, *49*, 745–749.

14. Pabbaraju, K.; Tokaryk, K.L.; Wong, S.; Fox, J.D. Comparison of the Luminex xTAG respiratory viral panel with in-house nucleic acid amplification tests for diagnosis of respiratory virus infections. *J. Clin. Microbiol.* **2008**, *46*, 3056–3062.

15. Lee, B.E.; Mukhi, S.N.; May-Hadford, J.; Plitt, S.; Louie, M.; Drews, S.J. Determination of the relative economic impact of different molecular-based laboratory algorithms for respiratory viral pathogen detection, including Pandemic (H1N1), using a secure web based platform. *Virol. J.* **2011**, 8, 277–278. Available online: http://www.virologyj.com/content/8/1/277 (accessed on 31 October 2012).

16. Mukhi, S.N.; May-Hadford, J.; Plitt, S.; Preiksaitis, J.; Lee, B.E. DIAL: A Platform for real-time Laboratory Surveillance. *Online J. Public Health Inform.* **2010**, *2*, doi:10.5210/ojphi.v2i3.3041.

17. Pabbaraju, K.; Wong, S.; McMillan, T.; Lee, B.E.; Fox, J.D. Diagnosis and epidemiological studies of human metapneumovirus using real-time PCR. *J. Clin. Virol.* **2007**, *40*, 186–192.

18. Boivin, G.; De, S.G.; Cote, S.; Gilca, R.; Abed, Y.; Rochette, L.; Bergeron, M.G.; Dery, P. Human metapneumovirus infections in hospitalized children. *Emerg. Infect. Dis.* **2003**, *9*, 634–640.

19. Kuypers, J.; Wright, N.; Corey, L.; Morrow, R. Detection and quantification of human metapneumovirus in pediatric specimens by real-time RT-PCR. *J. Clin. Virol.* **2005**, *33*, 299–305.

20. Wolf, D.G.; Greenberg, D.; Kalkstein, D.; Shemer-Avni, Y.; Givon-Lavi, N.; Saleh, N.; Goldberg, M.D.; Dagan, R. Comparison of human metapneumovirus, respiratory syncytial virus and influenza A virus lower respiratory tract infections in hospitalized young children. *Pediatr. Infect. Dis. J.* **2006**, *25*, 320–324.

21. Sung, C.C.; Chi, H.; Chiu, N.C.; Huang, D.T.; Weng, L.C.; Wang, N.Y.; Huang, F.Y. Viral etiology of acute lower respiratory tract infections in hospitalized young children in Northern Taiwan. *J. Microbiol. Immunol. Infect.* **2011**, *44*, 184–190.

22. Xiao, N.G.; Xie, Z.P.; Zhang, B.; Yuan, X.H.; Song, J.R.; Gao, H.C.; Zhang, R.F.; Hou, Y.D.; Duan, Z.J. Prevalence and clinical and molecular characterization of human metapneumovirus in children with acute respiratory infection in China. *Pediatr. Infect. Dis. J.* **2010**, *29*, 131–134.

23. Martin, E.T.; Kuypers, J.; Wald, A.; Englund, J.A. Multiple *versus* single virus respiratory infections: Viral load and clinical disease severity in hospitalized children. *Influenza. Other Respir. Viruses* **2012**, *6*, 71–77.

24. Esper, F.P.; Spahlinger, T.; Zhou, L. Rate and influence of respiratory virus co-infection on pandemic (H1N1) influenza disease. *J. Infect.* **2011**, *63*, 260–266.

25. Thiberville, S.D.; Ninove, L.; Vu Hai, V; Botelho-Nevers, E.; Gazin, C.; Thirion, L.; Salez, N.; de Lamballerie, X.; Charrel, R.; Brouqui, P. The viral etiology of an influenza-like illness during the 2009 pandemic. *J. Med. Virol.* **2012**, *84*, 1071–1079.

26. Bitko, V.; Shulyayeva, O.; Mazumder, B.; Musiyenko, A.; Ramaswamy, M.; Look, D.C.; Barik, S. Nonstructural proteins of respiratory syncytial virus suppress premature apoptosis by an

NF-kappaB-dependent, interferon-independent mechanism and facilitate virus growth. *J. Virol.* **2007**, *81*, 1786–1795.

27. Spann, K.M.; Tran, K.C.; Chi, B.; Rabin, R.L.; Collins, P.L. Suppression of the induction of alpha, beta, and lambda interferons by the NS1 and NS2 proteins of human respiratory syncytial virus in human epithelial cells and macrophages [corrected]. *J. Virol.* **2004**, *78*, 4363–4369.

28. Ditt, V.; Lusebrink, J.; Tillmann, R.L.; Schildgen, V.; Schildgen, O. Respiratory infections by HMPV and RSV are clinically indistinguishable but induce different host response in aged individuals. *PLoS One* **2011**, *6*, e16314.

29. Franz, A.; Adams, O.; Willems, R.; Bonzel, L.; Neuhausen, N.; Schweizer-Krantz, S.; Ruggeberg, J.U.; Willers, R.; Henrich, B.; Schroten, H.; *et al.* Correlation of viral load of respiratory pathogens and co-infections with disease severity in children hospitalized for lower respiratory tract infection. *J. Clin. Virol.* **2010**, *48*, 239–245.

30. Hamelin, M.E.; Abed, Y.; Boivin, G. Human metapneumovirus: A new player among respiratory viruses. *Clin. Infect. Dis.* **2004**, *38*, 983–990.

31. Robinson, J.L.; Lee, B.E.; Bastien, N.; Li, Y. Seasonality and clinical features of human metapneumovirus infection in children in Northern Alberta. *J. Med. Virol.* **2005**, *76*, 98–105.

32. Bastien, N.; Ward, D.; Van, C.P.; Brandt, K.; Lee, S.H.; McNabb, G.; Klisko, B.; Chan, E.; Li, Y. Human metapneumovirus infection in the Canadian population. *J. Clin. Microbiol.* **2003**, *41*, 4642–4646.

33. Kahn, J.S. Newly discovered respiratory viruses: Significance and implications. *Curr. Opin. Pharmacol.* **2007**, *7*, 478–483.

5

Respiratory Syncytial Virus: Current Progress in Vaccine Development

Rajeev Rudraraju [1], **Bart G. Jones** [1], **Robert Sealy** [1], **Sherri L. Surman** [1] **and Julia L. Hurwitz** [1,2,*]

[1] Department of Infectious Diseases, St. Jude Children's Research Hospital,
262 Danny Thomas Place, Memphis, TN 38105, USA;
E-Mails: Rajeev.rudraraju@stjude.org (R.R.); bart.jones@stjude.org (B.G.J.);
robert.sealy@stjude.org (R.S.); sherri.surman@stjude.org (S.L.S.)

[2] Department of Microbiology, Immunology and Biochemistry,
University of Tennessee Health Science Center, 858 Madison Avenue, Memphis, TN 38163, USA

[*] Author to whom correspondence should be addressed; E-Mail: julia.hurwitz@stjude.org

Abstract: Respiratory syncytial virus (RSV) is the etiological agent for a serious lower respiratory tract disease responsible for close to 200,000 annual deaths worldwide. The first infection is generally most severe, while re-infections usually associate with a milder disease. This observation and the finding that re-infection risks are inversely associated with neutralizing antibody titers suggest that immune responses generated toward a first RSV exposure can significantly reduce morbidity and mortality throughout life. For more than half a century, researchers have endeavored to design a vaccine for RSV that can mimic or improve upon natural protective immunity without adverse events. The virus is herein described together with the hurdles that must be overcome to develop a vaccine and some current vaccine development approaches.

Keywords: respiratory syncytial virus; candidate vaccines; protective immunity

1. RSV, the Virus

Respiratory syncytial virus is a negative strand RNA virus in the family *Paramyxoviridae*, the subfamily *Pneumovirinae* and the genus *Pneumovirus*. RSV was first discovered in 1952 as the cause of a serious lower respiratory tract disease, most pronounced among children in their first year of life [1]. Other individuals who are susceptible to severe RSV disease include patients with cardiac and pulmonary disorders, patients with immunodeficiencies, and the elderly [2–6]. RSV infection generally presents as an upper respiratory tract (URT) infection which progresses for several days before virus traffics to the lung [1,7]. Most infants are able to clear virus without extreme adverse events, but in the United States approximately 2% require hospitalization [8,9]. Globally, RSV infections are estimated to result in up to 199,000 deaths annually in children younger than 5 years of age [10] and treatment options remain controversial. Re-infections can occur, but generally result in milder disease; risks of infection are inversely associated with RSV-specific serum neutralizing antibody titers [11,12]. For infants at risk for first infections, the passive transfer of monoclonal RSV F-specific antibodies is recommended, but this type of prophylaxis is expensive and unavailable for most individuals who need it [13]. A licensed vaccine, the single best health care solution to infectious disease, is unavailable in the RSV field.

The RSV genome consists of 11 coding sequences including NS1, NS2, N, P, M, SH, G, F, M2-1, M2-2 and L [1,14]. The predominant proteins on the outer membrane of the mature virus are G, F and SH. Initiation of infection is usually mediated by the interaction between RSV G, the major attachment glycoprotein, and the host cell membrane. The viral receptors for G (and F) proteins on mammalian cells are not fully defined, but G can bind highly sulfated heparin-like glycosaminoglycans [15] as well as the CX3CR1 fracktalkine chemokine receptor [16]. G attachment facilitates F-mediated membrane fusion, although F protein can bind cell membranes independently (e.g., via binding to cellular heparan sulfate and nucleolin [16,17]) and mediate virus infection in the absence of G [1,18]. Fusion occurs when the F1 subunit of F protein is inserted into the target membrane and the protein refolds into a hairpin structure bringing virus and cell membranes into close proximity [19]. Upon membrane fusion, virus material including a single negative strand RNA genome is released into the cell cytoplasm [19]. Viral RNA is then transcribed and replicated yielding viral mRNA and new virus genome. New virions are assembled at the cell membrane, bud using cell membranes as their outer coat, and then target new cells for additional rounds of infection. Non-structural proteins support virus production while down-regulating host cell growth and defense mechanisms [1].

2. Hurdles to Vaccine Development

A main hurdle for RSV vaccine development was encountered in the 1960s during the testing of a formalin-inactivated RSV vaccine (FI-RSV). Unfortunately, the vaccinated infants were not protected from RSV infection. Instead, an unusually large percentage of the vaccinated children, when subsequently exposed to RSV by natural causes, developed disease severe enough to require hospitalization and there were two vaccine-related deaths [20]. It is essential that such a scenario never be repeated, and because the reason for the vaccine-related adverse events has not been confirmed, scientists are unsure precisely how to proceed. There remains no licensed vaccine product after one-half century of additional research.

The cause of vaccine-related deaths remains a point of discussion. One potential explanation is as follows: The formalin treatment of RSV altered membrane proteins on the virus and in so doing, rendered a vaccine that induced antibody responses that were non-neutralizing [21,22]. The inactivated vaccine also failed to elicit robust CD8+ T cells, because these classical killers of virus-infected targets are best induced by endogenously expressed viral antigens. In the absence of robust neutralizing antibodies and CD8+ T cells, RSV persisted and induced an aggressive CD4+ T cell and cytokine response in the lower respiratory tract [23,24]. Uncontrolled RSV replication and persistent inflammation led to blockage of the small airways in infants, leading to substantial morbidity and mortality [1,4,14,25].

There is now debate as to which immune cell populations or effector molecules were responsible for disease [21,26–33]. In a murine model designed to recapitulate the clinical outcome with FI-RSV, it was demonstrated that a subset of RSV G-specific CD4+ Th2 cells and eosinophils associated with disease. [23,24,31,32,34,35]. Additional mouse experiments showed that inhibition of IL-4 and IL-10 Th2 cytokines abrogated pulmonary histopatholgy [24]. Some researchers argue that the induction of Th2 cells, or perhaps the induction of any RSV-specific T cells should be avoided [36], even though T cells may be key providers of help for B cells and cytotoxic T lymphocyte functions at the time of RSV exposure. Others argue that the large majority of granulocytes described in original clinical autopsy reports were neutrophils rather than eosinophils [37], questioning the absolute comparison between mouse and human responses to FI-RSV. The potential benefits provided under the appropriate conditions by Th2 cells, other CD4+ and CD8+ T cell subsets, and eosinophil populations are contemplated [37–42]. For example, it is noted that individuals who lack T cells can experience great difficulty in RSV clearance and suffer worse outcomes than their immunocompetent counterparts [4,14,43,44]. It is further noted that eosinophils can be beneficial in that their transfer to the lungs of RSV-infected mice can enhance RSV clearance and inhibit airway hyper-reactivity [45]. Until debates are resolved, researchers and regulatory boards struggle to define 'go' and 'no go' criteria for the advancement of candidate vaccines, particularly when clinical studies target the pediatric arena. It is possible that past RSV vaccine candidates may have proved safe and efficacious in children, but were never tested in seronegative, pediatric populations. Perhaps a solution resides in comprehensive data analyses, revealing the complexities of the immune system and that each lymphocyte subset need not be categorically designated as beneficial or injurious [46]. Rather, as is the case in most RSV-experienced adults, a variety of adaptive and innate immune effectors including B cells, CD4+ T helper cells and CD8+ cytotoxic T lymphocytes function synergistically to mediate safe elimination of virus and virus-infected cells.

Another issue pertinent to RSV vaccine development concerns the selection of an appropriate human test population. Vaccine studies in young infants are performed with hesitancy due to the devastating experience with the FI-RSV vaccine. One suggested possibility is that vaccines might be tested in seropositive adults including the elderly rather than in infants. A number of strategies are considered including: (i) standard vaccination of placebo and control groups with subsequent assessment of disease caused by natural RSV exposure; (ii) the use of an experimental RSV challenge virus [47]; and (iii) the vaccination of pregnant females to measure protection afforded to the infant at birth. One or more of these strategies may prove fruitful provided that attention is paid to a number of confounding variables. First, due to varying degrees of seropositivity in older individuals, immune responsiveness toward vaccination may be difficult to interpret. Individuals with high pre-existing immunity might be expected to show a boost in antibody titers following vaccination, but may instead clear vectors and antigens so rapidly that there is little opportunity for immune cells to re-activate. Second, vaccine safety data may be difficult to interpret due to frequent, unrelated disease complications in the oldest adults. One additional variable to be considered (upon design of either pediatric or adult vaccine protocols) is that individuals with poor diets or poor metabolism (e.g., vitamin deficiency) may exhibit general defects in immune responses toward respiratory virus vaccines [48,49]. With these considerations in mind, it has been proposed that RSV vaccine studies in the elderly are feasible, but would require the recruitment of thousands of participants to ensure fair vaccine assessment [50]. Another recent proposal has been that RSV vaccine studies might best be conducted not in the youngest infants or in adults, but in seronegative children who are at least 6 months of age [51]. Perhaps efficacy studies in older, seronegative children could assist vaccine licensure for a restricted age group while prompting additional clinical studies in the youngest infants.

3. Current RSV Vaccine Strategies

The first formal vaccine development effort occurred two centuries ago when Edward Jenner demonstrated that material from a cowpox lesion could serve as a vaccine for smallpox [52]. Successful vaccination, both then and now, relies on the safe introduction of a pathogen's antigenic determinants to the immune system. If the vaccine's antigenic determinants are well matched to those of the native pathogen (as was the case for cowpox and smallpox), the antigens will activate pathogen-specific lymphocytes. In the case of virus-specific B cells, some effectors will mature to the plasma cell stage and constitutively secrete antibodies into blood, lymph and mucosal secretions, while others will maintain memory status, capable of immediate re-activation upon pathogen exposure. Activated CD8+ T cells are classically known for their killing of virus infected cells, while CD4+ T cells, (including Th1, Th2, Th17, TFh, Treg, and other subsets) are known for their support and regulation of CD8+ and B cell activities [53–57]. The heightened or "primed" state of immune surveillance may last months or years to inhibit pathogen entry and pathogen-mediated damage to the host [58]. Generally, vaccines are developed by: (i) inactivating the virus; (ii) identifying a related virus in another species that is safe in humans (the Jennerian approach); (iii) attenuating the virus; or (iv) using recombinant technology to present viral antigens, often in the context of a replication competent or replication-incompetent vector. In the RSV vaccine field, because of the outcome of the FI-RSV vaccine study, the first approach is generally discouraged, even if candidate vaccines retain RSV neutralizing determinants. The second strategy, the Jennerian approach, has not been advanced due to an insufficient antigenic match between bovine and human RSV [59]. The third and fourth strategies are the topics of most current vaccine research, described in greater detail below. Preclinical testing of vaccine candidates is generally accomplished first in small animals and then in non-human primates. Most small animal studies use hamsters, BALB/c mice, or cotton rats [60–63] while non-human primate studies generally use African green monkeys, rhesus macaques and chimpanzees [64–66]. Each animal is at least semi-permissive for RSV infection and is therefore advantageous in that immune responses and immunopathological events can be measured, but no animal model fully predicts the course of immune responses and disease in humans. In one instance, for example, an attenuated RSV vaccine appeared to be safe in non-human primates, but proved unsafe when tested in seronegative children [67]. Again, the debates described above concerning: (i) interpretation of data from animal experiments; and (ii) selection of clinical trial target populations, must be considered to determine when and how to advance vaccine candidates from pre-clinical to clinical trials.

3.1. Attenuated Virus Vaccines: Testing Variant Mutations

One strategy for RSV vaccine development has been to attenuate virus by cold adaption [68,69]. An early product of this research was cpts-248/404 [70,71]. However, in the youngest infants, the vaccine caused URT congestion associated with peak virus recovery and was deemed unacceptable for further development. More recently the cpts-248/404/1030/ΔSH vaccine was developed by introducing further mutations and deleting the SH gene, resulting in a more satisfactory product [72]. In a recent clinical study with this candidate, post-vaccination nasal washes revealed viruses with partial loss of the temperature sensitive phenotype, often due to a tyrosine/asparagine substitution in the L gene at position 1321 [73]. Researchers corrected the problem by creating a reversion-resistant virus with an alternative attenuating codon at position 1321. However, they then discovered a compensatory mutation at position 1313, forcing a deletion of that position (Δ1313) to yield a safer vaccine. When the Δ1313 deletion was paired with an NS2 gene deletion and tested at incrementally increasing temperatures, another compensatory mutation was discovered, I1314T. Finally, a vaccine with a new combination of mutations (ΔNS2/Δ1313/1314L) is being developed for evaluation in phase I clinical trials [74]. Reverse genetics, a powerful technology that allows the manipulation of viral genomes and recovery of infectious, recombinant virus particles, has assisted the progress described above [75].

A number of attenuated RSV vaccines have now been tested clinically. Currently, a phase I clinical study in adults, seropositive children and seronegative children is in progress to test safety and immunogenicity of an intranasally (I.N.) delivered RSV M2-2 deletion mutant [73,76,77].

The development of live-attenuated vaccines presents significant challenges, particularly when vaccines are delivered by the respiratory route to neonates. A concern is that viruses with compensatory mutations in the live-attenuated vaccines may associate with reversion to pathogenic phenotypes and lead to increased frequencies of adverse reactions *in vivo*. There is also a difficulty related to manufacturing and distribution, as RSV is naturally sensitive to changes in temperature, and attenuated strains by definition are difficult to propagate to high titers.

3.2. Recombinant Protein Vaccines

Recombinant technology provides great flexibility both in terms of the RSV antigen(s) and the vector(s) with which the antigen is expressed. The major target antigens of recombinant vaccine technology are RSV G and F, as these are each capable of eliciting neutralizing antibodies as well as T cell responses. F is particularly attractive due to its considerable conservation among RSV isolates. Another antigen of recent interest is the small hydrophobic protein, SH [78].

As an example of progress in recombinant vaccine technology, Novartis is developing a postfusion RSV F trimer that elicits neutralizing antibodies and protection against RSV challenge in cotton rats [79]. Most researchers strive to match vaccine protein with pathogen protein to take advantage of polyclonal B and T cell responses that can work in unison to recognize and combat pathogen. Other researchers target particular epitopes such as a central conserved region of the G protein that induces antibodies to block the CX3C-CX3CR1 interaction. Mice vaccinated with fragments containing the CX3C motif have been shown to generate immune responses that can reduce lung virus titers and pulmonary inflammation following RSV challenge [80]. Still other researchers, as described above, propose that all T cell epitopes (and many B cell epitopes) should be removed from RSV vaccines [36,42]. Using computational design, epitope-scaffold vaccines have been developed to mimic an individual epitope on the F protein known to correspond with a neutralizing monoclonal antibody activity (motavizumab, [13]). In one case, several scaffolds were developed based on 13 discontinuous RSV F contact residues (xSxxLSxINDxxxxNDxKKLxSNx) for motavizumab. An automated search of protein structures supported the selection of three proteins as scaffolds: protein Z, a domain of protein A from *Staphylococcus aureus*, Cag-Z from *Helicobacter pylori* and the p26 capsid protein from equine infectious anemia virus. Amino acids outside of the motavizumab epitope were then modified or removed to optimize stability, solubility and motavizumab binding affinity. Critical to decisions concerning scaffold design are demonstrations that B cell and T cell determinants on viruses are often dependent on structural and spatial context, as regions outside the epitope affect 3-dimensional folding, post-translational modifications, and antigen processing [81–84]. For this reason, immune cells that respond to a protein fragment in one context (e.g., vaccine) do not necessarily recognize the same fragment when the context is changed (e.g., virus). When the *Stapylococcus aureus* protein A scaffold was fused to a pan-HLA DR binding epitope and tested for immunogenicity in mice, it induced RSV-binding antibodies, but these antibodies failed to neutralize RSV [36]. A separate study of a motavizumab-based scaffold in non-human primates illustrated neutralizing antibodies in a fraction of animals [85].

Most protein vaccines, whether designed to match unmanipulated viral proteins or targeted determinants, are combined with adjuvants. A plethora of adjuvants now exist including $W_{80}5EC$ [86], alum, 3-O-desacyl-4'-monophosphoryl lipid A (MPL), muramyl dipeptide (MDP), natural host defense peptides, CpG oligodeoxynucleotides (ODN) and polyphosphazenes. Polyphosphazenes are synthetic water-soluble polymers containing an inorganic backbone of alternating phosphorus and nitrogen atoms. Adjuvants are in some cases known to trigger cell molecules (e.g., toll-like receptors, TLR) to activate innate and adaptive immune responses. For example, MPL, CpG ODN, and MDP are ligands for TLR-4, TLR-9, and NOD2, respectively. The $W_{80}5EC$ product can serve both as an adjuvant and as a virus-inactivation method [86]. While adjuvant choices are many, U.S. Food and Drug Administration (FDA)-approved and licensed adjuvants are limited (alum and MPL). There is also a large variety of combinations for formulations of liposomes, nanoparticles or microparticles (synthetic particles and/or particles encompassing bacterial or viral components [87]) for the delivery of RSV proteins, peptides, and/or adjuvants. As an example, a truncated, secreted, trimeric F protein has been formulated for I.N. delivery with combinations of a TLR agonist (CpG ODN), an innate defense regulator peptide (IDR1002-VQRWLIVWRIRK), and polyphosphazene as nano- or microparticles, to induce RSV protective immunity [88,89]. Yet another example is Novavax's near-full length F glycoprotein formulated as a nanoparticle vaccine. This vaccine has been tested in healthy adults and has been shown to induce significant increases in the anti-F antibody response, including micro-neutralizing activities and competitive activity against the neutralizing monoclonal antibody Palivizumab [13,90–92]. An additional use of adjuvant has been with MPL combined not with a recombinant protein or particle, but with virosomes comprising membranes from RSV [93].

3.3. Replication Competent, Recombinant Viral Vaccines

Reverse genetics has assisted the development of recombinant viral vaccines that can serve as delivery systems for RSV antigens. One such vaccine, which has been well advanced in clinical trials, is MedImmune's MEDI-534 [94,95]. This vaccine is a replication-competent vaccine that expresses RSV F [75,96]. The backbone is based on a bovine parainfluenza virus type 3 with substituted human PIV3 F and HN glycoproteins. MEDI-534 was tested in non-human primates and also in a phase I study in young children between the ages of 6 months and <24 months. Doses of 10,000, 100,000 and 1,000,000 $TCID_{50}$ were tested in the clinical trial and RSV specific antibody responses were noted in 50% of vaccinees administered three 1,000,000 $TCID_{50}$ doses of vaccine with two month intervals. Virus that was shed from study participants revealed genetic changes that were associated with reduced RSV F protein expression. A close analysis of the MEDI-534 vaccine then demonstrated that some of the same genetic variants were minor components of the administered vaccine [97]. The implication of these sequence variants is a current topic of discussion.

Another promising candidate is St. Jude's recombinant, replication competent vaccine (SeVRSV), also developed with reverse genetics technology [75]. Sendai virus (SeV), a mouse parainfluenza virus type I with a high sequence and antigenic similarity to human parainfluenza virus type I (hPIV-1), was used as the vaccine's backbone [98–102]. SeV is an attractive vaccine candidate and vaccine backbone, because there has never been a confirmed case of SeV-associated disease in humans. The species specificity of Sendai virus is attributed in part to its unique sensitivity to human type I interferon [103]. In small animals a single I.N. dose of SeV induced B and T cell responses within days after immunization that lasted for the animal's lifetime without need for a booster [62]. The SeVRSV recombinant carries the RSV F gene and thereby instructs its expression in infected cells [104]. When tested in cotton rats, SeVRSV protected animals from challenge with both A and B RSV isolates. SeVRSV could also be mixed with two additional SeV-based vaccines in a single I.N.

inoculation to protect against four different challenge viruses: RSV, hPIV-1, hPIV-2 and hPIV-3 [62]. When SeVRSV was tested as a vaccine in African green monkeys with non-recombinant SeV as a control, it safely and fully prevented infection of the lower airways following RSV challenge [66]. The non-recombinant SeV has already entered clinical trials as a hPIV-1 vaccine and has been well tolerated in adults [105] and 3–6 year old children. SeVRSV is now being manufactured for testing in an age de-escalation clinical trial. Previous pre-clinical and clinical data suggest that SeVRSV will safely protect children from both RSV and hPIV-1 infections. When compared to the live-attenuated RSV vaccines, SeV based vaccines benefit from their relative stability to temperature changes and ease of growth to high titers in chicken eggs and cell cultures, a boon for manufacturing and vaccine distribution.

3.4. A Variety of New Vectors and Concepts in the RSV Vaccine Field

A great number of additional recombinant vaccines are in stages of pre-clinical testing. Vectors include Semliki Forest virus [106], Venezuelan equine encephalitis virus [107,108], adenovirus from humans or non-human primates [109,110], influenza virus [111], measles virus [112], Newcastle disease virus like particles (VLPs [113]) and plasmid DNA [114,115]. Other vaccine delivery systems are based not on viruses, but bacteria, yeast or plants [116], such as the Mucosis SynGEM® vaccine, an I.N. vaccine that presents native trimeric F protein formulated in a non-living bacterium-like particle (BLP) [117]. There have also been combination prime-boost strategies using one form of recombinant vaccine followed by another. For example a recombinant vaccine prime based on replication-defective chimpanzee adenovirus can be followed with a boost based on modified vaccinia Ankara (MVA) [118], or a recombinant DNA prime can be followed by recombinant adenoviral vector boosts [119]. This article describes a portion, but not all of the vaccine candidates that are currently under investigation. Table 1 provides a short list as a sampling of vaccine strategies with references and review articles. It is quite likely that one or more than one of the current vaccine candidates will prove successful. The advanced development and licensure of a safe and effective RSV vaccine will indeed be momentous, a long-awaited milestone for the prevention of the significant sickness and death caused by RSV infections.

Table 1. Sample respiratory syncytial virus (RSV) vaccine references and review articles.

Vaccine Type	Sample references
Attenuated RSV	[73,74]
Inactivated RSV	[86,120]
RSV protein(s) adjuvanted and/or as micro/nano-particles	[79,89]
Epitope scaffold	[36]
Virosome	[93,121]
Virus like particle (VLP)	[113,122]
Replication competent virus-based vector	[66,94,95,97]
Bacteria-based vector	[123–125]
Plant-based vector	[116]
Prime-boost with heterologous vectors	[118,119].
Related review articles	**[1,4,14,25,115,126]**

Acknowledgments

This work was supported in part by NIH, NIAID grants P01-AI-054955, R01-AI088729, and R01-AI78819, NCI grant P30-CA21765 and the American Lebanese Syrian Associated Charities. Acknowledgement is given to S. Varga, N. Lukacs and K. Harrod for organizing the 8th International Respiratory Syncytial Virus Symposium in 2012.

References

1.   Collins, P.L.; Crowe, J.E. Respiratory Syncytial Virus and Metapneumovirus. In *Fields Virology*, 5th ed.; Knipe, D.M., Howley, P.M, Griffin, D.E., Lamb, R.A., Martin, M.A., Roizman B., *et al.*, Eds.; Lippincott Williams&Wilkins: Philadelphia, PA, USA, 2007; pp. 1601–1646.

2.   Groothuis, J.R.; Gutierrez, K.M.; Lauer, B.A. Respiratory syncytial virus infection in children with bronchopulmonary dysplasia. *Pediatrics* **1988**, *82*, 199–203.

3.   Falsey, A.R.; Hennessey, P.A.; Formica, M.A.; Cox, C.; Walsh, E.E. Respiratory syncytial virus infection in elderly and high-risk adults. *N. Engl. J. Med.* **2005**, *352*, 1749–1759.

4.   Collins, P.L.; Melero, J.A. Progress in understanding and controlling respiratory syncytial virus: Still crazy after all these years. *Virus Res.* **2011**, *162*, 80–99.

5.   El Saleeby, C.M.; Somes, G.W.; DeVincenzo, J.P.; Gaur, A.H. Risk factors for severe respiratory syncytial virus disease in children with cancer: The importance of lymphopenia and young age. *Pediatrics* **2008**, *121*, 235–243.

6.   Madhi, S.A.; Schoub, B.; Simmank, K.; Blackburn, N.; Klugman, K.P. Increased burden of respiratory viral associated severe lower respiratory tract infections in children infected with human immunodeficiency virus type-1. *J. Pediatr.* **2000**, *137*, 78–84.

7.   Wright, P.F.; Gruber, W.C.; Peters, M.; Reed, G.; Zhu, Y.; Robinson, F.; Coleman-Dockery, S.; Graham, B.S. Illness severity, viral shedding, and antibody responses in infants hospitalized with bronchiolitis caused by respiratory syncytial virus. *J. Infect. Dis.* **2002**, *185*, 1011–1018.

8.   Zhou, H.; Thompson, W.W.; Viboud, C.G.; Ringholz, C.M.; Cheng, P.Y.; Steiner, C.; Abedi, G.R.; Anderson, L.J.; Brammer, L.; Shay, D.K. Hospitalizations associated with influenza and respiratory syncytial virus in the United States, 1993–2008. *Clin. Infect. Dis.* **2012**, *54*, 1427–1436.

9.   Thompson, W.W.; Shay, D.K.; Weintraub, E.; Brammer, L.; Cox, N.; Anderson, L.J.; Fukuda, K. Mortality associated with influenza and respiratory syncytial virus in the United States. *JAMA* **2003**, *289*, 179–186.

10.   Nair, H.; Nokes, D.J.; Gessner, B.D.; Dherani, M.; Madhi, S.A.; Singleton, R.J.; O'Brien, K.L.; Roca, A.; Wright, P.F.; Bruce, N.; *et al.* Global burden of acute lower respiratory infections due to respiratory syncytial virus in young children: A systematic review and meta-analysis. *Lancet* **2010**, *375*, 1545–1555.

11. Glezen, W.P.; Taber, L.H.; Frank, A.L.; Kasel, J.A. Risk of primary infection and reinfection with respiratory syncytial virus. *Am. J. Dis. Child.* **1986**, *140*, 543–546.

12. Shinoff, J.J.; O'Brien, K.L.; Thumar, B.; Shaw, J.B.; Reid, R.; Hua, W.; Santosham, M.; Karron, R.A. Young infants can develop protective levels of neutralizing antibody after infection with respiratory syncytial virus. *J. Infect. Dis.* **2008**, *198*, 1007–1015.

13. Fernandez, P.; Trenholme, A.; Abarca, K.; Griffin, M.P.; Hultquist, M.; Harris, B.; Losonsky, G.A. A phase 2, randomized, double-blind safety and pharmacokinetic assessment of respiratory syncytial virus (RSV) prophylaxis with motavizumab and palivizumab administered in the same season. *BMC. Pediatr.* **2010**, *10*, 38.

14. Collins, P.L.; Graham, B.S. Viral and host factors in human respiratory syncytial virus pathogenesis. *J. Virol.* **2008**, *82*, 2040–2055.

15. Feldman, S.A.; Hendry, R.M.; Beeler, J.A. Identification of a linear heparin binding domain for human respiratory syncytial virus attachment glycoprotein G. *J. Virol.* **1999**, *73*, 6610–6617.

16. Harcourt, J.L.; Karron, R.A.; Tripp, R.A. Anti-G protein antibody responses to respiratory syncytial virus infection or vaccination are associated with inhibition of G protein CX3C-CX3CR1 binding and leukocyte chemotaxis. *J. Infect. Dis.* **2004**, *190*, 1936–1940.

17. Tayyari, F.; Marchant, D.; Moraes, T.J.; Duan, W.; Mastrangelo, P.; Hegele, R.G. Identification of nucleolin as a cellular receptor for human respiratory syncytial virus. *Nat. Med.* **2011**, *17*, 1132–1135.

18. Techaarpornkul, S.; Collins, P.L.; Peeples, M.E. Respiratory syncytial virus with the fusion protein as its only viral glycoprotein is less dependent on cellular glycosaminoglycans for attachment than complete virus. *Virology* **2002**, *294*, 296–304.

19. Russell, C.J.; Luque, L.E. The structural basis of paramyxovirus invasion. *Trends Microbiol.* **2006**, *14*, 243–246.

20. Chin, J.; Magoffin, R.L.; Shearer, L.A.; Schieble, J.H.; Lennette, E.H. Field evaluation of a respiratory syncytial virus vaccine and a trivalent parainfluenza virus vaccine in a pediatric population. *Am. J. Epidemiol.* **1969**, *89*, 449–463.

21. Murphy, B.R.; Prince, G.A.; Walsh, E.E.; Kim, H.W.; Parrott, R.H.; Hemming, V.G.; Rodriguez, W.J.; Chanock, R.M. Dissociation between serum neutralizing and glycoprotein antibody responses of infants and children who received inactivated respiratory syncytial virus vaccine. *J. Clin. Microbiol.* **1986**, *24*, 197–202.

22. Murphy, B.R.; Walsh, E.E. Formalin-inactivated respiratory syncytial virus vaccine induces antibodies to the fusion glycoprotein that are deficient in fusion-inhibiting activity. *J. Clin. Microbiol.* **1988**, *26*, 1595–1597.

23. Varga, S.M.; Wang, X.; Welsh, R.M.; Braciale, T.J. Immunopathology in RSV infection is mediated by a discrete oligoclonal subset of antigen-specific CD4(+) T cells. *Immunity* **2001**, *15*, 637–646.

24. Connors, M.; Giese, N.A.; Kulkarni, A.B.; Firestone, C.Y.; Morse, H.C., III; Murphy, B.R. Enhanced pulmonary histopathology induced by respiratory syncytial virus (RSV) challenge of formalin-inactivated RSV-immunized BALB/c mice is abrogated by depletion of interleukin-4 (IL-4) and IL-10. *J. Virol.* **1994**, *68*, 5321–5325.

25. Blanco, J.C.; Boukhvalova, M.S.; Shirey, K.A.; Prince, G.A.; Vogel, S.N. New insights for development of a safe and protective RSV vaccine. *Hum. Vaccines* **2010**, *6*, 482–492.

26. Delgado, M.F.; Coviello, S.; Monsalvo, A.C.; Melendi, G.A.; Hernandez, J.Z.; Batalle, J.P.; Diaz, L.; Trento, A.; Chang, H.Y.; Mitzner, W.; *et al.* Lack of antibody affinity maturation due to poor Toll-like receptor stimulation leads to enhanced respiratory syncytial virus disease. *Nat. Med.* **2009**, *15*, 34–41.

27. Shaw, C.A.; Otten, G.; Wack, A.; Palmer, G.A.; Mandl, C.W.; Mbow, M.L.; Valiante, N.; Dormitzer, P.R. Antibody affinity maturation and respiratory syncytial virus disease. *Nat. Med.* **2009**, *15*, 725–726.

28. Polack, F.P.; Teng, M.N.; Collins, P.L.; Prince, G.A.; Exner, M.; Regele, H.; Lirman, D.D.; Rabold, R.; Hoffman, S.J.; Karp, C.L.; *et al.* A role for immune complexes in enhanced respiratory syncytial virus disease. *J. Exp. Med.* **2002**, *196*, 859–865.

29. Polack, F.P. Atypical measles and enhanced respiratory syncytial virus disease (ERD) made simple. *Pediatr. Res.* **2007**, *62*, 111–115.

30. Kakuk, T.J.; Soike, K.; Brideau, R.J.; Zaya, R.M.; Cole, S.L.; Zhang, J.Y.; Roberts, E.D.; Wells, P.A.; Wathen, M.W. A human respiratory syncytial virus (RSV) primate model of enhanced pulmonary pathology induced with a formalin-inactivated RSV vaccine but not a recombinant FG subunit vaccine. *J. Infect. Dis.* **1993**, *167*, 553–561.

31. Walzl, G.; Matthews, S.; Kendall, S.; Gutierrez-Ramos, J.C.; Coyle, A.J.; Openshaw, P.J.; Hussell, T. Inhibition of T1/ST2 during respiratory syncytial virus infection prevents T helper cell type 2 (Th2)- but not Th1-driven immunopathology. *J. Exp. Med.* **2001**, *193*, 785–792.

32. Rosenberg, H.F.; Dyer, K.D.; Domachowske, J.B. Respiratory viruses and eosinophils: Exploring the connections. *Antiviral Res.* **2009**, *83*, 1–9.

33. Becker, Y. Respiratory syncytial virus (RSV) evades the human adaptive immune system by skewing the Th1/Th2 cytokine balance toward increased levels of Th2 cytokines and IgE, markers of allergy—A review. *Virus Genes* **2006**, *33*, 235–252.

34. Srikiatkhachorn, A.; Braciale, T.J. Virus-specific CD8+ T lymphocytes downregulate T helper cell type 2 cytokine secretion and pulmonary eosinophilia during experimental murine respiratory syncytial virus infection. *J. Exp. Med.* **1997**, *186*, 421–432.

35. Legg, J.P.; Hussain, I.R.; Warner, J.A.; Johnston, S.L.; Warner, J.O. Type 1 and type 2 cytokine imbalance in acute respiratory syncytial virus bronchiolitis. *Am. J Respir. Crit. Care Med.* **2003**, *168*, 633–639.

36. McLellan, J.S.; Correia, B.E.; Chen, M.; Yang, Y.; Graham, B.S.; Schief, W.R.; Kwong, P.D. Design and characterization of epitope-scaffold immunogens that present the motavizumab epitope from respiratory syncytial virus. *J Mol. Biol.* **2011**, *409*, 853–866.

37. Prince, G.A.; Curtis, S.J.; Yim, K.C.; Porter, D.D. Vaccine-enhanced respiratory syncytial virus disease in cotton rats following immunization with Lot 100 or a newly prepared reference vaccine. *J. Gen. Virol.* **2001**, *82*, 2881–2888.

38. Chu, V.T.; Frohlich, A.; Steinhauser, G.; Scheel, T.; Roch, T.; Fillatreau, S.; Lee, J.J.; Lohning, M.; Berek, C. Eosinophils are required for the maintenance of plasma cells in the bone marrow. *Nat. Immunol.* **2011**, *12*, 151–159.

39. Olson, M.R.; Varga, S.M. CD8 T cells inhibit respiratory syncytial virus (RSV) vaccine-enhanced disease. *J. Immunol.* **2007**, *179*, 5415–5424.

40. Power, U.F.; Plotnicky, H.; Blaecke, A.; Nguyen, T.N. The immunogenicity, protective efficacy and safety of BBG2Na, a subunit respiratory syncytial virus (RSV) vaccine candidate, against RSV-B. *Vaccine* **2003**, *22*, 168–176.

41. Graham, B.S. Biological challenges and technological opportunities for respiratory syncytial virus vaccine development. *Immunol. Rev.* **2011**, *239*, 149–166.

42. McLellan, J.S. F Protein Structures and Their Implications for Humoral Immunity. Presented at the 8th Respiratory Syncytial Virus Symposium, Santa Fe, NM, 2012.

43. Fishaut, M.; Tubergen, D.; McIntosh, K. Cellular response to respiratory viruses with particular reference to children with disorders of cell-mediated immunity. *J. Pediatr.* **1980**, *96*, 179–186.

44. Hall, C.B.; Powell, K.R.; MacDonald, N.E.; Gala, C.L.; Menegus, M.E.; Suffin, S.C.; Cohen, H.J. Respiratory syncytial viral infection in children with compromised immune function. *N. Engl. J Med.* **1986**, *315*, 77–81.

45. Phipps, S.; Lam, C.E.; Mahalingam, S.; Newhouse, M.; Ramirez, R.; Rosenberg, H.F.; Foster, P.S.; Matthaei, K.I. Eosinophils contribute to innate antiviral immunity and promote clearance of respiratory syncytial virus. *Blood* **2007**, *110*, 1578–1586.

46. Welliver, R.C., Sr. The immune response to respiratory syncytial virus infection: Friend or foe? *Clin. Rev. Allergy Immunol.* **2008**, *34*, 163–173.

47. DeVincenzo, J.; Lambkin-Williams, R.; Wilkinson, T.; Cehelsky, J.; Nochur, S.; Walsh, E.; Meyers, R.; Gollob, J.; Vaishnaw, A. A randomized, double-blind, placebo-controlled study of an RNAi-based therapy directed against respiratory syncytial virus. *Proc. Natl. Acad. Sci. USA* **2010**, *107*, 8800–8805.

48. Rudraraju, R.; Surman, S.L.; Jones, B.G.; Sealy, R.; Woodland, D.L.; Hurwitz, J.L. Reduced frequencies and heightened CD103 expression among virus-induced CD8(+) T cells in the respiratory tract airways of vitamin A-deficient mice. *Clin. Vaccine Immunol.* **2012**, *19*, 757–765.

49. Surman, S.L.; Rudraraju, R.; Sealy, R.; Jones, B.; Hurwitz, J.L. Vitamin A deficiency disrupts vaccine-induced antibody-forming cells and the balance of IgA/IgG isotypes in the upper and lower respiratory tract. *Viral Immunol.* **2012**, *25*, 341–344.

50. Falsey AR. RSV In Adults: What Do We Know? What Do We Need to Know? Where Are We Going? In Proceedings of the 7th International Respiratory Syncytial Virus Symposium, Rotterdam, The Netherlands, 2 December 2010.

51. Graham, B.S. Future of RSV vaccine development. Presented at the 8th Respiratory Syncytial Virus Symposium, Santa Fe, NM, USA, 2012.

52. Moss, B. Smallpox vaccines: Targets of protective immunity. *Immunol. Rev.* **2011**, *239*, 8–26.

53. Murphy, K.; Travers, P.; Walport, M. *Janeway's Immunobiology*, 7th ed.; Garland Science: New York, NY, USA, 2008.

54. Peters, A.; Lee, Y.; Kuchroo, V.K. The many faces of Th17 cells. *Curr. Opin. Immunol.* **2011**, *23*, 702–706.

55. Kelso, A. Th1 and Th2 subsets: Paradigms lost? *Immunol. Today* **1995**, *16*, 374–379.

56. Mosmann, T.R.; Cherwinski, H.; Bond, M.W.; Giedlin, M.A.; Coffman, R.L. Two types of murine helper T cell clone. I. Definition according to profiles of lymphokine activities and secreted proteins. *J. Immunol.* **1986**, *136*, 2348–2357.

57. Crotty, S. Follicular helper CD4 T cells (TFH). *Annu. Rev. Immunol.* **2011**, *29*, 621–663.

58. Crotty, S.; Felgner, P.; Davies, H.; Glidewell, J.; Villarreal, L.; Ahmed, R. Cutting edge: Long-term B cell memory in humans after smallpox vaccination. *J Immunol.* **2003**, *171*, 4969–4973.

59. Lerch, R.A.; Anderson, K.; Amann, V.L.; Wertz, G.W. Nucleotide sequence analysis of the bovine respiratory syncytial virus fusion protein mRNA and expression from a recombinant vaccinia virus. *Virology* **1991**, *181*, 118–131.

60. Schmidt, A.C.; McAuliffe, J.M.; Murphy, B.R.; Collins, P.L. Recombinant bovine/human parainfluenza virus type 3 (B/HPIV3) expressing the respiratory syncytial virus (RSV) G and F proteins can be used to achieve simultaneous mucosal immunization against RSV and HPIV3. *J. Virol.* **2001**, *75*, 4594–4603.

61. Stevens, W.W.; Sun, J.; Castillo, J.P.; Braciale, T.J. Pulmonary eosinophilia is attenuated by early responding CD8(+) memory T cells in a murine model of RSV vaccine-enhanced disease. *Viral Immunol.* **2009**, *22*, 243–251.

62. Jones, B.; Zhan, X.; Mishin, V.; Slobod, K.S.; Surman, S.; Russell, C.J.; Portner, A.; Hurwitz, J.L. Human PIV-2 recombinant Sendai virus (rSeV) elicits durable immunity and combines with two additional rSeVs to protect against hPIV-1, hPIV-2, hPIV-3, and RSV. *Vaccine* **2009**, *27*, 1848–1857.

63. Zhan, X.; Slobod, K.S.; Krishnamurthy, S.; Luque, L.E.; Takimoto, T.; Jones, B.; Surman, S.; Russell, C.J.; Portner, A.; Hurwitz, J.L. Sendai virus recombinant vaccine expressing hPIV-3 HN or F elicits protective immunity and combines with a second recombinant to prevent hPIV-1, hPIV-3 and RSV infections. *Vaccine* **2008**, *26*, 3480–3488.

64. Crowe, J.E., Jr.; Randolph, V.; Murphy, B.R. The live attenuated subgroup B respiratory syncytial virus vaccine candidate RSV 2B33F is attenuated and immunogenic in chimpanzees, but exhibits partial loss of the ts phenotype following replication *in vivo*. *Virus Res.* **1999**, *59*, 13–22.

65. De, W.L.; Power, U.F.; Yuksel, S.; Van, A.G.; Nguyen, T.N.; Niesters, H.G.; de Swart, R.L.; Osterhaus, A.D. Evaluation of BBG2Na in infant macaques: Specific immune responses after vaccination and RSV challenge. *Vaccine* **2004**, *22*, 915–922.

66. Jones, B.G.; Sealy, R.E.; Rudraraju, R.; Traina-Dorge, V.L.; Finneyfrock, B.; Cook, A.; Takimoto, T.; Portner, A.; Hurwitz, J.L. Sendai virus-based RSV vaccine protects African green monkeys from RSV infection. *Vaccine* **2012**, *30*, 959–968.

67. Karron, R.A.; Wright, P.F.; Crowe, J.E., Jr.; Clements-Mann, M.L.; Thompson, J.; Makhene, M.; Casey, R.; Murphy, B.R. Evaluation of two live, cold-passaged, temperature-sensitive respiratory syncytial virus vaccines in chimpanzees and in human adults, infants, and children. *J. Infect. Dis.* **1997**, *176*, 1428–1436.

68. Friedewald, W.T.; Forsyth, B.R.; Smith, C.B.; Gharpure, M.A.; Chanock, R.M. Low-temperature-grown RS virus in adult volunteers. *JAMA* **1968**, *204*, 690–694.

69. Schickli, J.H.; Kaur, J.; Tang, R.S. Nonclinical phenotypic and genotypic analyses of a Phase 1 pediatric respiratory syncytial virus vaccine candidate MEDI-559 (rA2cp248/404/1030DeltaSH) at permissive and non-permissive temperatures. *Virus Res.* **2012**, *169*, 38–47.

70. Wright, P.F.; Karron, R.A.; Belshe, R.B.; Thompson, J.; Crowe, J.E., Jr.; Boyce, T.G.; Halburnt, L.L.; Reed, G.W.; Whitehead, S.S.; Anderson, E.L.; *et al.* Evaluation of a live, cold-passaged, temperature-sensitive, respiratory syncytial virus vaccine candidate in infancy. *J. Infect. Dis.* **2000**, *182*, 1331–1342.

71. Firestone, C.Y.; Whitehead, S.S.; Collins, P.L.; Murphy, B.R.; Crowe, J.E., Jr. Nucleotide sequence analysis of the respiratory syncytial virus subgroup A cold-passaged (cp) temperature sensitive (ts) cpts-248/404 live attenuated virus vaccine candidate. *Virology* **1996**, *225*, 419–422.

72. Karron, R.A.; Wright, P.F.; Belshe, R.B.; Thumar, B.; Casey, R.; Newman, F.; Polack, F.P.; Randolph, V.B.; Deatly, A.; Hackell, J. Identification of a recombinant live attenuated respiratory syncytial virus vaccine candidate that is highly attenuated in infants. *J. Infect. Dis.* **2005**, *191*, 1093–1104.

73. Buchholz, U.J.; Luongo, C.; Winter, C.C.; Tang, R.S.; Karron, R.A.; Schickli, J.H.; Collins, P.L. Live-Attenuated RSV Vaccine Candidates for Clinical Studies: Improving Genetic Stability and Backup Plans. Presented at the 8th Respiratory Syncytial Virus Symposium, Santa Fe, NM, USA, 2012.

74. Luongo, C.; Winter, C.C.; Collins, P.L.; Buchholz, U.J. Respiratory syncytial virus modified by deletions of the NS2 gene and amino acid S1313 of the L polymerase protein is a temperature sensitive live-attenuated vaccine candidate that is phenotypically stable at physiological temperature. *J. Virol.* **2012**, *87*, 1985–96.

75. Nagai, Y.; Kato, A. Paramyxovirus reverse genetics is coming of age. *Microbiol. Immunol.* **1999**, *43*, 613–624.

76. Jin, H.; Zhou, H.; Cheng, X.; Tang, R.; Munoz, M.; Nguyen, N. Recombinant respiratory syncytial viruses with deletions in the NS1, NS2, SH, and M2-2 genes are attenuated *in vitro* and *in vivo*. *Virology* **2000**, *273*, 210–218.

77. Cheng, X.; Zhou, H.; Tang, R.S.; Munoz, M.G.; Jin, H. Chimeric subgroup A respiratory syncytial virus with the glycoproteins substituted by those of subgroup B and RSV without the M2-2 gene are attenuated in African green monkeys. *Virology* **2001**, *283*, 59–68.

78. Schepens, B.; de Baets, S.; Sedyen, K.; Bogaert, P.; Gilbert, B.; Piedra, P.A.; Fiers, W.; Saelens, X. She's a novel target for RSV vaccination. Presented at the 8th Respiratory Syncytial Virus Symposium, Santa Fe, NM, USA, 2012.

79. Swanson, K.A.; Settembre, E.C.; Shaw, C.A.; Dey, A.K.; Rappuoli, R.; Mandl, C.W.; Dormitzer, P.R.; Carfi, A. Structural basis for immunization with postfusion respiratory syncytial virus fusion F glycoprotein (RSV F) to elicit high neutralizing antibody titers. *Proc. Natl. Acad. Sci. USA* **2011**, *108*, 9619–9624.

80. Zhang, W.; Choi, Y.; Haynes, L.M.; Harcourt, J.L.; Anderson, L.J.; Jones, L.P.; Tripp, R.A. Vaccination to induce antibodies blocking the CX3C-CX3CR1 interaction of respiratory syncytial virus G protein reduces pulmonary inflammation and virus replication in mice. *J. Virol.* **2010**, *84*, 1148–1157.

81. Sealy, R.; Chaka, W.; Surman, S.; Brown, S.A.; Cresswell, P.; Hurwitz, J.L. Target peptide sequence within infectious human immunodeficiency virus type 1 does not ensure envelope-specific T-helper cell reactivation: Influences of cysteine protease and gamma interferon-induced thiol reductase activities. *Clin. Vaccine Immunol.* **2008**, *15*, 713–719.

82. Colman, P.M.; Laver, W.G.; Varghese, J.N.; Baker, A.T.; Tulloch, P.A.; Air, G.M.; Webster, R.G. Three-dimensional structure of a complex of antibody with influenza virus neuraminidase. *Nature* **1987**, *326*, 358–363.

83. Arnold, P.Y.; La Gruta, N.L.; Miller, T.; Vignali, K.M.; Adams, P.S.; Woodland, D.L.; Vignali, D.A. The majority of immunogenic epitopes generate CD4+ T cells that are dependent on MHC class II-bound peptide-flanking residues. *J. Immunol.* **2002**, *169*, 739–749.

84. Moudgil, K.D.; Sercarz, E.E.; Grewal, I.S. Modulation of the immunogenicity of antigenic determinants by their flanking residues. *Immunol. Today* **1998**, *19*, 217–220.

85. Correia, B.E.; Bates, J.T.; Loomis, R.; Connell, M.J.; Baneyx, G.; Jardine, J.G.; Rupert, P.; Correnti, C.; Vittal, V.; Kalyuzhniy, O.; *et al.* A Computationally Designed Experimental RSV F Protein Epitope Vaccine that Induces Potent Neutralizing Antibodies in Nonhuman Primates. Presented at the 8th Respiratory Syncytial Virus Symposium, Santa Fe, NM, USA, 2012.

86. Makidon, P.E.; Bitko, V.; Simon, J.K.; Lukacs, N.W.; Hamouda, T.; O'Konek, J.J.; Fattom, A.; Baker, J.R., Jr. Immunogenicity and Efficacy of Line 19 RSV Vaccine in Cotton Rats. Presented at the 8th Respiratory Syncytial Virus Symposium, Santa Fe, NM, 2012.

87. Grasso, S.; Santi, L. Viral nanoparticles as macromolecular devices for new therapeutic and pharmaceutical approaches. *Int. J. Physiol. Pathophysiol. Pharmacol.* **2010**, *2*, 161–178.

88. Garg, R.; Brownlie, R.; Latimer, L.; Connor, W.; Simko, E.; Gerdts, V.; Babiuk, L.A.; Potter, A.; van Drunen Littel-van den Hurk, S. Intranasal immunization with the RSV fusion protein formulated with novel combination adjuvants induces protective immunity. Presented at the 8th Respiratory Syncytial Virus Symposium, Santa Fe, NM, USA, 2012.

89. Garlapati, S.; Garg, R.; Brownlie, R.; Latimer, L.; Simko, E.; Hancock, R.E.; Babiuk, L.A.; Gerdts, V.; Potter, A.; van Drunen Littel-van den Hurk, S. Enhanced immune responses and protection by vaccination with respiratory syncytial virus fusion protein formulated with CpG oligodeoxynucleotide and innate defense regulator peptide in polyphosphazene microparticles. *Vaccine* **2012**, *30*, 5206–5214.

90. Glenn, G.M.; Smith, G.; Raghunandan, R.; Li, H.; Zhou, B.; Thomas, D.N.; Fries, L. Immunogenicity of an Sf9 insect cell-derived respiratory syncytial virus fusion protein nanoparticle vaccine: Insights into pathogenicity. Presented at the 8th Respiratory Syncytial Virus Symposium, Santa Fe, NM, USA, 2012.

91. Smith, G.; Raghunandan, R.; Wu, Y.; Liu, Y.; Massare, M.; Nathan, M.; Zhou, B.; Lu, H.; Boddapati, S.; Li, J.; Respiratory syncytial virus fusion glycoprotein expressed in insect cells form protein nanoparticles that induce protective immunity in cotton rats. *PLoS One* **2012**, *7*, e50852.

92. Simoes, E.A.; Groothuis, J.R.; Carbonell-Estrany, X.; Rieger, C.H.; Mitchell, I.; Fredrick, L.M.; Kimpen, J.L. Palivizumab prophylaxis, respiratory syncytial virus, and subsequent recurrent wheezing. *J. Pediatr.* **2007**, *151*, 34–42.

93. Kamphuis, T.; Meijerhof, T.; Stegmann, T.; Lederhofer, J.; Wilschut, J.; De, H.A. Immunogenicity and protective capacity of a virosomal respiratory syncytial virus vaccine adjuvanted with monophosphoryl lipid A in mice. *PLoS One* **2012**, *7*, e36812.

94. Bernstein, D.I.; Malkin, E.; Abughali, N.; Falloon, J.; Yi, T.; Dubovsky, F. Phase 1 study of the safety and immunogenicity of a live, attenuated respiratory syncytial virus and parainfluenza virus type 3 vaccine in seronegative children. *Pediatr. Infect. Dis. J.* **2012**, *31*, 109–114.

95. Tang, R.S.; Spaete, R.R.; Thompson, M.W.; MacPhail, M.; Guzzetta, J.M.; Ryan, P.C.; Reisinger, K.; Chandler, P.; Hilty, M.; Walker, R.E.; *et al.* Development of a PIV-vectored RSV vaccine: Preclinical evaluation of safety, toxicity, and enhanced disease and initial clinical testing in healthy adults. *Vaccine* **2008**, *26*, 6373–6382.

96. Tang, R.S.; MacPhail, M.; Schickli, J.H.; Kaur, J.; Robinson, C.L.; Lawlor, H.A.; Guzzetta, J.M.; Spaete, R.R.; Haller, A.A. Parainfluenza virus type 3 expressing the native or soluble fusion (F) Protein of Respiratory Syncytial Virus (RSV) confers protection from RSV infection in African green monkeys. *J. Virol.* **2004**, *78*, 11198–11207.

97. Tang, R.S.; Malkin, E.; Stillman, E.; Nelson, C.; Yang, C.-F.; Song, E.; Liang, B.; Shambaugh, C.; Zuo, F.; Liem, A.; *et al.* Implication of genetic changes observed in Phase 1 evaluation of MEDI-534, a live attenuated chimeric bovine human parainfluenza type 3 vectored RSV vaccine. Presented at the 8th Respiratory Syncytial Virus Symposium, Santa Fe, NM, USA 2012.

98. Power, U.F.; Ryan, K.W.; Portner, A. Sequence characterization and expression of the matrix protein gene of human parainfluenza virus type 1. *Virology* **1992**, *191*, 947–952.

99. Lyn, D.; Gill, D.S.; Scroggs, R.A.; Portner, A. The nucleoproteins of human parainfluenza virus type 1 and Sendai virus share amino acid sequences and antigenic and structural determinants. *J. Gen. Virol.* **1991**, *72*, 983–987.

100. Sangster, M.; Smith, F.S.; Coleclough, C.; Hurwitz, J.L. Human parainfluenza virus-type 1 immunization of infant mice protects from subsequent Sendai virus infection. *Virology* **1995**, *212*, 13–19.

101. Dave, V.P.; Allan, J.E.; Slobod, K.S.; Smith, S.F.; Ryan, K.; Powell, U.; Portner, A.; Hurwitz, J.L. Viral cross-reactivity and antigenic determinants recognized by human parainfluenza virus type 1-specific cytotoxic T-cells. *Virology* **1994**, *199*, 376–383.

102. Smith, F.S.; Portner, A.; Leggiadro, R.J.; Turner, E.V.; Hurwitz, J.L. Age-related development of human memory T-helper and B-cell responses toward parainfluenza virus type-1. *Virology* **1994**, *205*, 453–461.

103. Bousse, T.; Chambers, R.L.; Scroggs, R.A.; Portner, A.; Takimoto, T. Human parainfluenza virus type 1 but not Sendai virus replicates in human respiratory cells despite IFN treatment. *Virus Res.* **2006**, *121*, 23–32.

104. Zhan, X.; Hurwitz, J.L.; Krishnamurthy, S.; Takimoto, T.; Boyd, K.; Scroggs, R.A.; Surman, S.; Portner, A.; Slobod, K.S. Respiratory syncytial virus (RSV) fusion protein expressed by recombinant Sendai virus elicits B-cell and T-cell responses in cotton rats and confers protection against RSV subtypes A and B. *Vaccine* **2007**, *25*, 8782–8793.

105. Slobod, K.S.; Shenep, J.L.; Lujan-Zilbermann, J.; Allison, K.; Brown, B.; Scroggs, R.A.; Portner, A.; Coleclough, C.; Hurwitz, J.L. Safety and immunogenicity of intranasal murine parainfluenza virus type 1 (Sendai virus) in healthy human adults. *Vaccine* **2004**, *22*, 3182–3186.

106. Chen, M.; Hu, K.F.; Rozell, B.; Orvell, C.; Morein, B.; Liljestrom, P. Vaccination with recombinant alphavirus or immune-stimulating complex antigen against respiratory syncytial virus. *J. Immunol.* **2002**, *169*, 3208–3216.

107. Mok, H.; Lee, S.; Utley, T.J.; Shepherd, B.E.; Polosukhin, V.V.; Collier, M.L.; Davis, N.L.; Johnston, R.E.; Crowe, J.E., Jr. Venezuelan equine encephalitis virus replicon particles encoding respiratory syncytial virus surface glycoproteins induce protective mucosal responses in mice and cotton rats. *J. Virol.* **2007**, *81*, 13710–13722.

108. Elliott, M.B.; Chen, T.; Terio, N.B.; Chong, S.Y.; Abdullah, R.; Luckay, A.; Egan, M.A.; Boutilier, L.A.; Melville, K.; Lerch, R.A.; *et al.* Alphavirus replicon particles encoding the fusion or attachment glycoproteins of respiratory syncytial virus elicit protective immune responses in BALB/c mice and functional serum antibodies in rhesus macaques. *Vaccine* **2007**, *25*, 7132–7144.

109. Kohlmann, R.; Schwannecke, S.; Tippler, B.; Ternette, N.; Temchura, V.V.; Tenbusch, M.; Uberla, K.; Grunwald, T. Protective efficacy and immunogenicity of an adenoviral vector vaccine encoding the codon-optimized F protein of respiratory syncytial virus. *J. Virol.* **2009**, *83*, 12601–12610.

110. Johnson, T.R.; Rangel, D.; Liao, G.; Eastman, E.M.; Gall, J.G. Induction of Broadly Neutralizing Humoral Responses by Immunization with Respiratory Syncytial Virus F Expressing Adenovirus Vectors. Presented at the 8th Respiratory Syncytial Virus Symposium, Santa Fe, NM, USA, 2012.

111. De Baets, S.; Schepens, B.; Sedeyn, K.; Schotsaert, M.; Bogaert, P.; Fiers, W.; Saelens, X. Recombinant influenza virus carrying an RSV CTL epitope protects mice against respiratory syncytial virus infection. Presented at the 8th Respiratory Syncytial Virus Symposium, Santa Fe, NM, USA, 2012.

112. Sawada, A.; Komase, K.; Nakayama, T. AIK-C measles vaccine expressing fusion protein of respiratory syncytial virus induces protective antibodies in cotton rats. *Vaccine* **2011**, *29*, 1481–1490.

113. McGinnes, L.W.; Gravel, K.A.; Finberg, R.W.; Kurt-Jones, E.A.; Massare, M.J.; Smith, G.; Schmidt, M.R.; Morrison, T.G. Assembly and immunological properties of Newcastle disease virus-like particles containing the respiratory syncytial virus F and G proteins. *J. Virol.* **2011**, *85*, 366–377.

114. Andersson, C.; Liljestrom, P.; Stahl, S.; Power, U.F. Protection against respiratory syncytial virus (RSV) elicited in mice by plasmid DNA immunisation encoding a secreted RSV G protein-derived antigen. *FEMS Immunol. Med. Microbiol.* **2000**, *29*, 247–253.

115. Hurwitz, J.L. Respiratory syncytial virus vaccine development. *Expert. Rev. Vaccines* **2011**, *10*, 1415–1433.

116. Lau, J.M.; Korban, S.S. Transgenic apple expressing an antigenic protein of the human respiratory syncytial virus. *J. Plant Physiol.* **2010**, *167*, 920–927.

117. Haijema, B.J.; Leenhouts, K.; Widjaja, I.; Rigter, A.; de Haan, X.; Rottier, P. Intranasal administration of bacterium-like particles carrying RSV F antigen (SynGEM) induces a safe and protective RSV-specific immune response. Presented at the 8th Respiratory Syncytial Virus Symposium, Santa Fe, NM, USA, 2012.

118. Taylor, G.; Thom, M.; Herbert, B.; Pierantoni, A.; Capone, S.; Nicosia, A.; Vitelli, A. Novel replication-defective chimpanzee adenovirus (ChAD) and modified vaccinia Ankara (MVA) vectors expressing human (H)RSV antigens protect calves against BRSV infection. Presented at the 8th Respiratory Syncytial Virus Symposium, Santa Fe, NM, USA, 2012.

119. Grunwald, T.; Tenbusch, M.; Schulte, R.; Franz, M.; Hannaman, D.; Tippler, B.; de Swart, R.L.; Steinman, R.; Stahl-Hennig, C.; Uberla, K. Immunogenicity and efficacy of genetic RSV vaccines in rhesus monkeys. Presented at the 8th Respiratory Syncytial Virus Symposium, Santa Fe, NM, USA, 2012.

120. Shafique, M.; Wilschut, J.; De, H.A. Induction of mucosal and systemic immunity against respiratory syncytial virus by inactivated virus supplemented with TLR9 and NOD2 ligands. *Vaccine* **2012**, *30*, 597–606.

121. Stegmann, T.; Kamphuis, T.; Meijerhof, T.; Goud, E.; De, H.A.; Wilschut, J. Lipopeptide-adjuvanted respiratory syncytial virus virosomes: A safe and immunogenic non-replicating vaccine formulation. *Vaccine* **2010**, *28*, 5543–5550.

122. Murawski, M.R.; McGinnes, L.W.; Finberg, R.W.; Kurt-Jones, E.A.; Massare, M.J.; Smith, G.; Heaton, P.M.; Fraire, A.E.; Morrison, T.G. Newcastle disease virus-like particles containing respiratory syncytial virus G protein induced protection in BALB/c mice, with no evidence of immunopathology. *J. Virol.* **2010**, *84*, 1110–1123.

123. Cautivo, K.M.; Bueno, S.M.; Cortes, C.M.; Wozniak, A.; Riedel, C.A.; Kalergis, A.M. Efficient lung recruitment of respiratory syncytial virus-specific Th1 cells induced by recombinant bacillus Calmette-Guerin promotes virus clearance and protects from infection. *J. Immunol.* **2010**, *185*, 7633–7645.

124. Xie, C.; He, J.S.; Zhang, M.; Xue, S.L.; Wu, Q.; Ding, X.D.; Song, W.; Yuan, Y.; Li, D.L.; Zheng, X.X.; *et al.* Oral respiratory syncytial virus (RSV) DNA vaccine expressing RSV F protein delivered by attenuated Salmonella typhimurium. *Hum. Gene Ther.* **2007**, *18*, 746–752.

125. Falcone, V.; Mihm, D.; Neumann-Haefelin, D.; Costa, C.; Nguyen, T.; Pozzi, G.; Ricci, S. Systemic and mucosal immunity to respiratory syncytial virus induced by recombinant Streptococcus gordonii surface-displaying a domain of viral glycoprotein G. *FEMS Immunol. Med. Microbiol.* **2006**, *48*, 116–122.

126. Schickli, J.H.; Dubovsky, F.; Tang, R.S. Challenges in developing a pediatric RSV vaccine. *Hum. Vaccin.* **2009**, *5*, 582–591.

6

Diversity in Glycosaminoglycan Binding Amongst hMPV G Protein Lineages

Penelope Adamson [1,2,*], Sutthiwan Thammawat [1], Gamaliel Muchondo [1], Tania Sadlon [1,2] and David Gordon [1,2]

[1] Department of Microbiology and Infectious Diseases, Flinders University, Flinders Medical Centre, Bedford Park, SA 5042, Australia; E-Mails: ant3714@hotmail.com (S.T.); gamaliel.muchondo@health.sa.gov.au (G.M.); tania.sadlon@health.sa.gov.au (T.S.); d.gordon@flinders.edu.au (D.G.)

[2] Department of Microbiology and Infectious Diseases, SA Pathology, Flinders Medical Centre, Bedford Park, SA 5042, Australia

* Author to whom correspondence should be addressed;
E-Mail: penelope.adamson@health.sa.gov.au

Abstract: We have previously shown that hMPV G protein (B2 lineage) interacts with cellular glycosaminoglycans (GAGs). In this study we examined subtypes A1, A2 and B1 for this interaction. GAG-dependent infectivity of available hMPV strains was demonstrated using GAG-deficient cells and heparin competition. We expressed the G protein ectodomains from all strains and analysed these by heparin affinity chromatography. In contrast to the B2 lineage, neither the A2 or B1 G proteins bound to heparin. Sequence analysis of these strains indicated that although there was some homology with the B2 heparin-binding domains, there were less positively charged residues, providing a likely explanation for the lack of binding. Although sequence analysis did not demonstrate well defined positively charged domains in G protein of the A1 strain, this protein was able to bind heparin, albeit with a lower affinity than G protein of the B2 strain. These results indicate diversity in GAG interactions between G proteins of different lineages and suggest that the GAG-dependency of all strains may be mediated by interaction with an alternative surface protein, most probably the conserved fusion (F) protein. Analysis of both native and recombinant F protein confirmed that F protein binds heparin, supporting this conclusion.

Keywords: human metapneumovirus (hMPV); Glycosaminoglycan (GAG); G protein; F protein; infectivity

---

1. Introduction

Human metapneumovirus (hMPV) is responsible for causing serious respiratory illness, most commonly in infants and young children, but also in the elderly and immunocompromised patients [1–5]. hMPV is a member of the genus *Metapneumovirus* within the family *Paramyxoviridae*. Avian pnuemovirus is the only other member of this genus [5]. Respiratory syncytial virus (RSV), a member of the genus *Pneumovirus*, also within the family *Paramyxoviridae*, is the most closely related human pathogen to hMPV and as such they share many of the same symptoms [6–9]. These range from mild upper respiratory tract disease to severe lower tract diseases such as bronchiolitis and pneumonia [5] and together, hMPV and RSV, are responsible for at least 50% of all respiratory viral infections requiring hospitalisation in children [10,11].

hMPV is an enveloped, single stranded, negative-sense RNA virus which contains 3 envelope glycoproteins, the fusion (F), attachment (G) and the small hydrophobic (SH) protein. It is the organisation of the genome and the lack of non structural genes which separates hMPV from other paramyxoviruses, such as RSV [5,8]. Phylogenetic analysis of the nucleotide sequence of several hMPV genes has shown that hMPV is divided into two major groups, A and B, both of which can be further divided into two minor subgroups, 1 and 2 [12–16]. hMPV resembles other members of the *Paramyxoviridae* family genetically and morphologically, as determined by electron microscopy [17].

Whilst the fusion protein of hMPV is highly conserved, immunogenic and induces protective antibodies, the other surface glycoproteins, G and SH, unlike most other *Paramyxoviridae*, have been shown to be only weakly or negligibly immunogenic [18–22]. The G protein of hMPV is a type II membrane protein consisting of extracellular, transmembrane and intracellular domains [8] and is highly glycosylated [12,23]. It is highly variable, particularly the extracellular domain [13]. This diversity along with its extensive glycosylation probably aids in its evasion of the immune system [12]. The role of the G protein has not been fully elucidated, however previous studies indicate that it likely plays a role in viral attachment [24] and replication [25].

Glycosaminoglycans (GAGs) are linear polysaccharides which are comprised of repeating disaccharide units. The repeat units of GAGs consist of an amino sugar (N-acetylglucosamine or N-acetylgalactosamine) and uronic acid (glucuronic or iduronic acid) or galactose which are variably sulphated, except hyaluronic acid which lacks sulphate groups [26]. They are covalently attached to core proteins to form proteoglycans which are found in tissue, the extracellular matrix (ECM) and on the inside and the surface of most cell types [26].

A number of viruses, including other paramyxoviruses, have been shown to interact with cell surface GAGs to facilitate cellular attachment and subsequent entry into cells [27–30]. Past studies of RSV and our previous study of hMPV have shown that infection is markedly or completely inhibited by the presence of soluble GAGs such as heparin, by removing GAGs from the surface of cells enzymatically or with the use of GAG deficient cells [24,31,32].

We have shown previously that attachment of hMPV to cells may be mediated by a G protein-GAG interaction. This initial work was carried out using G protein of the B2 lineage. Due to the high variability of G protein between strains we investigated if this is consistent for all hMPV strains. Using recombinantly expressed G protein we demonstrated that, other that the B2 strain, only the A1 strain binds to GAGs. By truncating the G proteins of the A1 and B2 subtypes, we have further characterised the functional domains within each protein involved in these interactions. Furthermore, using hMPV infected cell lysates and recombinant F protein, we show binding of the F protein to GAGs suggesting that this protein is also involved in virus attachment to the cell surface, and providing an explanation for the GAG-dependency of all hMPV strains.

2. Results and Discussion

2.1. Susceptibility of hMPV Primary Isolates to Inhibition of Infection by Heparin

To date our investigations have focused on G protein from the hMPV B2 strain. To determine if the infectivity of other strains is also GAG-dependent, we incubated primary isolates of hMPV A2, B1 and B2 strains with and without heparin before inoculation of LLC-MK2 cells. Infectivity was determined using quantitative real time PCR. Primary isolates were used to preclude the possibility that heparin binding was an adaptation of the virus during cell culture. hMPV A1 strain is not represented in these experiments as a primary isolate could not be obtained during the specimen collection period. Infection with all available hMPV strains was markedly or completely inhibited by heparin pre-incubation (Table 1).

Table 1. Susceptibility of hMPV primary isolates to inhibition of infection by heparin [1].

Isolate	Subtype	Ct value [2]	
		Heparin Pre-treated	**Untreated virus**
V47041	B2	Negative	24.1
V52283	A2	30.2	16.6
V50569	B1	Negative	13.1

[1] LLC-MK2 cells were inoculated with primary isolates of hMPV, ±50 IU heparin pre-treatment. Infectivity was determined by a quantitative real-time RT-PCR for nucleoprotein gene. [2] Results are represented as a cycle threshold (Ct) value. Higher or negative Ct values after heparin pretreatment of the virus indicate reduced viral infectivity.

2.2. GAG-Deficient CHO Cells Are Resistant to hMPV Infection

As soluble heparin was able to reduce or completely inhibit infection of LLC-MK2 cells, we examined the ability of the 3 primary isolates to infect CHO-K1 and CHO-pgsA 745 cells. CHO-pgsA 745 cells lack xylosyltransferase activity and therefore are deficient in cellular GAGs [33]. The CHO-K1 and CHO-pgsA cells were incubated for 2 weeks with nasopharyngeal aspirates positive for hMPV by PCR. As the viral titres from CHO cultures were low, the wild type and mutant CHO-K1 cell supernatants were tested for infectious hMPV by subsequent incubation with LLC-MK2 cells followed by cell ELISA. Infectivity of all three strains, hMPV A2, B1 and B2, was dependent on GAGs as GAG deficient CHO-K1 cells had negligible evidence of infection (Figure 1).

Figure 1. Primary isolates of hMPV utilise GAGs to mediate infection. CHO-K1 and CHO-pgsA 745 cells were inoculated with hMPV PCR positive nasopharyngeal aspirates. LLC-MK2 cells were inoculated with the CHO cell supernatants and infectivity determined by cell ELISA using a hMPV matrix protein mAb. Data represent mean values ± SD of triplicate wells.

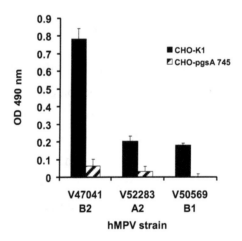

2.3. Binding of hMPV G Glycoprotein to Immobilised Heparin

Previous studies carried out in our laboratory demonstrated the binding of G protein of hMPV B2 strain to cellular GAGs [24]. To determine if this is consistent for all strains of hMPV, we expressed the extracellular domain of the G protein for the A1, A2 and B1 strains in the yeast *Pichia pastoris* X33. The recombinant B1 G protein migrated at an apparent molecular weight of 60 kDa which is comparable to the recombinant B2 ectodomain, however the apparent molecular weights for the A1 and A2 protein migration were 100 kDa and 75 kDa, respectively (Figure 2). The purified recombinant proteins were applied to heparin agarose columns and after extensive washing were eluted with a stepwise salt gradient. The recombinant G ectodomains of hMPV strains B2 and A1 bound to the heparin column while strains A2 and B1 did not (Figure 2). The recombinant hMPV B2 G protein appears to have a higher affinity for heparin than the recombinant hMPV A1 G protein as it requires a higher salt concentration for elution.

Figure 2. Heparin agarose affinity chromatography of recombinant G ectodomain for A1, A2, B1 and B2 hMPV strains. The start (S), flow through (FT), final wash (W) and salt elution fractions were analyzed by 10% SDS-PAGE under reducing conditions and western blot analysis using anti-c-Myc monoclonal antibody. A1, A2, B1 and B2 indicate the strain type.

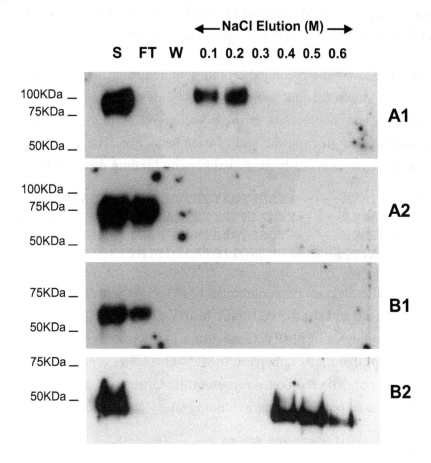

2.4. Functional Domains in hMPV G A1 Protein Involved in GAG Interactions

We have previously identified 2 adjacent regions of highly charged amino acids within the extracellular region of the B2 G protein which are important for heparin binding [24]. These domains are less well defined in other hMPV strains (Figure 3) and certainly appear to be lacking in the A1 and B1 strains. Despite this, the A1 strain G protein still interacts with heparin, perhaps due to the high number of positively charged residues adjacent to this region.

To identify the regions of A1 strain G protein involved in binding to heparin, we constructed 8 fragments of the hMPV G A1 ectodomain (Figure 4a), particularly targeting the region previously shown to be important for binding in hMPV G B2 strain (Figure 4b). These recombinant truncations migrated at sizes on SDS PAGE which varied depending on the length of the hMPV G (A1) fragment expressed. The purified hMPV G A1 fragments were applied to a heparin agarose column and following extensive washing were eluted with a stepwise salt gradient. hMPV-G A1 F3 and F4, but none of the other fragments, bound to heparin agarose (Figure 5, some data not shown). hMPV-G A1

F4 (residues 93–142 of the extracellular domain) is the smallest fragment which binds heparin. A smaller fragment, hMPV-G A1 F6 (residues 108–142), was unable to bind heparin, which indicates that residues 93–108 are crucial for the interaction of hMPV-G A1 F4 with heparin. However, since the non-binding hMPV-G A1 F2 (residues 1–115) also incorporates residues 93–108, there must be additional residues required for the heparin-G protein interaction between residues 115 and 142. These results indicate that the region of GAG binding in hMPV G A1 is similar to that identified in hMPV G B2 despite the fact that there are no well defined positively charged clusters in this protein.

Figure 3. Comparison of the predicted amino acid sequence for representatives of each strain of hMPV G protein (residues 98–136/137/142 of the extracellular domain). Strains are shown in blue and number of positively charged residues (shown in red in the sequence) is indicated in green at the end of each sequence. The yellow highlights in the B2 sequence indicate the previously identified heparin binding domains [24].

```
A1  98  TKNNPRTSSR------TRSPPRATTRSVRRTTTLHTSSIRKRPPT  136  11
A2  98  EKKPTGATTK-----KEKETTTRTTSTAATQTLNTTNQTSNGREA  137   7
B1  98  IRNNLSTASS------TQSSPRAATKAIRRATTFRMSSTGRRPTT  136   8
B2  98  EKKKTRATTQRRGKGKENTNQTTSTAATQTTNTTNQIRNASETIT  142   9
```

Figure 4. A schematic diagram of recombinant hMPV G protein from (**a**) the A1 strain and the fragments produced and (**b**) the B2 strain. hMPV-G A1 F1, F2, F3, F4, F5, F6, F7 and F8 indicate the 8 fragments of hMPV G A1 strain that were engineered. The sequence of the smallest fragment that binds to heparin (hMPV-G A1 F4) is shown with the positively charged residues in red. The red boxes represent the clusters of positively charged amino acids that are considered potential heparin binding sites.

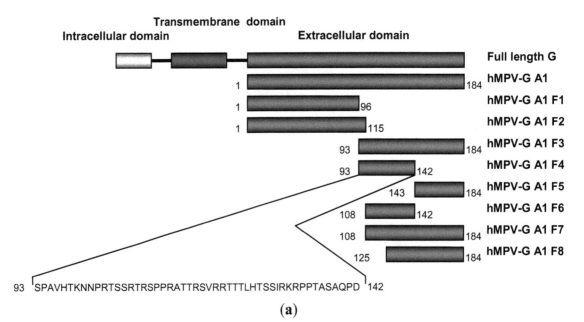

(a)

Figure 4. *Cont.*

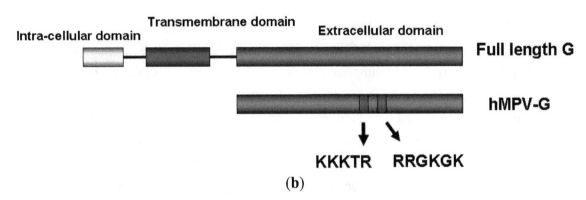

(b)

Figure 5. Heparin agarose affinity chromatography of recombinant F2, F3, F4, and F6 fragments of the hMPV G A1 strain ectodomain. The start (S), flow through (FT), final wash (W) and salt elution fractions were analysed by 10%–14% SDS-PAGE under reducing conditions and western blot analysis using anti-c-Myc MAb.

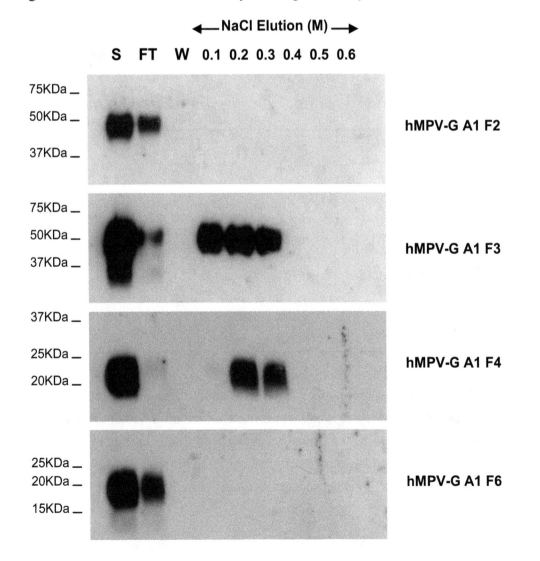

2.5. Binding of hMPV F Protein to Immobilised Heparin

The results of the infection experiments indicate that infection with the available strains of hMPV is dependent on the presence of GAGs; however not all of the hMPV G recombinant proteins bind to immobilised heparin (Figure 2). This implies that there are interactions occurring between GAGs and other surface exposed proteins on hMPV. An alternative to the attachment (G) protein is the fusion (F) protein which is highly conserved across all strains of hMPV. Fusion protein binding to GAGs was demonstrated by incubating hMPV infected cell lysates with heparin agarose and elution with salt (Figure 6). Both the precursor F protein, F_0, and the biologically active cleaved F_1 protein bound to heparin. No proteins were detected when uninfected cell lysate was subjected to heparin affinity precipitation (Figure 6).

Figure 6. Binding of native hMPV F protein to heparin. Start material (ST), flow through (FT), wash (W) and 2M NaCl elution (E) fractions were analysed by 10% SDS-PAGE under reducing conditions and western blot analysis using anti-hMPV F antibody. Arrows indicate bands corresponding to the predicted sizes of full length precursor hMPV-F (F_0) and the cleavage fragment hMPV F_1. Molecular weight markers are shown in kDa.

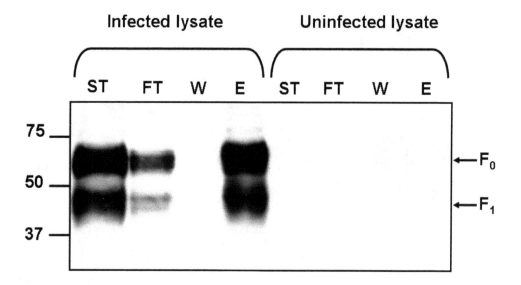

Additionally, the extracellular domain of F protein was cloned and expressed in a mammalian expression system. This resulted in a recombinant protein which migrated on SDS PAGE according to the predicted molecular weight of the uncleaved precursor form (F_0). Binding of soluble recombinant F protein to GAGs was investigated by heparin affinity chromatography. Recombinant hMPV-F protein bound to heparin with high affinity as demonstrated by protein elution with a high salt concentration (Figure 7).

Figure 7. Heparin agarose affinity chromotography of recombinant soluble hMPV-F protein. Start material (ST), flow through (FT), wash (W) and elution (E) fractions, with 0.5M NaCl (E1 & E2), 1M NaCl (E3 & E4) and 1.5M NaCl (E5 & E6), were analysed by 10% SDS-PAGE under reducing conditions and western blot analysis using anti-hMPV F antibody. Molecular weight markers are shown in kDa.

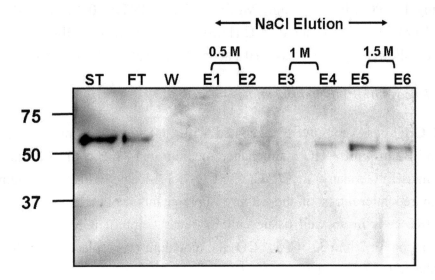

3. Experimental Section

3.1. Cells and Viruses

The rhesus monkey kidney cells (LLC-MK2) and the human epithelial tumour cell line (HEp-2) were grown in medium 199 (Invitrogen, Carlsbad, CA, USA) supplemented with 10% foetal bovine serum (FBS). Wild type Chinese hamster ovary cells (CHO-K1) and GAG-deficient CHO-pgsA745 cells [33] were grown in Hams F12 medium (Invitrogen) supplemented with 10% FBS.

The A2 (V52283), B1 (V50569) and B2 (V47041) strains of hMPV were isolated from clinical samples by the Virology Laboratory, Flinders Medical Centre (FMC). These samples were positive only for hMPV and were not coinfected with influenza A, influenza B, RSV, adenovirus or parainfluenza 1, 2 or 3. Stocks of hMPV were prepared by inoculating LLC-MK2 cells with the hMPV strains and incubating for 14 to 21 days at 37 °C in 5% CO_2. Stocks were stored at−70 °C until use. RNA extracted from the hMPV A1 strain was kindly provided to us by Dr. I. Mackay (Queensland Paediatric Infectious Diseases Laboratory, Sir Albert Sakzewski Virus Research Centre, Royal Children's Hospital, Queensland, Australia). hMPV strain subtyping was based on the Ishiguro classification [14].

3.2. Heparin Inhibition of hMPV Infection

Primary isolates of hMPV, A2, B1 and B2 strains (A1 was not available as it was not detected in South Australia during the collection period for these isolates), were pre-treated with or without heparin (50 IU/mL heparin) at 37 °C for 30 min before inoculation of LLC-MK2 cells. The cultures were incubated for 14 days with the maintenance medium changed every 3 days. Infectivity was determined after 14 days by a quantitative real-time RT-PCR for a 163 bp region of the nucleoprotein gene of hMPV [34]. Viral RNA extracted from the cultures was reverse transcribed using 50 U MMLV reverse transcriptase and 1 μM NL-N-reverse following the manufacturer's protocol. Five μL cDNA was amplified using a Rotor Gene RG-3000 (Corbett Research, Sydney, Australia) in a 25 μL reaction containing 1 × PCR buffer, 5 mM $MgCl_2$, 200 μM dNTPs, 0.4 μM NL-N-forward, 0.2 μM NL-N-reverse, 0.1 μM NL-N-probe and 0.75 U HotStar Taq polymerase (QIAGEN) with a 15 min Taq activation at 95 °C followed by 55 cycles of 10 s at 95 °C, 15 s at 55 °C and 15 s at 72 °C.

3.3. GAG Dependence of hMPV Primary Isolates

CHO-K1 and CHO-pgsA cells were incubated with 200 μL of the primary hMPV isolates for strains A2, B1 and B2 in 1 mL CHO maintenance medium in 14 mL conical tubes (Cellstar, Greiner Bio-one, Frickenhausen, Germany) at 37 °C, 5% CO_2 for 14 days with the medium changed every 3 days. Two hundred microlitres of the culture supernatants, collected on day 14, were used to inoculate LLC-MK2 cells in 96 well tissue culture plates (Linbro, ICN Biomedicals, Aurora, OH, USA). After incubation for 2 h in 37 °C, 5% CO_2 the inoculum was replaced with 200 μL maintenance medium and incubated for 7 days at 37 °C, 5% CO_2.

Infectivity was assessed using a cell based enzyme linked immunosorbent assay (ELISA) [24]. Briefly, confluent monolayers of Hep-2 cells in 96 well plates were inoculated with day 7 LLC-MK2 cell supernatants and incubated for 2 h at 37 °C, 5% CO_2. Unbound virus was removed by washing with medium 199 and the cells were cultured in medium 199 containing 1 μg/mL trypsin at 37 °C, 5% CO_2. After 48 h the cells were fixed with 1% paraformaldehyde in phosphate buffered saline (PBS) for 30 min at room temperature. Cells were washed twice with PBS, permeabilised with 0.02% Triton X-100/PBS for 30 min at 4 °C and then washed twice with PBS. The cells were blocked with 5% skim milk/PBS for 1 h before incubation with 1/320 (v/v) hMPV matrix protein monoclonal antibody (Chemicon, Temecula, CA, USA) in 0.5% Tween 20/PBS followed by 1/10,000 (v/v) horseradish peroxidase (HRP) conjugated sheep anti-mouse immunoglobulin G (Chemicon) in 0.5% Tween 20/PBS. All incubations were 1 h at 37 °C and the wells were washed four times with PBS after each step. The wells were developed by incubating with O-phenylenediamine substrate (Sigma, St. Louis, MO, USA) for 30 min. Reactions were stopped with 1N H_2SO_4 and the absorbance at 490 nm was determined. Wells were inoculated in triplicate and each experiment carried out at least twice.

3.4. Construction and Expression of Recombinant hMPV G Proteins

The ectodomains of A1, A2 and B1 were cloned and expressed for this study using similar methods as that described for the construction and expression of the extracellular domain of the G protein of the B2 strain of hMPV [24]. Briefly, RNA was extracted from hMPV (subtype A2 and B1) infected LLC-MK2 cells using the QIAamp Viral RNA purification kit (QIAGEN, Hilden, Germany) following the manufacturer's protocol. cDNA was synthesised using 500 μM GB1R or GA2R, as appropriate, or

50 ng random primer (Promega, Madison, WI, USA) for the A1 strain, using 200 U Moloney murine leukaemia virus (MMLV) reverse transcriptase (Invitrogen) according to the manufacturer's conditions. The ectodomain of hMPV G protein was amplified using 0.8 µM forward and reverse primers (Table 2) for individual strains of hMPV or the region of the G protein to be expressed. PCR was carried out in a reaction containing 1 × PCR buffer, 1 × Q-Solution, 1.5 mM $MgCl_2$, 400 µM dNTPs and 0.75 U HotStar Taq Polymerase (QIAGEN) and 5 µL cDNA. Forward and reverse primers incorporated restriction sites compatible with those in the multiple cloning site of the pPICZαA plasmid (Invitrogen) as underlined in Table 2. This allowed cloning of the PCR products downstream of the yeast α factor signal sequence, resulting in the secretion of the expressed protein into the growth medium. The PCR products were cloned in frame with the C-terminal tags, c-Myc and 6 × HIS, for ease of detection and purification. Following transformation into *Pichia pastoris* X33 yeast, expression of the soluble recombinant protein was induced with methanol over 3–4 days. The hMPV G proteins were purified using immobilised metal affinity chromatography (IMAC) over HP fast flow chelating columns (GE Life Sciences, Uppsala, Sweden) loaded with nickel chloride. The sequence of each construct was verified prior to transformation into *P. pastoris* X33.

Table 2. Primers used to amplify the extracellular region of the hMPV strains A1, A2, B1 and B2, hMPV-G A1 strain fragments and the hMPV F extracellular region. Restriction sites incorporated for ease of cloning are underlined; EcoRI (GAATTC), MluI (ACGCGT) and XbaI (TCTAGA). Bases incorporated to remain in frame with the C-terminal tags are shown in italics.

Primer Name	hMPV Strains	Primer Sequence
GB2F	B2	5'-GGGGAATTCGATCATGCAACATTAAGAAACATG-3'
GB2R	B2	5'-GGGTCTAGAGCTCCTGCACCTCYCCGTGCAT-3'
GB1F	B1	5'-AGAATTCGAATCAGAACATCACACCAG-3'
GB1R	B1	5'-ATCTAGAGCTGTGCTTGCAGATGCCTG-3'
GA2F	A2	5'-AGAATTCGATTATGCAACATTAAAAAACATG-3'
GA2R	A2	5'-ATCTAGAGCACTACTTAGAGAAGATGTGTC-3'
GA1F	A1	5'-AGAATTCAACTATAMAATGCAARAAAACTCCGA-3'
GA1R	A1	5'-TTCTAGAGCACTAGTTTGGTTGTATGTTGTTGA-3'
GA1F2	A1	5'-AGAATTCAGCCCAGCAGTCCACACAAAAAC-3'
GA1R1	A1	5'-TTCTAGATCGACTGCTGGGCTTGTCTTTGTTC-3'
GA1R2	A1	5'-TTCTAGATCTGTTGTTGCCCGTGGTGGGGAAC-3'
GA1F3	A1	5'-AGAATTCGACAGCAGCGCAACAATCC-3'
GA1F4	A1	5'-AGAATTCACACGTTCCCCACCACG-3'
GA1F5	A1	5'-AGAATTCCTCCACACAAGCAGCATAAG-3'
GA1R4	A1	5'-TTCTAGAGCGTCTGGTTGGGCTGATGC-3'
FMPV-for	B2	5'-GGGACGCGTCTTAAAGAGAGCTAYYTAGAAG-3'
FMPV-r2B	B2	5'-GGGTCTAGAGCRCCAGTGTTTCCTTTTTCTGC-3'

3.5. Heparin Agarose Affinity Chromatography

Heparin agarose chromatography was carried out in 50 mM sodium phosphate buffer pH 7.4 (PB) using 1 mL heparin agarose columns (Pierce Chemical Corporation, Rockford, IL, USA and Sigma). Recombinant proteins were dialysed into phosphate buffer overnight and then passed over the column 4–6 times. The columns were extensively washed with phosphate buffer and then eluted in a step-wise NaCl gradient. Start, flow-through, wash and elutions were all analysed using SDS-PAGE and western blotting.

3.6. Detection of hMPV G Protein by Western Blot

Proteins were separated by 10%–14% SDS PAGE (depending on the expected size of the protein) under reducing conditions and transferred onto Amersham^{TM} Hybond^{TM}-ECL membrane (GE Healthcare). Membranes were blocked with 5% skim milk/PBS and incubated with 1/5 (v/v) anti-c-Myc monoclonal antibody (from in-house hybridoma cell line 9E10) followed by 1/2,000 (v/v) HRP conjugated sheep anti-mouse immunoglobulin G. The proteins were visualised using enhanced chemiluminescence (ECL).

3.7. Heparin Binding Studies Using hMPV Infected Cell Lysates

Monolayers of LLC-MK2 cells were infected with hMPV (over 10 days) or virus/Chlamydia transport medium (VCTM), as a "mock" inoculum control. Cells were washed twice with PBS and lysed with 250 µL 60 mM n-octyl β-B-glucopyranoside (Sigma), 1 × protease inhibitor cocktail tablet (Roche, Mannheim, Germany) in PBS. After 20 min on ice, cell debris was removed by centrifugation at 13,000 × g for 15 min at 4 °C and the supernatant collected. Infected and uninfected cell lysates were diluted 1:2 (v/v) in PB and incubated with heparin agarose, washed and eluted with salt. Fractions were analysed by SDS-PAGE and western blotting.

3.8. Detection of hMPV F Protein by Western Blot

Proteins were separated by 10% SDS PAGE under reducing conditions and transferred onto Amersham^{TM} Hybond^{TM}-ECL membrane. Membranes were blocked with 5% skim milk/PBS and incubated with 1/2,000 (v/v) hamster polyclonal anti-hMPV F antibody (MedImmune, Gaithersburg, MD, USA) followed by 1/2,000 (v/v) HRP conjugated goat anti-Armenian hamster immunoglobulin (Rockland Immunochemicals, Gilbertsville, PA, USA). The proteins were visualised using ECL.

3.9. Construction and Expression of hMPV F Protein

The extracellular domain of the F gene of hMPV (B2 strain) was amplified as described previously using the primers shown in Table 2 and amplification conditions as described for amplification of hMPV G protein. The PCR product was cloned into the mammalian expression vector, BSRαEN [35] downstream of the factor H (fH) signal sequence. The hMPV F/BSRαEN construct was verified by sequencing. CHO-K1 cells were transiently transfected with hMPV F/BSRαEN using Lipofectamine 2000 (Invitrogen) then grown in OPTI-MEM (Invitrogen) for 72 h. Supernatant was harvested and analysed for protein expression using SDS PAGE and western blotting with anti-hMPV F antibody.

4. Conclusions

In this study we investigated whether sequence variability between different strains of hMPV G protein would affect the ability of their attachment proteins to interact with GAGs. Although infection with all strains tested (A2, B1 and B2) was inhibited by soluble heparin and required cell surface GAGs for infection, only recombinant G proteins from the A1 and B2 strains bound heparin agarose. Some viruses, including Sindbis and Ross River virus have been shown to adapt during cell culture to bind to heparin [36–38]. Sequence analysis of these serially cultured viruses, show the introduction of amino acid substitutions which are likely to create heparin binding domains to better adapt to cell culture and to expand the host range of the viruses. However, this may abrogate the ability of these viruses to retain their pathogenicity as has been shown in culture-adapted Sindbis virus [38]. We confirmed that the GAG dependency of each hMPV strain was not an artifact of serial cell culture passage by using non-passaged primary isolates for these experiments and also by sequencing the G gene of a series of primary isolates (data not shown).

We observed differences in the apparent molecular weight of the G proteins expressed for each strain. The proteins expressed for the B1 and B2 strains migrated on SDS PAGE at apparent molecular weights of approximately 60 kDa and 50 kDa, respectively, however A1 and A2 recombinant G protein migrated at approximately 100 kDa and 75 kDa, respectively. This could be due to varying lengths of the hMPV G ectodomains expressed and/or differences in glycosylation between strains. It has been demonstrated that differential glycosylation of RSV G protein, dependent on the cell line of origin, results in changes in electrophoretic mobility on SDS PAGE [39]. Yeast expression systems, such as *Saccharomyces cerevisiae*, are known to hyperglycosylate secreted proteins, however this is less likely in glycoproteins expressed by *Pichia pastoris* which are thought to resemble those of higher eukaryotes [40].

The interactions between hMPV G protein and GAGs are most likely mediated by electrostatic interactions between positively charged residues in the G ectodomain and negatively charged sulphates on the GAGs rather than at specific recognition sites. It appears from our results that hMPV B2 G protein has a higher affinity for heparin than hMPV A1 G protein. This could be due to the availability of positively charged residues on the protein surface after folding, the number of positively charged residues or the spacing of the residues. The conformation of Kaposi's sarcoma-associated herpesvirus complement control protein (KCP) is important in the formation of a strong positive patch on the KCP which is then available to bind to heparin. Using docking simulations, Mark *et al.* [41] showed that the extended conformation of this protein presented a more favourable docking site than could be found in the bent conformation. Differences in conformation of the G protein in each strain, due to high sequence variability, may explain the reduced affinity for heparin of hMPV A1 G protein compared to G protein of the B2 strain. To investigate regions of positively charged residues we produced a series of truncations of hMPV G (A1) strain which were tested for binding to heparin agarose. The results indicated a region between residues 93 and 142 may be responsible for G protein-GAG interactions. This domain contained a greater concentration of positively charged residues and is not dissimilar to the region identified for the B2 strain [24]. When the amino acid sequence of G protein from each hMPV strain is compared (Figure 3), GAG-binding strains had a higher number of positively charged residues in the tentative binding region (residues 98–136/137/142). The increased affinity of the G protein of the B2 strain is probably not due to the total number of positively charged residues, as the A1 strain has more in this region, but more likely the clustering of the residues seen in the B2 strain. Consensus motifs, XBBXBX, XBBBXXBX and TXXBXXTBXXXTBB (where B is the probability of basic residues, X is an uncharged hydrophobic residue and T is an amino acid in a turn) have been proposed [42,43] to mediate GAG recognition however these do not hold true for every heparin binding protein, including factor H. This suggests that the orientation and spacing of amino acids, as described by Margalit et al. [44], and the local absence of a negative charge are important. Although it is apparent from our previous study [24] that hMPV infection is inhibited by a wide range of GAGs, other viruses, such as RSV, Dengue virus and yellow fever virus, have a far more limited repertoire of cell surface GAGs [45,46]. It may be possible that different strains of hMPV are also this discriminatory and hence do not bind heparin, although our infection experiments suggest that this is unlikely. A complex interaction between the number and clustering of charged residues is ultimately likely to determine GAG-binding characteristics. Further mutagenesis of the A1 strain or engineering additional positively charged residues into this region within the non-binding strains may provide a greater insight into the residues involved.

We have shown that the dependency of hMPV infection on GAGs is not explained by a common interaction of G protein with GAGs. There is debate that the G protein of hMPV is not essential for virus infectivity. Replication of a mutant hMPV virus which was lacking the G protein was shown to be as efficient in cell culture as wild type virus, however replication in vivo was markedly reduced [25,47]. Similarly this has been investigated for RSV [48]; however the effect of deleting RSV G protein appears to be cell specific [49] and replication of mutant RSV in the respiratory tract of mice is highly restricted. We have shown in this study, and previously, that both hMPV infectivity and G protein binding can be mediated by GAGs, however it is unlikely that the mechanism of infection is solely reliant on the ability of G protein to bind GAGs. There is evidence that some viruses recognise more than one receptor to gain entry to target host cells [50,51]. Wickham et al. [51] described the use of multiple receptors in adenovirus which firstly binds to the cell with a high affinity interaction through the fibre protein and then to integrins via RGD sequences present in the penton base. Another example is the cascade of interactions involved in the entry of HSV into cells which involves several virion glycoproteins, some of which interact with heparin sulphate [52–57]. Our results indicate a mechanism similar to that described for adenovirus. The inhibition of infection of the two strains not shown to bind heparin agarose via their attachment proteins, can be explained by the ability of the highly conserved F protein to bind to heparin. We showed that F protein, either in its native form, as part of a hMPV infected cell lysate, or expressed recombinantly, was able to bind to heparin with high affinity.

This indicates that the GAG dependency of all hMPV strains for infectivity may be mediated by F protein-GAG interactions. These results have recently been confirmed by Chang *et al.* [58] who demonstrated that interactions between the hMPV F protein (of the A2 subtype) and the glycosaminoglycan heparan sulphate was essential for efficient binding of virus to cell surfaces and is most likely the initial step in virus binding and infection. Virus attachment and entry appears to require a combination of GAG binding with, or as a precursor to, other interactions, including integrin binding. Recently an integrin binding recognition Arg-Gly-Asp (RGD) sequence was identified in the F protein of hMPV which is conserved across all strains [19]. The F protein was shown to interact with the integrin $\alpha v \beta 1$ and this was suggested as a potential route for viral entry. Subsequently the same group has demonstrated that F protein not only binds $\alpha v \beta 1$ but will interact with a range of integrins known to bind RGD sequences [59]. Although not essential for virus attachment the interaction between the fusion protein and integrins is critical for efficient infection [58,59].

It is still unclear as to whether the binding of hMPV to GAGs is specific, however it is more likely due to non-specific electrostatic interactions and may represent the first step in a multivalent receptor process. In summary, we have shown that diversity exists in GAG binding amongst hMPV G protein lineages and that there is a high affinity interaction between GAGs and the hMPV fusion protein which could explain the dependency of hMPV on glycosaminoglycans.

Acknowledgments

The authors would like to thank Ian Mackay, Queensland Paediatric Infectious Diseases Laboratory, Sir Albert Sakzewski Virus Research Centre, Royal Children's Hospital, Queensland, Australia for kindly providing us with RNA extracted from the hMPV A1 strain. This work was supported by the Channel 7 Children's Research Foundation, the Flinders Medical Centre Foundation and SA Pathology. ST was supported by a Royal Thai Government Ph.D. scholarship.

References

1. Boivin, G.; Abed, Y.; Pelletier, G.; Ruel, L.; Moisan, D.; Cote, S.; Peret, T.C.; Erdman, D.D.; Anderson, L.J. Virological features and clinical manifestations associated with human metapneumovirus: A new paramyxovirus responsible for acute respiratory-tract infections in all age groups. *J. Infect. Dis.* **2002**, *186*, 1330–1334.

2. Boivin, G.; de Serres, G.; Cote, S.; Gilca, R.; Abed, Y.; Rochette, L.; Bergeron, M.G.; Dery, P. Human metapneumovirus infections in hospitalized children. *Emerg. Infect. Dis.* **2003**, *9*, 634–640.

3. Osterhaus, A.; Fouchier, R. Human metapneumovirus in the community. *Lancet* **2003**, *361*, 890–891.

4. Peret, T.C.; Boivin, G.; Li, Y.; Couillard, M.; Humphrey, C.; Osterhaus, A.D.; Erdman, D.D.; Anderson, L.J. Characterization of human metapneumoviruses isolated from patients in North America. *J. Infect. Dis.* **2002**, *185*, 1660–1663.

5. Van den Hoogen, B.G.; de Jong, J.C.; Groen, J.; Kuiken, T.; de Groot, R.; Fouchier, R.A.; Osterhaus, A.D. A newly discovered human pneumovirus isolated from young children with respiratory tract disease. *Nat. Med.* **2001**, *7*, 719–724.

6. Kahn, J.S. Epidemiology of human metapneumovirus. *Clin. Microbiol. Rev.* **2006**, *19*, 546–557.

7. King, A.M.; Lefkowitz, E.; Adams, M.J.; Carstens, E.B. Virus taxonomy: Ninth report of the international committee on taxonomy of viruses; Ninth Report; Academic Press, Elsevier: Oxford, UK, 2012; pp. 672–682. Available online: http://ictvonline.org/virusTaxonomy.asp?version=2009 (accessed on 14 February 2012).

8. Van den Hoogen, B.G.; Bestebroer, T.M.; Osterhaus, A.D.; Fouchier, R.A. Analysis of the genomic sequence of a human metapneumovirus. *Virology* **2002**, *295*, 119–132.

9. Van den Hoogen, B.G.; van Doornum, G.J.; Fockens, J.C.; Cornelissen, J.J.; Beyer, W.E.; de Groot, R.; Osterhaus, A.D.; Fouchier, R.A. Prevalence and clinical symptoms of human metapneumovirus infection in hospitalized patients. *J. Infect. Dis.* **2003**, *188*, 1571–1577.

10. Cilla, G.; Onate, E.; Perez-Yarza, E.G.; Montes, M.; Vicente, D.; Perez-Trallero, E. Hospitalization rates for human metapneumovirus infection among 0- to 3-year-olds in Gipuzkoa (Basque Country), Spain. *Epidemiol. Infect.* **2009**, *137*, 66–72.

11. Ordas, J.; Boga, J.A.; Alvarez-Arguelles, M.; Villa, L.; Rodriguez-Dehli, C.; de Ona, M.; Rodriguez, J.; Melon, S. Role of metapneumovirus in viral respiratory infections in young children. *J. Clin. Microbiol.* **2006**, *44*, 2739–2742.

12. Bastien, N.; Liu, L.; Ward, D.; Taylor, T.; Li, Y. Genetic variability of the G glycoprotein gene of human metapneumovirus. *J. Clin. Microbiol.* **2004**, *42*, 3532–3537.

13. Biacchesi, S.; Skiadopoulos, M.H.; Boivin, G.; Hanson, C.T.; Murphy, B.R.; Collins, P.L.; Buchholz, U.J. Genetic diversity between human metapneumovirus subgroups. *Virology* **2003**, *315*, 1–9.

14. Ishiguro, N.; Ebihara, T.; Endo, R.; Ma, X.; Kikuta, H.; Ishiko, H.; Kobayashi, K. High genetic diversity of the attachment (G) protein of human metapneumovirus. *J. Clin. Microbiol.* **2004**, *42*, 3406–3414.

15. Ludewick, H.P.; Abed, Y.; van Niekerk, N.; Boivin, G.; Klugman, K.P.; Madhi, S.A. Human metapneumovirus genetic variability, South Africa. *Emerg. Infect. Dis.* **2005**, *11*, 1074–1078.

16. Van den Hoogen, B.G.; Herfst, S.; Sprong, L.; Cane, P.A.; Forleo-Neto, E.; de Swart, R.L.; Osterhaus, A.D.; Fouchier, R.A. Antigenic and genetic variability of human metapneumoviruses. *Emerg. Infect. Dis.* **2004**, *10*, 658–666.

17. Feuillet, F.; Lina, B.; Rosa-Calatrava, M.; Boivin, G. Ten years of human metapneumovirus research. *J. Clin. Virol.* **2012**, *53*, 97–105.

18. Chanock, R.M.; Murphy, B.R.; Collins, P.L. Parainfluenza Viruses. In *Fields Virology*, 4th ed.; Knipe, D.M., Howley, P.M., Griffin, D.E., Martin, M.A., Lamb, R.A., Roizman, B., Straus, S.E., Eds.; Lippincott Williams and Wilkins: Philadelphia, PA, USA, 2001; Volume 1, pp. 1341–1379.

19. Cseke, G.; Maginnis, M.S.; Cox, R.G.; Tollefson, S.J.; Podsiad, A.B.; Wright, D.W.; Dermody, T.S.; Williams, J.V. Integrin αvβ1 promotes infection by human metapneumovirus. *Proc. Natl. Acad. Sci. USA* **2009**, *106*, 1566–1571.

20. Skiadopoulos, M.H.; Biacchesi, S.; Buchholz, U.J.; Amaro-Carambot, E.; Surman, S.R.; Collins, P.L.; Murphy, B.R. Individual contributions of the human metapneumovirus F, G, and SH surface glycoproteins to the induction of neutralizing antibodies and protective immunity. *Virology* **2006**, *345*, 492–501.

21. Skiadopoulos, M.H.; Biacchesi, S.; Buchholz, U.J.; Riggs, J.M.; Surman, S.R.; Amaro-Carambot, E.; McAuliffe, J.M.; Elkins, W.R.; St Claire, M.; Collins, P.L.; *et al.* The two major human metapneumovirus genetic lineages are highly related antigenically, and the fusion (F) protein is a major contributor to this antigenic relatedness. *J. Virol.* **2004**, *78*, 6927–6937.

22. Tang, R.S.; Mahmood, K.; Macphail, M.; Guzzetta, J.M.; Haller, A.A.; Liu, H.; Kaur, J.; Lawlor, H.A.; Stillman, E.A.; Schickli, J.H.; *et al.* A host-range restricted parainfluenza virus type 3 (PIV3) expressing the human metapneumovirus (hMPV) fusion protein elicits protective immunity in African green monkeys. *Vaccine* **2005**, *23*, 1657–1667.

23. Liu, L.; Bastien, N.; Li, Y. Intracellular processing, glycosylation, and cell surface expression of human metapneumovirus attachment glycoprotein. *J. Virol.* **2007**, *81*, 13435–13443.

24. Thammawat, S.; Sadlon, T.A.; Hallsworth, P.G.; Gordon, D.L. Role of cellular glycosaminoglycans and charged regions of viral G protein in human metapneumovirus infection. *J. Virol.* **2008**, *82*, 11767–11774.

25. Biacchesi, S.; Pham, Q.N.; Skiadopoulos, M.H.; Murphy, B.R.; Collins, P.L.; Buchholz, U.J. Infection of nonhuman primates with recombinant human metapneumovirus lacking the SH, G, or M2-2 protein categorizes each as a nonessential accessory protein and identifies vaccine candidates. *J. Virol.* **2005**, *79*, 12608–12613.

26. Esko, J.D.; Kimata, K.; Lindahl, U. Proteoglycans and Sulfated Glycosaminoglycans. In *Essentials of Glycobiology*, 2nd ed.; Cold Spring Harbor Laboratory Press: Cold Spring Harbor, NY, USA, 2009; Chapter 16.

27. Baba, M.; Snoeck, R.; Pauwels, R.; de Clercq, E. Sulfated polysaccharides are potent and selective inhibitors of various enveloped viruses, including herpes simplex virus, cytomegalovirus, vesicular stomatitis virus, and human immunodeficiency virus. *Antimicrob. Agents Chemother.* **1988**, *32*, 1742–1745.

28. Feldman, S.A.; Hendry, R.M.; Beeler, J.A. Identification of a linear heparin binding domain for human respiratory syncytial virus attachment glycoprotein G. *J. Virol.* **1999**, *73*, 6610–6617.

29. Hosoya, M.; Balzarini, J.; Shigeta, S.; de Clercq, E. Differential inhibitory effects of sulfated polysaccharides and polymers on the replication of various myxoviruses and retroviruses, depending on the composition of the target amino acid sequences of the viral envelope glycoproteins. *Antimicrob. Agents Chemother.* **1991**, *35*, 2515–2520.

30. Zhu, Z.; Gershon, M.D.; Ambron, R.; Gabel, C.; Gershon, A.A. Infection of cells by varicella zoster virus: Inhibition of viral entry by mannose 6-phosphate and heparin. *Proc. Natl. Acad. Sci. USA* **1995**, *92*, 3546–3550.

31. Krusat, T.; Streckert, H.J. Heparin-dependent attachment of respiratory syncytial virus (RSV) to host cells. *Arch. Virol.* **1997**, *142*, 1247–1254.

32. Wyde, P.R.; Moylett, E.H.; Chetty, S.N.; Jewell, A.; Bowlin, T.L.; Piedra, P.A. Comparison of the inhibition of human metapneumovirus and respiratory syncytial virus by NMSO3 in tissue culture assays. *Antivir. Res.* **2004**, *63*, 51–59.

33. Esko, J.D.; Stewart, T.E.; Taylor, W.H. Animal cell mutants defective in glycosaminoglycan biosynthesis. *Proc. Natl. Acad. Sci. USA* **1985**, *82*, 3197–3201.

34. Maertzdorf, J.; Wang, C.K.; Brown, J.B.; Quinto, J.D.; Chu, M.; de Graaf, M.; van den Hoogen, B.G.; Spaete, R.; Osterhaus, A.D.; Fouchier, R.A. Real-time reverse transcriptase PCR assay for detection of human metapneumoviruses from all known genetic lineages. *J. Clin. Microbiol.* **2004**, *42*, 981–986.

35. Shenoy-Scaria, A.M.; Gauen, L.K.; Kwong, J.; Shaw, A.S.; Lublin, D.M. Palmitylation of an amino-terminal cysteine motif of protein tyrosine kinases p56^{lck} and p59^{fyn} mediates interaction with glycosyl-phosphatidylinositol-anchored proteins. *Mol. Cell Biol.* **1993**, *13*, 6385–6392.

36. Byrnes, A.P.; Griffin, D.E. Binding of sindbis virus to cell surface heparan sulfate. *J. Virol.* **1998**, *72*, 7349–7356.

37. Heil, M.L.; Albee, A.; Strauss, J.H.; Kuhn, R.J. An amino acid substitution in the coding region of the E2 glycoprotein adapts Ross River virus to utilize heparan sulfate as an attachment moiety. *J. Virol.* **2001**, *75*, 6303–6309.

38. Klimstra, W.B.; Ryman, K.D.; Johnston, R.E. Adaptation of Sindbis virus to BHK cells selects for use of heparan sulfate as an attachment receptor. *J. Virol.* **1998**, *72*, 7357–7366.

39. Garcia-Beato, R.; Martinez, I.; Franci, C.; Real, F.X.; Garcia-Barreno, B.; Melero, J.A. Host cell effect upon glycosylation and antigenicity of human respiratory syncytial virus G glycoprotein. *Virology* **1996**, *221*, 301–309.

40. Cregg, J.M.; Vedvick, T.S.; Raschke, W.C. Recent advances in the expression of foreign genes in *Pichia pastoris. Biotechnology* **1993**, *11*, 905–910.

41. Mark, L.; Lee, W.H.; Spiller, O.B.; Villoutreix, B.O.; Blom, A.M. The Kaposi's sarcoma-associated herpesvirus complement control protein (KCP) binds to heparin and cell surfaces via positively charged amino acids in CCP1-2. *Mol. Immunol.* **2006**, *43*, 1665–1675.

42. Cardin, A.D.; Weintraub, H.J. Molecular modeling of protein-glycosaminoglycan interactions. *Arteriosclerosis* **1989**, *9*, 21–32.

43. Hileman, R.E.; Fromm, J.R.; Weiler, J.M.; Linhardt, R.J. Glycosaminoglycan-protein interactions: Definition of consensus sites in glycosaminoglycan binding proteins. *Bioessays* **1998**, *20*, 156–167.

44. Margalit, H.; Fischer, N.; Ben-Sasson, S.A. Comparative analysis of structurally defined heparin binding sequences reveals a distinct spatial distribution of basic residues. *J. Biol. Chem.* **1993**, *268*, 19228–19231.

45. Germi, R.; Crance, J.M.; Garin, D.; Guimet, J.; Lortat-Jacob, H.; Ruigrok, R.W.; Zarski, J.P.; Drouet, E. Heparan sulfate-mediated binding of infectious dengue virus type 2 and yellow fever virus. *Virology* **2002**, *292*, 162–168.

46. Hallak, L.K.; Spillmann, D.; Collins, P.L.; Peeples, M.E. Glycosaminoglycan sulfation requirements for respiratory syncytial virus infection. *J. Virol.* **2000**, *74*, 10508–10513.

47. Biacchesi, S.; Skiadopoulos, M.H.; Yang, L.; Lamirande, E.W.; Tran, K.C.; Murphy, B.R.; Collins, P.L.; Buchholz, U.J. Recombinant human metapneumovirus lacking the small hydrophobic SH and/or attachment G glycoprotein: Deletion of G yields a promising vaccine candidate. *J. Virol.* **2004**, *78*, 12877–12887.

48. Karron, R.A.; Buonagurio, D.A.; Georgiu, A.F.; Whitehead, S.S.; Adamus, J.E.; Clements-Mann, M.L.; Harris, D.O.; Randolph, V.B.; Udem, S.A.; Murphy, B.R.; *et al.* Respiratory syncytial virus (RSV) SH and G proteins are not essential for viral replication *in vitro*: Clinical evaluation and molecular characterization of a cold-passaged, attenuated RSV subgroup B mutant. *Proc. Natl. Acad. Sci. USA* **1997**, *94*, 13961–13966.

49. Teng, M.N.; Whitehead, S.S.; Collins, P.L. Contribution of the respiratory syncytial virus G glycoprotein and its secreted and membrane-bound forms to virus replication *in vitro* and *in vivo*. *Virology* **2001**, *289*, 283–296.

50. Haywood, A.M. Virus receptors: Binding, adhesion strengthening, and changes in viral structure. *J. Virol.* **1994**, *68*, 1–5.

51. Wickham, T.J.; Mathias, P.; Cheresh, D.A.; Nemerow, G.R. Integrins $\alpha_v\beta_3$ and $\alpha_v\beta_5$ promote adenovirus internalization but not virus attachment. *Cell* **1993**, *73*, 309–319.

52. Fuller, A.O.; Lee, W.C. Herpes simplex virus type 1 entry through a cascade of virus-cell interactions requires different roles of gD and gH in penetration. *J. Virol.* **1992**, *66*, 5002–5012.

53. Herold, B.C.; Visalli, R.J.; Susmarski, N.; Brandt, C.R.; Spear, P.G. Glycoprotein C-independent binding of herpes simplex virus to cells requires cell surface heparan sulphate and glycoprotein B. *J. Gen. Virol.* **1994**, *75*, 1211–1222.

54. Herold, B.C.; WuDunn, D.; Soltys, N.; Spear, P.G. Glycoprotein C of herpes simplex virus type 1 plays a principal role in the adsorption of virus to cells and in infectivity. *J. Virol.* **1991**, *65*, 1090–1098.

55. Johnson, R.M.; Spear, P.G. Herpes simplex virus glycoprotein D mediates interference with herpes simplex virus infection. *J. Virol.* **1989**, *63*, 819–827.

56. McClain, D.S.; Fuller, A.O. Cell-specific kinetics and efficiency of herpes simplex virus type 1 entry are determined by two distinct phases of attachment. *Virology* **1994**, *198*, 690–702.

57. WuDunn, D.; Spear, P.G. Initial interaction of herpes simplex virus with cells is binding to heparan sulfate. *J. Virol.* **1989**, *63*, 52–58.

58. Chang, A.; Masante, C.; Buchholz, U.J.; Dutch, R.E. Human metapneumovirus (HMPV) binding and infection are mediated by interactions between the HMPV fusion protein and heparan sulphate. *J. Virol.* **2012**, *86*, 3230–3243.

59. Cox, R.G.; Livesay, S.B.; Johnson, M.; Ohi, M.D; Williams, J.V. The human metapneumovirus fusion protein mediates entry via an interaction with RGD-binding integrins. *J. Virol.* **2012**, *86*, 12148–12160.

7

Human Metapneumovirus Antagonism of Innate Immune Responses

Deepthi Kolli [1], Xiaoyong Bao [1] and Antonella Casola [1,2,3,]*

[1] Departments of Pediatrics, University of Texas Medical Branch, Galveston, TX 77550, USA;
E-Mails: dekolli@utmb.edu (D.K.); xibao@utmb.edu (X.B.)

[2] Microbiology and Immunology, University of Texas Medical Branch, Galveston, TX 77550, USA

[3] Sealy Center for Molecular Medicine, University of Texas Medical Branch, Galveston,
TX 77550, USA

* Author to whom correspondence should be addressed; E-Mail: ancasola@utmb.edu

Abstract: Human metapneumovirus (hMPV) is a recently identified RNA virus belonging to the *Paramyxoviridae* family, which includes several major human and animal pathogens. Epidemiological studies indicate that hMPV is a significant human respiratory pathogen with worldwide distribution. It is associated with respiratory illnesses in children, adults, and immunocompromised patients, ranging from upper respiratory tract infections to severe bronchiolitis and pneumonia. Interferon (IFN) represents a major line of defense against virus infection, and in response, viruses have evolved countermeasures to inhibit IFN production as well as IFN signaling. Although the strategies of IFN evasion are similar, the specific mechanisms by which paramyxoviruses inhibit IFN responses are quite diverse. In this review, we will present an overview of the strategies that hMPV uses to subvert cellular signaling in airway epithelial cells, the major target of infection, as well as in primary immune cells.

Keywords: metapneumovirus; viral proteins; innate immune system; interferon antagonism

1. Human Metapneumovirus (hMPV): A Recently Discovered Human Viral Pathogen

The *Paramyxoviridae* family includes enveloped, negative-sense, single-stranded RNA viruses, which are major and ubiquitous disease causing pathogens of humans and animals [1]. Among them are important viruses that cause acute respiratory morbidity, particularly in infancy, elderly and in immunocompromised subjects of any age. The family is taxonomically divided into two subfamilies, the *Paramyxovirinae*, with five genera, and the *Pneumovirinae*, which includes two genera (Table 1). The classification of these viruses is based on their genome organization, morphological and biological characteristics, and sequence relationship of the encoded proteins. The pneumoviruses can be distinguished from the *Paramyxovirinae* members morphologically because they contain narrower nucleocapsids [1]. In addition, pneumoviruses have differences in genome organization, the number of encoded proteins and an attachment protein that is different from that of members of the subfamily *Paramyxovirinae*. There are two genera in the *Pneumovirinae* family, the *Pneumovirus* genus that includes human and bovine respiratory syncytial virus (RSV) and the *Metapneumovirus* genus that includes human metapneumovirus (hMPV) and avian metapneumovirus (APV) (Table 1). Human RSV encodes 11 separate proteins, while hMPV encodes nine proteins that generally correspond to those of RSV, except that hMPV lacks the non-structural proteins NS1 and NS2 and the gene order is different from that of pneumoviruses (Figure 1).

Table 1. Representative members of the *Paramyxoviridae* family.

Subfamily	Genus	Virus
Paramyxovirinae		
	Henipavirus	Hendravirus
		Nipah virus
	Morbillivirus	Measles virus (MeV)
	Respirovirus	Sendai virus (SeV)
		Human parainfluenza virus type 1 (hPIV1)
		Human parainfluenza virus type 3 (hPIV3)
		Bovine parainfluenza virus type 3 (BPIV3)
	Rubulavirus	Parainfluenza virus type 5 (PIV5)
		Mumps virus (MuV)
		Human parainfluenza virus type 2 (hPIV2)
Pneumovirinae		
	Pneumovirus	Human respiratory syncytial virus (hRSV)
		Bovine respiratory syncytial virus (BRSV)
	Metapneumovirus	Avian pneumovirus (APV)
		Human metapneumovirus (hMPV)

Figure 1. Genomic organization of *Pneumovirinae*.

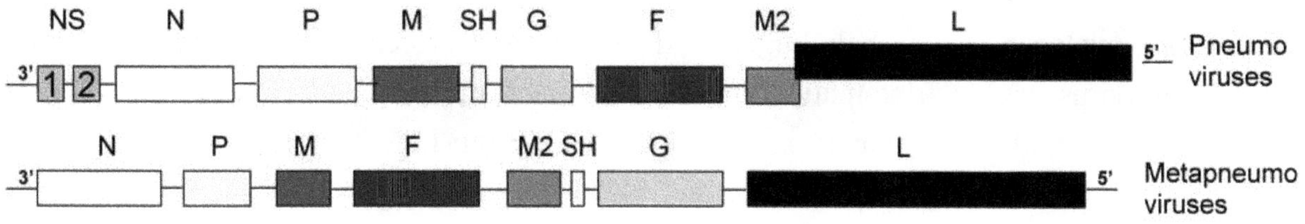

Since its first identification in 2001, hMPV has been isolated from individuals of all ages with acute respiratory tract infection worldwide [2]. Virtually, all children older than five years show 100% serologic evidence of infection [3]. Around 12% of all respiratory tract infections in children are caused by hMPV, second only to RSV [2,4–6]. HMPV also accounts for 10% of all hospitalizations of elderly patients with respiratory tract infections and it has been isolated from respiratory samples of a single winter season as often as parainfluenza [7]. Phylogenetic analysis of strains from many countries demonstrates two distinct hMPV genotypes, A and B, which can be divided in two subgroups: A1, A2, B1 and B2 [2,4]. The clinical features associated with hMPV in children are similar to those of RSV. hMPV is associated with both upper and lower respiratory tract infections. Fever, cough, tachypnea, wheezing and hypoxia are frequently observed in infected children. Chest radiographs demonstrate focal infiltrates and peribronchial cuffing. Many children have a clinical syndrome consistent with bronchiolitis. A significant proportion of symptomatic children who tested positive for hMPV had co-morbidities such as a history of prematurity, chronic lung disease or complex congenital heart diseases [8]. These findings suggest that the populations of children prone to severe RSV disease may be also prone to hMPV disease. Although RSV and hMPV share similar clinic features, hMPV induces a different spectrum of immune mediators compared to RSV [9–11], suggesting that the host cell responses and likely the pathogenesis of lung disease are viral specific.

2. Pattern Recognition Receptors (PRRs) in hMPV-Induced Signaling

The innate immune response represents a critical component of the host defense against viruses and is coordinated at the cellular level by activation of transcription factors that regulate the expression of inducible gene products with antiviral and/or inflammatory activity. Viruses contain conserved structural moieties, known as pathogen associated molecular pattern (PAMPs), that are recognized by several families of PRRs, in particular Toll-Like Receptors (TLR) and RNA helicases. Their relative contribution in virus-triggered cellular signaling is stimulus- and cell-type-dependent (Reviewed in [12]). So far, 10 members of TLRs have been identified in humans, and 13 in mice. Among those, TLR3, 4, 7, 8 and 9 have been shown to be more commonly involved in the innate response to viral infections [13,14]. TLR3 recognizes double-stranded RNA (ds-RNA) that is produced during viral replication [12]. Recently, RSV has been shown to relocate TLR3 from endosomes to cytoplasmic membrane in infected airway epithelial cells, resulting in increased chemokine production after an initial phase that is dependent on RSV replication [15,16]. However, we did not find a similar role of

TLR3 in hMPV-induced cellular signaling either in airway epithelial cells [17] or in primary immune cells, such as dendritic cells (DCs) [18].

Several viral envelop proteins, including RSV F protein and proteins of mammary tumor virus, murine leukemia virus, vesicular stomatitis virus [19–21], and more recently Ebola virus [22], have been shown to activate TLR4 in primary immune cells. Similar to LPS, the primary ligand of TLR4, RSV F protein requires the presence of CD14 and MD-2 for signaling [23,24]. TLR4 signaling has been shown to play an important role in controlling paramyxovirus infection. TLR4-deficient mice challenged with RSV exhibited impaired natural killer (NK) cell and CD14+ cell pulmonary trafficking, diminished NK cell function, and impaired IL-12 induction, in addition to impaired RSV clearance [20]. In a model of alveolar macrophage depletion of TLR4-defective C3H/HeJ mice, we have shown that the early NF-κB response that occurs in the lung after RSV infection, is dependent upon alveolar macrophages and TLR4 [25]. Furthermore, both TLR4 and the adaptor molecule MyD88 have been shown to be required for optimal protection against viral challenge in a mouse model of RSV infection [26]. Our recent investigations have shown that down regulation of TLR4 expression in human DCs or lack of functional TLR4 in mouse bone marrow-derived DCs result in significantly reduced expression of hMPV-induced cytokine, chemokine, and type I IFN secretion, indicating an important role of this TLR in the activation of cellular signaling following hMPV infection [18]. In addition, mice lacking TLR4 showed less clinical disease, significantly lower levels of cytokines and chemokines, compared to the wild type. Accordingly, inflammatory cell recruitment in the BAL, lungs, as well as in lymph nodes, was also significantly reduced [27]. These results indicate that TLR4 is important for activation of the innate immune response to hMPV infection, however, it also contributes to disease pathogenesis.

TLR7 and 8 share highest homology to each other among the TLR family and both of them recognize single-stranded RNA (ss-RNA) [28,29], while TLR9 recognize viral CpG DNA motif [30,31]. In case of hMPV, it has been shown that induction of cytokines and type I Interferon (IFN) is TLR7-dependent [32], using TLR7-deficient mice and TLR7 specific oligonucleotide-based inhibitor ISS661. While a similar requirement in RSV infection of pDCs has not been demonstrated yet, recently a critical role for TLR7 and MyD88 in the recognition and development of innate inflammatory responses necessary to limit pneumovirus infection has been reported [33]. No direct involvement of TLR9 in innate immune cellular signaling in response to either RSV or hMPV has been reported yet.

After recognition of their own PAMPs, following viral infection, TLRs trigger intracellular signaling pathways that are necessary to the induction of inflammatory cytokines, chemokines, as well as type I IFN. Three structural domains, *i.e.*, a Leucine Rich Region (LRR) in the N-terminal ectodomain, a transmembrane region, and a Toll/IL-1R resistance (TIR) domain in the intracellular region, are structural hallmarks of all known Toll/TLRs. Differential utilization of four TIR-containing adapter molecules (*i.e.*, MyD88, TIRAP, TRIF, and TRAM) by distinct TLRs leads to activation of downstream signaling pathways, findings based largely on studies in adapter knockout mice. Two major TLR signaling pathways have been identified, *i.e.*, one that is MyD88-dependent, and gives rise to strong and early activation of the transcription factor NF-κB, and a TRIF-dependent, MyD88-independent pathway that primarily drives strong activation of IRF-3, with later activation of NF-κB. The MyD88-dependent pathway results in induction of highly NF-κB-dependent, proinflammatory genes (TNF-α, IL-1β, IL-6), while the MyD88-independent pathway leads to gene induction that is highly IRF-3-dependent (IFN-β, RANTES). TLR4 activates both pathways for gene expression, as it is the only TLR that uses both adapter proteins (Figure 2) [13,34,35].

Figure 2. Toll-Like Receptors (TLR) signaling pathway involved in hMPV-induced gene expression in primary immune cells. Upon binding of their specific viral PAMP, TLR4 and 7 lead to activation of NF-κB- and IRF-dependent gene expression by engaging the adaptor MyD88 alone (TLR7) or in combination with TRIF (TLR4). Ub indicates ubiquitination; P indicates phosphorylation.

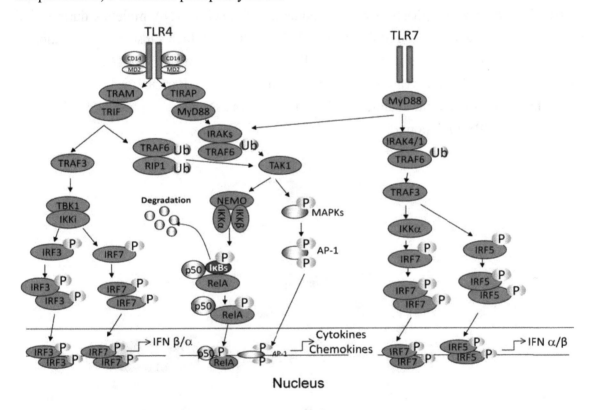

Aside from the recognition of viral RNA through the TLRs, two DExD/H box RNA helicases, retinoic acid inducible gene (RIG)-I and melanoma differentiation-associated gene (MDA)-5, have been identified to be essential for IFN induction by several viruses including Newcastle, Sendai, hepatitis C, influenza and RSV [16,36–39]. Both RIG-I and MDA-5 share two homologous CARD domains and a helicase domain that is required for its interaction with viral RNA [36,40]. The CARD domains of the RNA helicases mediate its interaction with the CARD domain of the mitochondrial protein MAVS (also known as IPS-1/VISA/Cardif), leading to subsequent activation of downstream signaling molecules, such as IRFs, NF-κB and AP-1 [41,42–44]. Viral RNA signaling mediated by RIG-I is independent from TLRs, as dominant negative RIG-I does not block TLR-mediated signaling [41,43]. Generation of RIG-I and MDA-5 knock-out mice has identified a major antiviral role for RNA helicases in several cell types, including macrophages and conventional DCs, but not in plasmacytoid DCs (pDCs), which instead require TLR7 and/or TLR9 to mount an effective antiviral response (Reviewed in [44]). We have recently shown that hMPV infection of airway epithelial cells induces the expression RIG-I and MDA-5 and that RIG-I, but not MDA-5, plays a fundamental role in hMPV-induced cellular signaling, as inhibition of RIG-I expression significantly decreases activation of IRF and NF-κB transcription factors and production of type I IFN and proinflammatory cytokines and chemokines [17]. MAVS was also necessary for hMPV-induced cellular signaling, as expression of a dominant negative mutant MAVS significantly reduced IFN-β and chemokine gene transcription, in response to hMPV infection. RIG-I-dependent signaling was necessary to induce a cellular antiviral state, as reduction of RIG-I expression resulted in enhanced hMPV replication (Figure 3) [17].

Figure 3. RIG-I/MAVS signaling pathway regulating hMPV-induced NF-κB and IRF activation in airway epithelial cells. Production of specific RNA moieties during viral replication leads to activation of the RIG-I-MAVs pathway, which subsequent activation of the IKK complex, which is upstream NF-κB activation, and of the TBK1/IKKβ complex, which regulates IRF-3 activation, leading to proinflammatory/immune gene expression. P indicates phosphorylation; ? indicates the unknown kinase that phosphorylates NF-κB in response to hMPV infection.

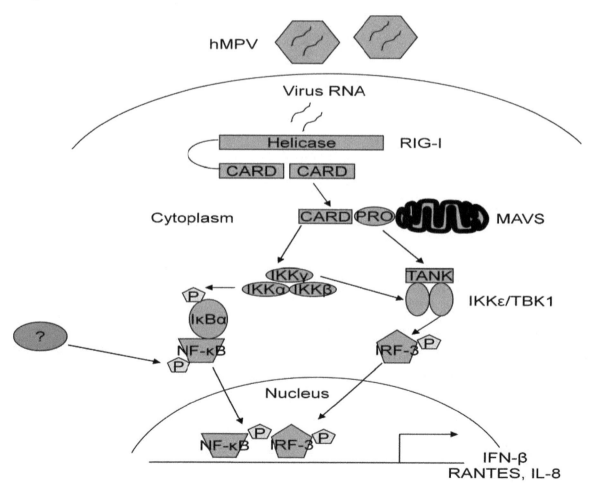

3. Inhibition of TLR Signaling

Dendritic cells are professional antigen-presenting cells that can be generally divided into myeloid CD11c[+] "conventional" DCs (cDCs) or pDCs [45]. Both subsets specialize in detecting viruses and initiating innate and adaptive immune responses that lead to viral elimination or control [46]. Under baseline conditions, these cells reside in the peripheral tissue in an immature, resting state scattered throughout the respiratory mucosal wall [47] and express several receptors for recognizing viruses [48] such as TLRs. These DCs are often the first immune cells to come in contact with infecting viruses after infection, particularly after mucosal exposure, and can became primary targets of infection. After detection, uptake, and degradation of viruses, DCs initiate immune responses via the secretion of interferon, chemokines, and proinflammatory cytokines, and the upregulation of a variety of costimulatory molecules and receptors, a process globally known as cell maturation. The central role of DC in initiating and shaping the immune response, together with their presence at and recruitment to the site of infection and concomitant exposure to infectious virus, makes them obvious candidates for viral manipulation of the host immune response.

We and others have reported that hMPV can infect monocyte-derived DCs (moDCs), resulting in viral antigen expression [10,49,50] and maturation (increased expression of MHC II, CD86) [10,50]. HMPV can also infect pDCs, although less efficiently than moDCs [10]. In recent investigations we have shown that hMPV infection inhibits TLR-dependent signaling both *in vitro* and *in vivo*. Type I IFN production in isolated moDCs, following stimulation with TLR3 and 4 agonists, and in pDCs, in response to a TLR9 agonist, was significantly reduced by hMPV infection in a replication-dependent manner [10,18]. Furthermore, prior infection of BALB/c mice with hMPV completely suppressed IFN-α production induced by intranasal application of poly-ICLC (TLR3 ligand) or a synthetic CpG-ODN (TLR9 ligand) in mice lung [51], indicating that hMPV interferes with one or multiple signal transduction pathways activated in response to TLR stimulation in a variety of cell types.

4. Interferon Signaling Antagonism

IFNs are a group of cytokines that activate an array of cellular genes that are critical in restricting viral replication and modulating adaptive immunity. Production of IFNs is an important feature of the host response to viral infections. Type I IFNs (IFN-α and -β) are the key mediators produced by airway epithelial cells infected with paramyxoviruses [36,52,53] including hMPV [54]. Secreted IFN-α/β bind to IFN-α/β receptors (IFNαR) leading to dimerization of the two subunits, IFNαR1 and IFNαR2. IFNαR1 and IFNαR2 then undergo conformational changes resulting in the activation of the Janus tyrosine kinase (Jak)/signal transducer and activator of transcription protein (STAT) pathway [55]. Tyrosine kinase 2 (Tyk2), a kinase belonging to the Jak family, is constitutively bound to IFNAR1. Tyk2 phosphorylates IFNAR1 at tyrosine residue 466 (Y466) and creates a docking site for STAT2 [56]. Subsequently, Tyk2 phosphorylates STAT2 at tyrosine 690 (Y690). Phosphorylation of STAT2 Y690 creates a new docking site for the SH2 domain of STAT1 [57,58], which is subsequently phosphorylated at Y701 by IFNAR2 bound-Jak1 [59]. Phosphorylated STAT1 and STAT2 then dimerize and bind to IRF-9 [60]. This newly formed heterotrimer, known as IFN-stimulated gene factor 3 (ISGF3), translocates into the nucleus to bind ISG gene promoter and activate transcription. ISGs induced by type I IFN signaling typically contain either interferon stimulated response elements (ISRE) or a gamma activated sequence (GAS) elements within their promoters, although there is a clear preference for genes containing an ISRE. Examples of ISRE-containing ISGs are ISG15, Myxovirus (influenza virus) resistance (Mx)1, 2'-5'-oligoadenylate synthetase (OAS)1, IRF-7 and protein kinase R (PKR) [61], while GAS-containing genes are IRF-1, IRF-2, IRF-8 and IRF-9 [62,63]. In addition to activating this canonical Jak/STAT pathway described above, stimulation of the IFNαR also activates several non canonical signaling events such as recruitment and phosphorylation of other STATs [61–63] and tyrosine phosphorylation of and activation of insulin receptor substrates 1 (IRS1) and 2 (IRS2) [63].

As IFN response is critical for a robust innate immune response, almost all mammalian viruses have developed strategies to interfere with IFN production and signaling and to disrupt innate host antiviral factors. These include directly targeting the pathways required for the induction of IFN production, targeting of signaling molecules belonging to the Jak/STAT signaling pathway, and increasing the expression or activity of endogenous cellular key regulators, such as suppressor of cytokine signaling (SOCS) proteins, protein tyrosine phosphatases (PTPs) and protein inhibitor of activated STATs (PIAS) [64,65]. Several members of the *Paramyxovirus* family have been shown to directly target STAT signaling through distinct mechanisms which include proteasomal degradation [66–68], sequestration in high-molecular-weight complexes [69,70] and inhibition of nuclear localization of STAT proteins [71]. The first description of hMPV capacity to interfere with IFN signaling came from Harrod *et al.* who tested the ability of hMPV to subvert IFN-α-dependent responses in airway epithelial cells using reporter gene assays. They showed that IFN-α-mediated induction of ISRE-driven luciferase activity was completely abolished in hMPV-infected A549 cells, as well as induction of ISGs, such OAS1, Mx1, RIG-I and MDA-5 [72]. This observation was paralleled by the inhibition of IFN-α-dependent tyrosine phosphorylation and subsequent nuclear translocation of STAT1 in hMPV-infected airway epithelial cells [72]. However, a mechanism responsible for the observed inhibition was not identified. Later, we have shown that hMPV infection affects several steps of the IFN signaling pathway, from inducing degradation of Jak1 and Tyk2 via a ubiquitin-proteasome-dependent pathway, to reducing IFNAR1 surface expression in infected cells, possibly due to increased internalization of the receptor as a result of viral-induced degradation of Tyk2 (Figure 4) [73]. Both phenomena were independent of type I IFN expression, since inhibition was also observed in Vero cells which do not produce type I IFN, and required *de novo* viral gene expression and/or viral RNA replication [73].

5. hMPV Proteins Identified as Antagonist of Host Innate Signaling Pathways

Among hMPV encoded proteins, phosphoprotein P, glycoprotein G, small hydrophobic protein (SH) and M2-2 have been shown to modulate hMPV-induced innate immune response, the first line of host defense against invading pathogens [18,32,74–76]. A discussion of the inhibitory function for each of these proteins is presented below.

Small hydrophobic (SH) glycoprotein. hMPV SH protein is a type II transmembrane glycoprotein [77]. It is the largest among the pneumoviruses (179 aa for the hMPV isolate CAN97-83 versus 175 aa for APV, 81 aa for BRSV, and 64 aa for HRSV) [77,78]. Even though it is substantially longer than RSV, it has similar characteristics to the one of RSV, including a high percentage of threonine and serine residues and a similar hydrophilicity profile [77,78]. HMPV SH protein is more prone to frequent frameshift and point mutations in culture presumably to give a selective advantage of the clinical isolates in culture [79] and does not appear to be required for virus growth *in vitro*. In fact, a recombinant hMPV virus lacking the SH protein (rhMPV-ΔSH) is viable, grows as well as the wild-type virus in MK2 cells and A549 cells [74,80] and is not significantly attenuated in animal models of infection [74,80,81]. Similar to the SH protein of several members of the *Paramyxoviridae* family such PIV5 and RSV [82,83], and more recently J paramyxovirus (JPV) [84] and mumps virus (MuV) [85], all of which have been shown to inhibit TNF-α-mediated NF-κB signaling, we have also reported an inhibitory role of hMPV SH protein in NF-κB activation [74]. Infection of airway epithelial cells with rhMPV-ΔSH led to increased interleukin 6 (IL-6), IL-8, and MCP-1 secretion, compared to rhMPV-WT [74]. Similarly, BALB/c mice infected with rhMPV-ΔSH showed enhanced production of TNF-α, IL-6, KC and MCP-1, compared to rhMPV-WT [74]. We observed significantly higher induction of IL-8 gene transcription in 293 cells infected with rhMPV-ΔSH compared to rhMPV-WT, and SH protein expression lead to inhibition of TNF-α induced IL-8 promoter activation, confirming a role of SH in inhibition of NF-κB-dependent gene transcription [74]. SH protein of hMPV affected NF-κB-dependent gene transcription by modulating NF-κB transcriptional activity and not by inhibiting nuclear translocation, and therefore the canonical pathway leading to NF-κB activation (Figure 4) [86]. Similar to Rep78 protein of adeno-associated virus type II, which targets PKA activation [87], hMPV SH might inhibit one of the kinases that phosphorylate NF-κB [74]. Our results indicate a possible novel mechanism by which paramyxovirus SH proteins can affect NF-κB activation, in addition to inhibiting TNF-induced NF-κB nuclear translocation, as it has been shown for RSV and PIV5 SH proteins [82,83]. Whether RSV, PIV5 and JPV SH proteins can also affect viral-induced NF-κB post-translational modifications will require further investigation.

Glycoprotein G. hMPV G protein is a type II mucin-like glycosylated protein [77]. The membrane anchor of G protein is proximal to the N terminus and their C terminus is oriented externally. Although the postulated function of G protein is for attachment, it has been shown that hMPV F protein alone is sufficient to mediate attachment and fusion in the absence of other surface proteins including G [80,81,88]. In addition, the interaction of F with cellular integrin receptors is independent of G protein [89], suggesting that G protein plays a minimal role in hMPV attachment. Although lack of G protein does not decrease significantly the ability of hMPV to replicate *in vitro*, a recombinant virus in which the G protein is deleted (rhMPV-ΔG) exhibits reduced replication in the upper and lower respiratory tract of Syrian hamsters and African green monkeys [80,81].

In the past few years, our laboratory has been focusing on the molecular mechanism(s) underlying the attenuation of rhMPV-ΔG. We discovered that hMPV G is an important virulence factor which inhibits cellular signaling both in airway epithelial cells and in primary immune cells [75,90]. The respiratory epithelium represents the principal and primary target site of respiratory viruses, including hMPV. We found that rhMPV-ΔG induces significantly higher amounts of the cytokines, chemokines and type I IFN than hMPV-WT in airway epithelial cells, due to enhanced activation of transcription factors belonging to the NF-κB (e.g., p65 and p50) and IRF families (e.g., IRF-3), demonstrated by increased nuclear translocation and/or phosphorylation [75]. As RIG-I and MAVS are central regulators of hMPV-induced cellular signaling in airway epithelial cells, we investigated whether G targeted the RIG-I/MAVS pathway and, indeed, we found that G protein physically interacts with RIG-I and inhibits RIG-I-, but not MAVS-dependent IFN-β gene transcription (Figure 4) [75].

Figure 4. Schematic diagram of sites of antagonism of cellular signaling and IFN production/responses by hMPV proteins. Major cellular targets of hMPV proteins in the TLR4, RIG-I/MAVS and type I IFN signaling pathways. P indicates phosphorylation.

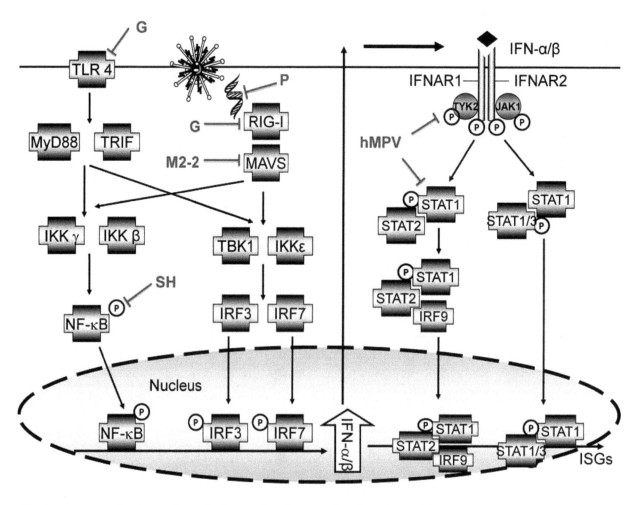

We have recently investigated the molecular mechanism by which G protein expression inhibits RIG-I activation. We found that the interaction of hMPV G with RIG-I occurs primarily through the

CARD domains of its N-terminus, preventing RIG-I association with the adaptor protein MAVS and RIG-I recruitment to mitochondria. HMPV G expression also prevented the interaction between mitochondria and mitochondria-associated membrane (MAM) component of the endoplasmic reticulum (ER), which contains Stimulator of IFN genes (STINGS), an important part of the viral-induced RIG-I/MAVS signaling pathway, leading in the end to the inhibition of cytokine, chemokine and type I interferon (IFN) expression. Mutagenesis analysis showed that hMPV G protein cytoplasmic domain played a major role in the observed inhibitory activity, and recombinant viruses expressing a G protein with amino acid substitution in position 2 and 3 recapitulated most of the phenotype observed with rhMPV-ΔG mutant upon infection of airway epithelial cells [91].

DCs play a pivotal role in shaping antiviral immune responses in the respiratory tract. They can efficiently sense invading pathogens by TLRs and, because of their strategic localization at mucosal sites, are involved in the response to viral infections [92,93]. We have recently demonstrated that moDCs infected with rhMPV-ΔG also produce higher levels of type I IFNs, cytokines and chemokines compared with cells infected with rhMPV-WT, suggesting that G protein plays an inhibitory role in viral-induced cellular responses of immune cells as well (Figure 4) [90]. As discussed above, TLR4 plays a major role in hMPV-induced activation of moDCs [90]. In our study, we found that G protein impaired TLR4-dependent signaling, as moDCs infection with rhMPV-ΔG inhibited LPS-induced production of cytokine and chemokines significantly less than rhMPV-WT, and treatment of moDCs with purified G protein resulted in significant inhibition of LPS-dependent signaling. Taken together, our results demonstrate that hMPV G protein plays an important role in inhibiting host innate immune responses in dendritic cells, possibly affecting adaptive immune responses as well. This is an important finding, as inadequate TLR stimulation, with subsequent lack of antibody affinity maturation has been recently identified as an important cause of vaccine failure and enhanced disease following administration of the formaline-inactivated RSV vaccine [94].

Inhibition of cellular signaling by surface glycoproteins has been demonstrated for other viruses as well. RSV G protein inhibits cytokine and chemokine secretion, as infection with a recombinant RSV lacking the full-length G protein (rRSV-ΔG) or the soluble part of G protein (rRSV-ΔsG) enhances production of IL-6 and IL-8 in monocytes [95], and IL-8 and RANTES secretion, and ICAM expression in airway epithelial cells [96]. RSV-ΔG also induces more immune mediator production, compared to WT virus, in a mouse model of infection [95]. Similarly, the surface glycoproteins of hantaviruses, in particular, those associated with hemorrhagic pulmonary syndrome (HPS), have been shown to affect IRF-3 activation and IFN production via interaction with RIG-I and TBK-1, a kinase responsible for viral-induced IRF-3 phosphorylation, and to inhibit IFN-mediated cellular responses [97,98]. Taken together, it could be a common feature of surface glycoproteins of enveloped single strand, negative strand RNA viruses to be inhibitory to antiviral signaling, consequently, leading to host immune evasion.

M2-2 protein. HMPV M2 encodes two overlapping proteins: M2-1 and M2-2. The M2-1 open reading frame (ORF) of strain CAN 97-83 is assumed to start with the first AUG at nucleotide position 14, and encodes a protein of 187 amino acids. The M2-2 ORF possibly initiates with the AUGs at positions 525 and 537, overlapping the M2-1 ORF by 53 or 41 nucleotides, respectively [77,99]. M2-1 protein is not essential for hMPV recovery using the reverse genetic system *in vitro*, in contrast to RSV M2-1 protein, which is essential for full viral replication [99–101]. The role of hMPV M2-2 protein in regulating viral RNA synthesis has been confirmed by our group and several others [81,99,102,103].

Similar to rhMPV-ΔG, recombinant rhMPV lacking M2-2 (rhMPV-ΔM2-2) is also listed as a live vaccine candidate, as it is attenuated, immunogenic and protective against hMPV challenge in both African green monkeys and hamsters [81,99,102]. Although the attenuation of rhMPV-ΔM2-2 could be explained by decreased viral genome accumulation by M2-2 deletion [99,102,103], we found that other mechanism(s) could be also associated with rhMPV-ΔM2-2 attenuation, as discussed below. We recently discovered that hMPV M2-2 is an important antagonist of host antiviral signaling, therefore, favoring hMPV replication. In fact, ΔM2-2-infected airway epithelial cells produced higher levels of IFN-β and other immune mediators, compared to rhMPV-WT-infected cells [76]. Although the expression of hMPV G protein was impaired due to a reduced ability of rhMPV-ΔM2-2 to replicate, which might contribute indirectly to the enhanced cellular responses observed following infection with the M2-2 deleted mutant, ectopic expression of G protein at levels comparable or higher than the one observed in WT-infected cells only partially reversed the enhancement in cellular responses observed with rhMPV-ΔM2-2, suggesting that M2-2 contributes to hMPV immune evasion as well. Indeed, in reporter gene assays, M2-2 protein, but not other soluble hMPV proteins, inhibited MAVS-induced IFN-β gene transcription, but not the induction mediated by downstream signaling molecules of the RIG-I/MAVS pathway, suggesting that MAVS is the target of M2-2 (Figure 4). Coimmunoprecipitation studies, both in an overexpression system or in the context of viral infection, showed a clear association of M2-2 with MAVS, supporting this concept [76].

We have also identified the domains of M2-2 responsible for the regulation of viral gene transcription, viral replication, and RIG-I-mediated signaling. We found that the first 25 amino acids of M2-2 are critical to promote viral gene transcription, but not involved in the regulation of viral replication and hMPV-induced signaling. In contrast, the domains spanning from amino acid 26 to 69 are dispensable for the regulation of viral gene transcription, but responsible for RIG-I signaling inhibition and viral replication facilitation [76].

In summary, hMPV uses both G and M2-2 protein to target the RIG-I/MAVS pathway. The mechanism by which viruses use two distinct viral proteins to target molecules belonging to the same cellular signaling pathway is becoming recognized as a common strategy to evade host immune defenses. For example, influenza virus uses its NS1 protein to target RIG-I [104,105], and its PB1-F2 and PB2 proteins to inhibit MAVS [106,107]. In case of RSV, NS2 protein of RSV antagonizes the activation of IFN-β transcription by interaction with RIG-I [108], and we recently found that NS1 protein inhibits IFN-β synthesis by associating with RIG-I downstream transcription factor IRF-3 and its transcriptional co-activator CBP [109].

Phosphoprotein (P). The P protein gene of the pneumoviruses, different from the one of paramyxovirinae, is monocistronic, encoding a single polypeptide with a predicted mass of 32.5 kDa [110], although production of multiple forms of phosphoprotein in infected cells has been reported [111]. Similar to other pneumoviruses, hMPV P protein is present within the helical ribonucleoprotein (RNP) complex. It has been shown that hMPV N and P proteins interact together and form cytoplasmic inclusion bodies [112].

Elegant studies conducted by Goutagny et al. [32], focusing on comparing the innate responses to hMPV A and B strains, showed that hMPV-B failed to elicit a type I IFN response in airway epithelial cells and in human monocytes, despite its ability to infect and replicate as efficiently as hMPV-A. Similar to our reports in epithelial cells [17], Goutagny and coworkers showed that hMPV A1 triggers RIG-I activation to induce type I IFN production while hMPV B1 did not [32]. They showed that in the context of the virus infection, the hMPV B viral RNA is prevented from being sensed by RIG-I and that the P protein is responsible for this inhibition (Figure 4). Since viral RNA is protected from free cellular RNases by RNP complex, proteins within the RNP, especially P protein in hMPV B1 probably could prevent the recognition of the viral RNA by the RIG-I pathway. This strain specific inhibition of RIG-I sensing by P protein has been ascribed to higher levels of expression of the P protein, as well as higher affinity for the RNA or other components of the RNP complex, during hMPV-B infection, compared to hMPV-A [32]. Moreover, the inhibitory effect of the hMPV-B P protein was restricted to the RIG-I pathway, because it did not prevent the induction of IFN-α/β in pDCs, which uses TLR7 pathway. In conclusion, this study suggests that in addition to other structural proteins such as G, SH and M2-2 proteins, RNP complex proteins might also play an important role in inhibition of viral- induced type I IFN expression.

In summary, hMPV antagonizes cellular responses and type I IFN secretion/signaling through a variety of mechanisms which involve the regulation of PRRs (both TLRs and RLR), as well as the key signaling molecules involved in the downstream signaling of IFN pathway such as STAT1, STAT2, Jak1 and Tyk2. The role of this inhibition of type I IFN signaling by hMPV in pathogenesis and severity of infection also needs to be investigated, as inhibition of IFN signaling may affect development of host adaptive immunity, leaving the host susceptible to reinfection. A better understanding of how hMPV inhibits cellular signaling and type I IFN pathway, and its consequences in regard to the innate and adaptive immune responses, is crucial for improving therapeutic approaches and the development of better vaccines against hMPV infection.

Acknowledgments

We would like to thank Allison Solari for her assistance in the manuscript submission.

References

1. Lamb, R.A.; Kolakofsky, D. Paramyxoviridae: The Viruses and Their Replication. In *Fundamental Virology*, 4th ed.; Knipe, D.M., Howley, P.M., Eds; Lippincott, Williams and Wilkins: Philadelphia, PA, USA, 2001; pp. 689–724.

2. Principi, N.; Bosis, S.; Esposito, S. Human metapneumovirus in paediatric patients. *Clin. Microbiol. Infect.* **2006**, *12*, 301–308.

3. Van den Hoogen, B.G.; de Jong, J.C.; Groen, J.; Kuiken, T.; de Groot, R.; Fouchier, R.A.; Osterhaus, A.D. A newly discovered human pneumovirus isolated from young children with respiratory tract disease. *Nat. Med.* **2001**, *7*, 719–724.

4. Kahn, J.S. Epidemiology of human metapneumovirus. *Clin. Microbiol. Rev.* **2006**, *19*, 546–557.

5. Williams, J.V.; Harris, P.A.; Tollefson, S.J.; Halburnt-Rush, L.L.; Pingsterhaus, J.M.; Edwards, K.M.; Wright, P.F.; Crowe, J.E., Jr. Human metapneumovirus and lower respiratory tract disease in otherwise healthy infants and children. *N. Engl. J. Med.* **2004**, *350*, 443–450.

6. Crowe, J.E., Jr. Human metapneumovirus as a major cause of human respiratory tract disease. *Pediatr. Infect. Dis. J.* **2004**, *23*, 215–221.

7. Boivin, G.; Abed, L.; Pelletier, G.; Ruel, L.; Moisan, D.; Cote', S.; Peret, T.C.; Erdman, D.D., Anderson, L.J. Virological features and clinical manifestations associated with the human metapneumovirus, a newly discovered paramyxovirus. *J. Infect. Dis.* **2002**, *186*, 1330–1334.

8. Esper, F.; Boucher, D.; Weibel, C.; Martinello, R.A.; Kahn, J.S. Human metapneumovirus infection in the United States: Clinical manifestations associated with a newly emerging respiratory infection in children. *Pediatrics* **2003**, *111*, 1407–1410.

9. Guerrero-Plata, A.; Casola, A.; Garofalo, R.P. Human metapneumovirus induces a profile of lung cytokines distinct from that of respiratory syncytial virus. *J. Virol.* **2005**, *79*, 14992–14997.

10. Guerrero-Plata, A.; Casola, A.; Suarez, G.; Yu, X.; Spetch, L.; Peeples, M.E.; Garofalo, R.P. Differential response of dendritic cells to human metapneumovirus and respiratory syncytial virus. *Am. J. Respir. Cell Mol. Biol.* **2006**, *34*, 320–329.

11. Bao, X.; Liu, T.; Spetch, L.; Kolli, D.; Garofalo, R.P.; Casola, A. Airway epithelial cell response to human metapneumovirus infection. *Virology* **2007**, *386*, 91–101.

12. Seth, R.B.; Sun, L.; Chen, Z.J. Antiviral innate immunity pathways. *Cell Res.* **2006**, *16*, 141–147.

13. Kawai, T.; Akira, S. TLR signaling. *Cell Death Differ.* **2006**, *13*, 816–825.

14. Takeda, K.; Akira, S. Toll-like receptors in innate immunity. *Int. Immunol.* **2005**, *17*, 1–14.

15. Groskreutz, D.J.; Monick, M.M.; Powers, L.S.; Yarovinsky, T.O.; Look, D.C.; Hunninghake, G.W. Respiratory syncytial virus induces TLR3 protein and protein kinase R, leading to increased double-stranded RNA responsiveness in airway epithelial cells. *J. Immunol.* **2006**, *176*, 1733–1740.

16. Liu, P.; Jamaluddin, M.; Li, K.; Garofalo, R.P.; Casola, A.; Brasier, A.R. Retinoic Acid-inducible gene I mediates early antiviral response and toll-like receptor 3 expression in respiratory syncytial virus-infected airway epithelial cells. *J. Virol.* **2007**, *81*, 1401–1411.

17. Liao, S.; Bao, X.; Liu, T.; Lai, S.; Li, K.; Garofalo, R.P.; Casola, A. Role of retinoic acid inducible gene-I in human metapneumovirus-induced cellular signalling. *J. Gen. Virol.* **2008**, *89*, 1978–1986.

18. Kolli, D.; Bao, X.; Liu, T.; Hong, C.; Wang, T.; Garofalo, R.P.; Casola, A. Human metapneumovirus glycoprotein G inhibits TLR4-dependent signaling in monocyte-derived dendritic cells. *J. Immunol.* **2011**, *187*, 47–54.

19. Beutler, B.; Hoebe, K.; Georgel, P.; Tabeta, K.; Du, X. Genetic analysis of innate immunity: Identification and function of the TIR adapter proteins. *Adv. Exp. Med. Biol.* **2005**, *560*, 29–39.

20. Haynes, L.M.; Moore, D.D.; Kurt-Jones, E.A.; Finberg, R.W.; Anderson, L.J.; Tripp, R.A. Involvement of toll-like receptor 4 in innate immunity to respiratory syncytial virus. *J. Virol.* **2001**, *75*, 10730–10737.

21. Rassa, J.C.; Meyers, J.L.; Zhang, Y.; Kudaravalli, R.; Ross, S.R. Murine retroviruses activate B cells via interaction with toll-like receptor 4. *Proc. Natl. Acad. Sci. USA* **2002**, *99*, 2281–2286.

22. Okumura, A.; Pitha, P.M.; Yoshimura, A.; Harty, R.N. Interaction between Ebola virus glycoprotein and host toll-like receptor 4 leads to induction of proinflammatory cytokines and SOCS1. *J. Virol.* **2010**, *84*, 27–33.

23. Kurt-Jones, E.A.; Popova, L.; Kwinn, L.; Haynes, L.M.; Jones, L.P.; Tripp, R.A.; Walsh, E.E.; Freeman, M.W.; Golenbock, D.T.; Anderson, L.J.; *et al.* Pattern recognition receptors TLR4 and CD14 mediate response to respiratory syncytial virus. *Nat. Immunol* **2000**, *1*, 398–401.

24. Lizundia, R.; Sauter, K.S.; Taylor, G.; Werling, D. Host species-specific usage of the TLR4-LPS receptor complex. *Innate Immun.* **2008**, *14*, 223–231.

25. Haeberle, H.; Takizawa, R.; Casola, A.; Brasier, A.R.; Dieterich, H.-J.; van Rooijen, N.; Gatalica, Z.; Garofalo, R.P. Respiratory syncytial virus-induced activation of NF-kB in the lung involves alveolar macrophages and Toll-like receptor 4-dependent pathways. *J. Infect. Dis.* **2002**, *186*, 1199–1206.

26. Cyr, S.L.; Angers, I.; Guillot, L.; Stoica-Popescu, I.; Lussier, M.; Qureshi, S.; Burt, D.S.; Ward, B.J. TLR4 and MyD88 control protection and pulmonary granulocytic recruitment in a murine intranasal RSV immunization and challenge model. *Vaccine* **2009**, *27*, 421–430.

27. Velayutham, T.S.; Kolli, D.; Ivanciuc, D.; Garofalo, R.P.; Casola, A. Critical role of Toll-like receptor 4 in human metapneumovirus innate immune responses and disease pathogenesis. *J. Infect. Dis.* **2012**, manuscript in submission.

28. Heil, F.; Hemmi, H.; Hochrein, H.; Ampenberger, F.; Kirschning, C.; Akira, S.; Lipford, G.; Wagner, H.; Bauer, S. Species-specific recognition of single-stranded RNA via toll-like receptor 7 and 8. *Science* **2004**, *303*, 1526–1529.

29. Jurk, M.; Heil, F.; Vollmer, J.; Schetter, C.; Krieg, A.M.; Wagner, H.; Lipford, G.; Bauer, S. Human TLR7 or TLR8 independently confer responsiveness to the antiviral compound R-848. *Nat. Immunol.* **2002**, *3*, 499.

30. Krug, A.; French, A.R.; Barchet, W.; Fischer, J.A.; Dzionek, A.; Pingel, J.T.; Orihuela, M.M.; Akira, S.; Yokoyama, W.M.; Colonna, M. TLR9-dependent recognition of MCMV by IPC and DC generates coordinated cytokine responses that activate antiviral NK cell function. *Immunity* **2004**, *21*, 107–119.

31. Krug, A.; Luker, G.D.; Barchet, W.; Leib, D.A.; Akira, S.; Colonna, M. Herpes simplex virus type 1 activates murine natural interferon-producing cells through toll-like receptor 9. *Blood* **2004**, *103*, 1433–1437.

32. Goutagny, N.; Jiang, Z.; Tian, J.; Parroche, P.; Schickli, J.; Monks, B.G.; Ulbrandt, N.; Ji, H.; Kiener, P.A.; Coyle, A.J.; *et al*. Cell type-specific recognition of human metapneumoviruses (HMPVs) by retinoic acid-inducible gene I (RIG-I) and TLR7 and viral interference of RIG-I ligand recognition by HMPV-B1 phosphoprotein. *J. Immunol.* **2010**, *184*, 1168–1179.

33. Davidson, S.; Kaiko, G.; Loh, Z.; Lalwani, A.; Zhang, V.; Spann, K.; Foo, S.Y.; Hansbro, N.; Uematsu, S.; Akira, S.; *et al*. Plasmacytoid dendritic cells promote host defense against acute pneumovirus infection via the TLR7-MyD88-dependent signaling pathway. *J. Immunol.* **2011**, *186*, 5938–5948.

34. Akira, S.; Uematsu, S.; Takeuchi, O. Pathogen recognition and innate immunity. *Cell* **2006**, *124*, 783–801.

35. Yamamoto, M.; Sato, S.; Hemmi, H.; Hoshino, K.; Kaisho, T.; Sanjo, H.; Takeuchi, O.; Sugiyama, M.; Okabe, M.; Takeda, K.; *et al*. Role of adaptor TRIF in the MyD88-independent toll-like receptor signaling pathway. *Science* **2003**, *301*, 640–643.

36. Andrejeva, J.; Childs, K.S.; Young, D.F.; Carlos, T.S.; Stock, N.; Goodbourn, S.; Randall, R.E. The V proteins of paramyxoviruses bind the IFN-inducible RNA helicase, mda-5, and inhibit its activation of the IFN-beta promoter. *Proc. Natl. Acad. Sci. USA* **2004**, *101*, 17264–17269.

37. Breiman, A.; Grandvaux, N.; Lin, R.; Ottone, C.; Akira, S.; Yoneyama, M.; Fujita, T.; Hiscott, J.; Meurs, E.F. Inhibition of RIG-I-dependent signaling to the interferon pathway during hepatitis C virus expression and restoration of signaling by IKKepsilon. *J. Virol.* **2005**, *79*, 3969–3978.

38. tenOever, B.R.; Sharma, S.; Zou, W.; Sun, Q.; Grandvaux, N.; Julkunen, I.; Hemmi, H.; Yamamoto, M.; Akira, S.; Yeh, W.C.; *et al*. Activation of TBK1 and IKKvarepsilon kinases by vesicular stomatitis virus infection and the role of viral ribonucleoprotein in the development of interferon antiviral immunity. *J. Virol.* **2004**, *78*, 10636–10649.

39. Siren, J.; Imaizumi, T.; Sarkar, D.; Pietila, T.; Noah, D.L.; Lin, R.; Hiscott, J.; Krug, R.M.; Fisher, P.B.; Julkunen, I.; *et al*. Retinoic acid inducible gene-I and mda-5 are involved in influenza A virus-induced expression of antiviral cytokines. *Microbes Infect.* **2006**, *8*, 2013–2020.

40. Pichlmair, A.; Schulz, O.; Tan, C.P.; Naslund, T.I.; Liljestrom, P.; Weber, F.; Reis e Sousa, C. RIG-I-mediated antiviral responses to single-stranded RNA bearing 5'-phosphates. *Science* **2006**, *314*, 997–1001.

41. Hiscott, J.; Lin, R.; Nakhaei, P.; Paz, S. MasterCARD: A priceless link to innate immunity. *Trends Mol. Med.* **2006**, *12*, 53–56.

42. Johnson, C.L.; Gale, M., Jr. CARD games between virus and host get a new player. *Trends Immunol.* **2006**, *27*, 1–4.

43. Kawai, T.; Takahashi, K.; Sato, S.; Coban, C.; Kumar, H.; Kato, H.; Ishii, K.J.; Takeuchi, O.; Akira, S. IPS-1, an adaptor triggering RIG-I- and Mda5-mediated type I interferon induction. *Nat. Immunol.* **2005**, *6*, 981–988.

44. Meylan, E.; Tschopp, J. Toll-like receptors and RNA helicases: Two parallel ways to trigger antiviral responses. *Mol. Cell* **2006**, *22*, 561–569.

45. Liu, Y.J.; Kanzler, H.; Soumelis, V.; Gilliet, M. Dendritic cell lineage, plasticity and cross-regulation. *Nat. Immunol.* **2001**, *2*, 585–589.

46. Rinaldo, C.R., Jr.; Piazza, P. Virus infection of dendritic cells: Portal for host invasion and host defense. *Trends Microbiol.* **2004**, *12*, 337–345.

47. Stumbles, P.A.; Upham, J.W.; Holt, P.G. Airway dendritic cells: Co-ordinators of immunological homeostasis and immunity in the respiratory tract. *APMIS* **2003**, *111*, 741–755.

48. Rescigno, M.; Borrow, P. The host-pathogen interaction: New themes from dendritic cell biology. *Cell* **2001**, *106*, 267–270.

49. Tan, M.C.; Battini, L.; Tuyama, A.C.; Macip, S.; Melendi, G.A.; Horga, M.A.; Gusella, G.L. Characterization of human metapneumovirus infection of myeloid dendritic cells. *Virology* **2007**, *357*, 1–9.

50. Le, N.C.; Munir, S.; Losq, S.; Winter, C.C.; McCarty, T.; Stephany, D.A.; Holmes, K.L.; Bukreyev, A.; Rabin, R.L.; Collins, P.L.; *et al.* Infection and maturation of monocyte-derived human dendritic cells by human respiratory syncytial virus, human metapneumovirus, and human parainfluenza virus type 3. *Virology* **2009**, *385*, 169–182.

51. Guerrero-Plata, A.; Baron, S.; Poast, J.S.; Adegboyega, P.A.; Casola, A.; Garofalo, R.P. Activity and regulation of alpha interferon in respiratory syncytial virus and human metapneumovirus experimental infections. *J. Virol.* **2005**, *79*, 10190–10199.

52. Horvath, C.M. Silencing STATs: Lessons from paramyxovirus interferon evasion. *Cytokine Growth Factor Rev.* **2004**, *15*, 117–127.

53. Horvath, C.M. Weapons of STAT destruction. Interferon evasion by paramyxovirus V protein. *Eur. J. Biochem.* **2004**, *271*, 4621–4628.

54. Bao, X.; Liu, T.; Spetch, L.; Kolli, D.; Garofalo, R.P.; Casola, A. Airway epithelial cell response to human metapneumovirus infection. *Virology* **2007**, *368*, 91–101.

55. Colamonici, O.R.; Uyttendaele, H.; Domanski, P.; Yan, H.; Krolewski, J.J. p135tyk2, an interferon-alpha-activated tyrosine kinase, is physically associated with an interferon-alpha receptor. *J. Biol. Chem.* **1994**, *269*, 3518–3522.

56. Colamonici, O.; Yan, H.; Domanski, P.; Handa, R.; Smalley, D.; Mullersman, J.; Witte, M.; Krishnan, K.; Krolewski, J. Direct binding to and tyrosine phosphorylation of the alpha subunit of the type I interferon receptor by p135tyk2 tyrosine kinase. *Mol. Cell Biol.* **1994**, *14*, 8133–8142.

57. Leung, S.; Qureshi, S.A.; Kerr, I.M.; Darnell, J.E., Jr.; Stark, G.R. Role of STAT2 in the alpha interferon signaling pathway. *Mol. Cell Biol.* **1995**, *15*, 1312–1317.

58. Qureshi, S.A.; Salditt-Georgieff, M.; Darnell, J.E., Jr. Tyrosine-phosphorylated Stat1 and Stat2 plus a 48-kDa protein all contact DNA in forming interferon-stimulated-gene factor 3. *Proc. Natl. Acad. Sci. USA* **1995**, *92*, 3829–3833.

59. Uze, G.; Schreiber, G.; Piehler, J.; Pellegrini, S. The receptor of the type I interferon family. *Curr. Top. Microbiol. Immunol.* **2007**, *316*, 71–95.

60. Li, X.; Leung, S.; Burns, C.; Stark, G.R. Cooperative binding of Stat1-2 heterodimers and ISGF3 to tandem DNA elements. *Biochimie* **1998**, *80*, 703–710.

61. Hata, N.; Sato, M.; Takaoka, A.; Asagiri, M.; Tanaka, N.; Taniguchi, T. Constitutive IFN-alpha/beta signal for efficient IFN-alpha/beta gene induction by virus. *Biochem. Biophys. Res. Commun.* **2001**, *285*, 518–525.

62. Trinchieri, G. Type I interferon: Friend or foe? *J. Exp. Med.* **2010**, *207*, 2053–2063.

63. Hervas-Stubbs, S.; Perez-Gracia, J.L.; Rouzaut, A.; Sanmamed, M.F.; Le, B.A.; Melero, I. Direct effects of type I interferons on cells of the immune system. *Clin. Cancer Res.* **2011**, *17*, 2619–2627.

64. Christophi, G.P.; Hudson, C.A.; Panos, M.; Gruber, R.C.; Massa, P.T. Modulation of macrophage infiltration and inflammatory activity by the phosphatase SHP-1 in virus-induced demyelinating disease. *J. Virol.* **2009**, *83*, 522–539.

65. Yasukawa, H.; Misawa, H.; Sakamoto, H.; Masuhara, M.; Sasaki, A.; Wakioka, T.; Ohtsuka, S.; Imaizumi, T.; Matsuda, T.; Ihle, J.N.; *et al.* The JAK-binding protein JAB inhibits Janus tyrosine kinase activity through binding in the activation loop. *EMBO J.* **1999**, *18*, 1309–1320.

66. Ramaswamy, M.; Shi, L.; Monick, M.M.; Hunninghake, G.W.; Look, D.C. Specific inhibition of type I interferon signal transduction by respiratory syncytial virus. *Am. J. Respir. Cell Mol. Biol.* **2004**, *30*, 893–900.

67. Didcock, L.; Young, D.F.; Goodbourn, S.; Randall, R.E. The V protein of simian virus 5 inhibits interferon signalling by targeting STAT1 for proteasome-mediated degradation. *J. Virol.* **1999**, *73*, 9928–9933.

68. Kubota, T.; Yokosawa, N.; Yokota, S.; Fujii, N. C terminal CYS-RICH region of mumps virus structural V protein correlates with block of interferon alpha and gamma signal transduction pathway through decrease of STAT 1-alpha. *Biochem. Biophys. Res. Commun.* **2001**, *283*, 255–259.

69. Rodriguez, J.J.; Cruz, C.D.; Horvath, C.M. Identification of the nuclear export signal and STAT-binding domains of the Nipah virus V protein reveals mechanisms underlying interferon evasion. *J. Virol.* **2004**, *78*, 5358–5367.

70. Rodriguez, J.J.; Parisien, J.P.; Horvath, C.M. Nipah virus V protein evades alpha and gamma interferons by preventing STAT1 and STAT2 activation and nuclear accumulation. *J. Virol.* **2002**, *76*, 11476–11483.

71. Takeuchi, K.; Kadota, S.I.; Takeda, M.; Miyajima, N.; Nagata, K. Measles virus V protein blocks interferon (IFN)-alpha/beta but not IFN-gamma signaling by inhibiting STAT1 and STAT2 phosphorylation. *FEBS Lett.* **2003**, *545*, 177–182.

72. Dinwiddie, D.L.; Harrod, K.S. Human Metapneumovirus Inhibits IFN-{alpha} Signaling Through Inhibition of STAT1 Phosphorylation. *Am. J. Respir. Cell Mol. Biol.* **2008**, *38*, 661–670.

73. Ren, J.; Kolli, D.; Liu, T.; Xu, R.; Garofalo, R.P.; Casola, A.; Bao, X. Human metapneumovirus inhibits IFN-beta signaling by downregulating Jak1 and Tyk2 cellular levels. *PLoS One* **2011**, *6*, e24496.

74. Bao, X.; Kolli, D.; Liu, T.; Shan, Y.; Garofalo, R.P.; Casola, A. Human metapneumovirus small hydrophobic protein inhibits NF-kappaB transcriptional activity. *J. Virol.* **2008**, *82*, 8224–8229.

75. Bao, X.; Liu, T.; Shan, Y.; Li, K.; Garofalo, R.P.; Casola, A. Human metapneumovirus glycoprotein G inhibits innate immune responses. *PLoS. Pathog.* **2008**, *4*, e1000077.

76. Ren, J.; Wang, Q.; Kolli, D.; Prusak, D.J.; Tseng, C.T.; Chen, Z.J.; Li, K.; Wood, T.G.; Bao, X. Human metapneumovirus M2-2 protein inhibits innate cellular signaling by targeting MAVS. *J. Virol.* **2012**, *86*, 13049–13061.

77. Van den Hoogen, B.G.; Bestebroer, T.M.; Osterhaus, A.D.; Fouchier, R.A. Analysis of the genomic sequence of a human metapneumovirus. *Virology* **2002**, *295*, 119–132.

78. Biacchesi, S.; Skiadopoulos, M.H.; Boivin, G.; Hanson, C.T.; Murphy, B.R.; Collins, P.L.; Buchholz, U.J. Genetic diversity between human metapneumovirus subgroups. *Virology* **2003**, *315*, 1–9.

79. Biacchesi, S.; Murphy, B.R.; Collins, P.L.; Buchholz, U.J. Frequent frameshift and point mutations in the SH gene of human metapneumovirus passaged in vitro. *J. Virol.* **2007**, *81*, 6057–6067.

80. Biacchesi, S.; Skiadopoulos, M.H.; Yang, L.; Lamirande, E.W.; Tran, K.C.; Murphy, B.R.; Collins, P.L.; Buchholz, U.J. Recombinant human Metapneumovirus lacking the small hydrophobic SH and/or attachment G glycoprotein: Deletion of G yields a promising vaccine candidate. *J. Virol.* **2004**, *78*, 12877–12887.

81. Biacchesi, S.; Pham, Q.N.; Skiadopoulos, M.H.; Murphy, B.R.; Collins, P.L.; Buchholz, U.J. Infection of nonhuman primates with recombinant human metapneumovirus lacking the SH, G, or M2-2 protein categorizes each as a nonessential accessory protein and identifies vaccine candidates. *J. Virol.* **2005**, *79*, 12608–12613.

82. Wilson, R.L.; Fuentes, S.M.; Wang, P.; Taddeo, E.C.; Klatt, A.; Henderson, A.J.; He, B. Function of small hydrophobic proteins of paramyxovirus. *J. Virol.* **2006**, *80*, 1700–1709.

83. Fuentes, S.; Tran, K.C.; Luthra, P.; Teng, M.N.; He, B. Function of the respiratory syncytial virus small hydrophobic protein. *J. Virol.* **2007**, *81*, 8361–8366.

84. Li, Z.; Xu, J.; Patel, J.; Fuentes, S.; Lin, Y.; Anderson, D.; Sakamoto, K.; Wang, L.F.; He, B. Function of the small hydrophobic protein of J paramyxovirus. *J. Virol.* **2011**, *85*, 32–42.

85. Xu, P.; Li, Z.; Sun, D.; Lin, Y.; Wu, J.; Rota, P.A.; He, B. Rescue of wild-type mumps virus from a strain associated with recent outbreaks helps to define the role of the SH ORF in the pathogenesis of mumps virus. *Virology* **2011**, *417*, 126–136.

86. Karin, M.; Delhase, M. The I kappa B kinase (IKK) and NF-kappa B: Key elements of proinflammatory signalling. *Semin. Immunol.* **2000**, *12*, 85–98.

87. Schmidt, M.; Chiorini, J.A.; Afione, S.; Kotin, R. Adeno-associated virus type 2 Rep78 inhibition of PKA and PRKX: Fine mapping and analysis of mechanism. *J. Virol.* **2002**, *76*, 1033–1042.

88. Schowalter, R.M.; Smith, S.E.; Dutch, R.E. Characterization of human metapneumovirus F protein-promoted membrane fusion: Critical roles for proteolytic processing and low pH. *J. Virol.* **2006**, *80*, 10931–10941.

89. Cox, R.G.; Livesay, S.B.; Johnson, M.; Ohi, M.D.; Williams, J.V. The human metapneumovirus fusion protein mediates entry via an interaction with RGD-binding integrins. *J. Virol.* **2012**, *86*, 12148–12160.

90. Kolli, D.; Bao, X.; Liu, T.; Hong, C.; Wang, T.; Garofalo, R.P.; Casola, A. Human metapneumovirus glycoprotein G inhibits TLR4-dependent signaling in monocyte-derived dendritic cells. *J. Immunol.* **2011**, *187*, 47–54.

91. Bao, X.; Kolli, D.; Ren, J.; Liu, T.; Garofalo, R.P.; Casola, A. Human metapneumovirus glycoprotein G targets RIG-I to inhibit airway epithelial cell responses. *J. Virol.* **2012**, manuscript in submission.

92. Pulendran, B.; Palucka, K.; Banchereau, J. Sensing pathogens and tuning immune responses. *Science* **2001**, *293*, 253–256.

93. Mellman, I.; Steinman, R.M. Dendritic cells: Specialized and regulated antigen processing machines. *Cell* **2001**, *106*, 255–258.

94. Delgado, M.F.; Coviello, S.; Monsalvo, A.C.; Melendi, G.A.; Hernandez, J.Z.; Batalle, J.P.; Diaz, L.; Trento, A.; Chang, H.Y.; Mitzner, W.; *et al.* Lack of antibody affinity maturation due to poor Toll-like receptor stimulation leads to enhanced respiratory syncytial virus disease. *Nat. Med.* **2009**, *15*, 34–41.

95. Polack, F.P.; Irusta, P.M.; Hoffman, S.J.; Schiatti, M.P.; Melendi, G.A.; Delgado, M.F.; Laham, F.R.; Thumar, B.; Hendry, R.M.; Melero, J.A.; *et al.* The cysteine-rich region of respiratory syncytial virus attachment protein inhibits innate immunity elicited by the virus and endotoxin. *Proc. Natl. Acad. Sci. USA* **2005**, *102*, 8996–9001.

96. Arnold, R.; Konig, B.; Werchau, H.; Konig, W. Respiratory syncytial virus deficient in soluble G protein induced an increased proinflammatory response in human lung epithelial cells. *Virology* **2004**, *330*, 384–397.

97. Alff, P.J.; Gavrilovskaya, I.N.; Gorbunova, E.; Endriss, K.; Chong, Y.; Geimonen, E.; Sen, N.; Reich, N.C.; Mackow, E.R. The pathogenic NY-1 hantavirus G1 cytoplasmic tail inhibits RIG-I- and TBK-1-directed interferon responses. *J. Virol.* **2006**, *80*, 9676–9686.

98. Geimonen, E.; LaMonica, R.; Springer, K.; Farooqui, Y.; Gavrilovskaya, I.N.; Mackow, E.R. Hantavirus pulmonary syndrome-associated hantaviruses contain conserved and functional ITAM signaling elements. *J. Virol.* **2003**, *77*, 1638–1643.

99. Buchholz, U.J.; Biacchesi, S.; Pham, Q.N.; Tran, K.C.; Yang, L.; Luongo, C.L.; Skiadopoulos, M.H.; Murphy, B.R.; Collins, P.L. Deletion of M2 gene open reading frames 1 and 2 of human metapneumovirus: Effects on RNA synthesis, attenuation, and immunogenicity. *J. Virol.* **2005**, *79*, 6588–6597.

100. Herfst, S.; de Graaf, M.; Schickli, J.H.; Tang, R.S.; Kaur, J.; Yang, C.F.; Spaete, R.R.; Haller, A.A.; van den Hoogen, B.G.; Osterhaus, A.D.; *et al.* Recovery of human metapneumovirus genetic lineages a and B from cloned cDNA. *J. Virol.* **2004**, *78*, 8264–8270.

101. Sutherland, K.A.; Collins, P.L.; Peeples, M.E. Synergistic effects of gene-end signal mutations and the M2-1 protein on transcription termination by respiratory syncytial virus. *Virology* **2001**, *288*, 295–307.

102. Schickli, J.H.; Kaur, J.; MacPhail, M.; Guzzetta, J.M.; Spaete, R.R.; Tang, R.S. Deletion of human metapneumovirus M2-2 increases mutation frequency and attenuates growth in hamsters. *Virol. J.* **2008**, *3*, 5–69.

103. Ren, J.; Wang, Q.; Kolli, D.; Prusak, D.J.; Tseng, C.T.; Li, K.; Wood, T.G.; Bao, X. Human metapneumovirus M2-2 protein inhibits the innate cellular signaling by targeting MAVS. *J. Virol.* **2012**, *86*, 13049–13061.

104. Guo, Z.; Chen, L.M.; Zeng, H.; Gomez, J.A.; Plowden, J.; Fujita, T.; Katz, J.M.; Donis, R.O.; Sambhara, S. NS1 protein of influenza A virus inhibits the function of intracytoplasmic pathogen sensor, RIG-I. *Am. J. Respir. Cell Mol. Biol.* **2007**, *36*, 263–269.

105. Opitz, B.; Rejaibi, A.; Dauber, B.; Eckhard, J.; Vinzing, M.; Schmeck, B.; Hippenstiel, S.; Suttorp, N.; Wolff, T. IFNbeta induction by influenza A virus is mediated by RIG-I which is regulated by the viral NS1 protein. *Cell Microbiol.* **2007**, *9*, 930–938.

106. Varga, Z.T.; Ramos, I.; Hai, R.; Schmolke, M.; Garcia-Sastre, A.; Fernandez-Sesma, A.; Palese, P. The influenza virus protein PB1-F2 inhibits the induction of type I interferon at the level of the MAVS adaptor protein. *PLoS. Pathog.* **2011**, *7*, e1002067.

107. Graef, K.M.; Vreede, F.T.; Lau, Y.F.; McCall, A.W.; Carr, S.M.; Subbarao, K.; Fodor, E. The PB2 subunit of the influenza virus RNA polymerase affects virulence by interacting with the mitochondrial antiviral signaling protein and inhibiting expression of beta interferon. *J. Virol.* **2010**, *84*, 8433–8445.

108. Ling, Z.; Tran, K.C.; Teng, M.N. Human respiratory syncytial virus nonstructural protein NS2 antagonizes the activation of beta interferon transcription by interacting with RIG-I. *J. Virol.* **2009**, *83*, 3734–3742.

109. Ren, J.; Liu, T.; Pang, L.; Li, K.; Garofalo, R.G.; Casola, A.; Bao, X. A novel mechanism for inhibition of IRF-3-dependent gene expression by human respiratory syncytial virus NS1 protein. *J. Gen. Virol.* **2011**, *92*, 2153–2159.

110. Bastien, N.; Normand, S.; Taylor, T.; Ward, D.; Peret, T.C.; Boivin, G.; Anderson, L.J.; Li, Y. Sequence analysis of the N, P, M and F genes of Canadian human metapneumovirus strains. *Virus Res.* **2003**, *93*, 51–62.

111. Tedcastle, A.B.; Fenwick, F.; Ingram, R.E.; King, B.J.; Robinson, M.J.; Toms, G.L. The characterization of monoclonal antibodies to human metapneumovirus and the detection of multiple forms of the virus nucleoprotein and phosphoprotein. *J. Med. Virolog.* **2012**, *84*, 1061–1070.

112. Derdowski, A.; Peters, T.R.; Glover, N.; Qian, R.; Utley, T.J.; Burnett, A.; Williams, J.V.; Spearman, P.; Crowe, J.E., Jr. Human metapneumovirus nucleoprotein and phosphoprotein interact and provide the minimal requirements for inclusion body formation. *J. Gen. Virol.* **2008**, *89*, 2698–2708.

8

RSV Fusion: Time for a New Model

Peter Mastrangelo and Richard G. Hegele *

Department of Laboratory Medicine and Pathobiology, University of Toronto, Toronto, ON M5S 1A8, Canada; E-Mail: peter.mastrangelo@utoronto.ca

* Author to whom correspondence should be addressed; E-Mail: richard.hegele@utoronto.ca

Abstract: In this review we propose a partially hypothetical model of respiratory syncytial virus (RSV) binding and entry to the cell that includes the recently discovered RSV receptor nucleolin, in an attempt to stimulate further inquiry in this research area. RSV binding and entry is likely to be a two-step process, the first involving the attachment of the virus to the cell membrane, which may be enhanced by electrostatic interactions with cellular glycoproteins/heparin and the viral G protein, and the second involving fusion to the cell membrane mediated by the viral F protein and a specific cellular fusion receptor. With our recent discovery of nucleolin as a functional fusion receptor for RSV, comes the possibility of a number of new approaches to the development of novel strategies for RSV prophylaxis and therapy, as well as raising some new questions concerning the pathobiology of RSV infection and tropism.

Keywords: RSV; nucleolin; receptor

1. Introduction

Human respiratory syncytial virus (RSV) is found ubiquitously and a major cause of acute lower respiratory tract infections in children leading to hospitalization and occasionally death [1]. RSV also causes disease in adults, particularly in the elderly and in the immunocompromised [2]. Treatment and prophylaxis, given primarily to infants, are limited to Ribavirin and Palivizumab, respectively [2]. RSV is a negative-polarity, enveloped, single-stranded RNA virus from the Paramyxoviridae family.

The viral genome encodes 11 proteins, three of which, small hydrophobic (SH), glycoprotein (G) and fusion (F) contribute to the viral coat. In spite of the fact that the virus was discovered in 1956, a safe, effective vaccine for RSV has remained elusive [3].

In this article we discuss aspects related to the discovery of nucleolin as a functional fusion receptor for RSV and propose a revised model for RSV fusion at the cell surface that incorporates nucleolin. Also, we discuss the implications this discovery has on the pathobiology of RSV infections and the development of novel prophylactic and therapeutic strategies.

2. Viral Envelope Proteins and Fusion

In order to understand attachment and fusion/entry into cells it is crucial to determine which viral envelope protein(s) are involved and what are their corresponding cellular ligands. The RSV G protein is a heterogeneous glycoprotein that defines the two subtypes of RSV (A and B). Besides its role in attachment of virus to the cell surface, the RSV G protein also helps the virus to elude the host immune system by mimicking cellular cytokines and through shedding [4]. Fusion of the virus to the cell membrane as well as the formation of syncytia, the characteristic cytopathic effect of RSV, is mediated by the viral F protein. The F protein unlike the G protein is homologous to both subtypes of RSV. SH, the remaining viral envelope protein, is not required for RSV attachment or entry [5].

As will be discussed in further detail below, we propose that RSV binding and entry into cells is likely to be at least a two-step process: first, attachment of the virus to the cell membrane mediated by electrostatic interactions with cellular glycoproteins/heparin and the viral G protein, and secondly, fusion to the cell membrane mediated by the viral F protein and a specific cellular fusion receptor.

3. Defining a Functional RSV Receptor

Molecules proposed to be the "RSV receptor" include intercellular adhesion molecule (ICAM)-1 [6], heparin [7], annexin II [8], toll-like receptor (TLR) 4 [9] and fractalkine (CX3CL1) receptor, CX3CR1 [10]. Prior to the discovery of nucleolin as a functional receptor of RSV, no candidate receptor molecule met all of the following criteria of being a functional receptor, including: (i) decreased infection through antibody neutralization, competition with soluble candidate receptor molecule or decreased receptor expression through RNA interference; (ii) increased infection of non-permissive cells after ectopic expression of the candidate receptor molecule on the cell surface [11]. Despite a lack of definitive validation of these various candidate receptor molecules by all of the above criteria to date, one or more of them could function as co-receptors or co-factors for RSV and nucleolin.

Binding of viral G protein in an electrostatic fashion to the cell surface may be the first step in efficient viral attachment prior to fusion via nucleolin. Heparin, for example, binds the RSV G protein [7] on HEp-2 cells, however it turns out that human airway epithelium does not express heparin on the apical surface, the site of RSV attachment and cellular entry [12]. Thus the binding to heparin by the G protein may simply serve to demonstrate that the G protein has a general affinity for negatively charged carbohydrates on the cell surface. Further, mutant forms of RSV that lack the G protein (RSVΔG) are capable of causing productive infections, albeit at much lower efficiency than wild-type RSV [13].

The RSV F protein is necessary for infection, as mutant RSV lacking F protein (RSVΔF) cannot infect cells on its own but rather requires a helper virus to gain entry into cells [14]. In contrast to RSV G, the F protein has a list of much more specific protein interactions. One example of such a protein interaction is RSV-F protein with intercellular adhesion molecule (ICAM)-1 expressed on the cell surface. Although it has not been definitively shown to be essential for viral fusion, ICAM-1 has been reported to bind the F protein and may as such still have a role in fusion [6]. Importantly, despite the apparently greater specificity of RSV F-protein interactions *vs.* RSV G, one must exercise caution over RSV F-protein interactions, as Toll-like receptor (TLR) 4 binds the purified RSV F protein, yet has no effect on viral infectivity in cell culture [9].

4. Nucleolin: A Functional Fusion Receptor of RSV [15]

4.1. Identifying Nucleolin as a Ligand of Intact RSV

To search for candidate RSV receptor molecules, we performed a number of preliminary experiments in which cell cultures from numerous mammalian species were treated with enzymes of cell surface components (protein, lipid, carbohydrate) and effects of enzyme pre-treatment on subsequent RSV infection were quantified. Results showed that pre-treatment of cells with trypsin, a protease, resulted in lower RSV infection than occurred in cells that did not undergo enzyme treatment, without affecting cell viability. These findings provided the rationale to use a Virus Overlay Protein Binding Assay (VOPBA) to identify candidate RSV receptor molecules [16]. VOPBA is essentially a modified Western blot where the virus substitutes for the primary antibody and is then detected with a virus-specific secondary. In protein extracts from various mammalian cell lines and numerous RSV isolates (including both laboratory-adapted and community strains of RSV A and RSV B), we reproducibly identified a VOPBA signal of approximately 100 kDa. As one would expect, a number of "hits" were obtained by mass spectrometry of this 100 kDa band, but nucleolin was the most consistent, being found in every extract and viral isolate tested, and it also satisfied the requirement of being found at the cell surface [17,18]. As noted above, RSV F and G are the envelope proteins primarily involved in cell surface binding. To determine if nucleolin binds to RSV F or G, immunoprecipitations (IPs) were performed. Nucleolin co-precipitated only with the viral F protein in every instance tested. Addition of excess heparin to the IPs did not interfere with the nucleolin-protein F interactions in IPs although we also saw, as have others, a decrease in RSV infection *in vitro* [13].

The biological plausibility of RSV-nucleolin interaction in infection was confirmed *in vitro* and *in vivo* through a series of experiments that included: visualization of RSV-nucleolin co-localization on the cell surface by use of confocal fluorescence microscopy; decreased RSV infection of cells pre-treated with nucleolin-specific antibody and when cellular nucleolin expression was silenced by use of RNA interference, or when virus was incubated with soluble recombinant nucleolin prior to being added to cell cultures; increased RSV infection of a non-permissive cell type (Sf9) [36] that had been transfected with the human nucleolin gene and which showed ectopic expression of human nucleolin protein on the cell surface; decreased RSV infection of mouse lung, in animals that were pre-treated with short-interfering RNA of mouse nucleolin, delivered intranasally prior to RSV challenge.

4.2. Nucleolin: Brief Overview

First described in 1973, nucleolin is a multifunction protein that is found throughout the cell but it is primarily localized within the nucleolus, contributing up to 10% of the total protein in that compartment [19,20]. Although its predicted molecular weight is 77–78 kDa (depending on the species), its relative molecular mobility in SDS-PAGE is 100–110 kDa [21], due to highly phosphorylated amino acids of the N-terminus [22]. Nucleolin has been shown to be more stable in proliferating cells due to inhibition of an auto-proteolytic activity more prominently found in quiescent cells [23]. Nucleolin is involved in diverse biological processes including cell proliferation, growth, cytokinesis, replication, embryogenesis and nucleogenesis and is considered necessary for cell survival and proliferation [24].

Nucleolin has a very high degree of evolutionary conservation [25] and can be divided into three structural/functional domains: (i) multiple acidic stretches in the N-terminus; (ii) multiple RNA recognition motifs (RRMs) in the central portion and (iii) a glycine/arginine rich domain in the C-terminal portion [21]. Although nucleolin is typically thought of first and foremost as an intranuclear protein [25], there is abundant evidence that it can also be found within the cytoplasm and on the cell surface and may play the role of a "molecular shuttle" between these compartments [24,26]. Nucleolin has a bipartite nuclear localization signal whose function is regulated by phosphorylation [27]. The actin cytoskeleton modulates the entry of substances via nucleolin into the cytoplasm [28]. The half-life of cell surface nucleolin is less than one hour and its expression is very sensitive to inhibition of transcription/translation, unlike nuclear nucleolin that has a half-life greater than eight hours [26].

In contrast to other cell surface proteins, nucleolin does not have a transmembrane domain or a glycosylphosphatidyl-inositol (GPI) anchor [26]; instead, nucleolin exists on the cell surface as part of a 500 kDa protein complex that includes other membrane proteins [29]. Nucleolin functions as a receptor for a number of different molecules including DNA nanoparticles [30], apoB/E-containing lipoproteins, laminin-1, viruses (see below) [24] and bacteria [31,32].

Nucleolin also plays a role in viral replication and intracellular trafficking of viral components. For example nucleolin is required for HSV-1 DNA replication [33] and also for trafficking of the viral protein US11 out of the nucleus [34]. It also has been shown to bind the RNA-dependent RNA polymerase of HCV (NS5B) [35]. In HCMV nucleolin helps to maintain the architecture of viral replication compartments [36]. Similarly, nucleolin has been shown to bind the 3' untranslated regions and protease-polymerase NS6/7 of feline calicivirus again having a role in viral replication [37]. That these roles in viral replication and trafficking are connected to nucleolin's role as a viral receptor has yet to be determined.

5. A New Model for RSV Fusion/Entry

In light of our findings of expression of cell surface nucleolin being sufficient for RSV infection, a revised model for RSV fusion can be generated. The present models for RSV fusion are in part inferred by analogy to data obtained for other enveloped viruses, particularly influenza virus [38,39]. The RSV F protein initially exists in a pre-fusion state that then undergoes conformational changes to a post-fusion form upon binding to receptor molecules expressed on the cell surface [31]. Current models reflect the fact that comparatively little is known about receptors or other factors involved in RSV fusion, and what triggers the conformational changes in the RSV F protein required for fusion. What seems evident from the results of our experiments is that nucleolin can allow this event to occur. We propose a model were nucleolin binds the pre-fusion conformation of the F protein possibly priming transition to the "extended" intermediate conformation [39]. Evidence that it is the pre-fusion form of RSV F that binds nucleolin is provided by results of our VOPBA experiments, in which live virus was shown to specifically bind nucleolin immobilized on a membrane in the absence of any cells [13]. It follows that this interaction would be with the pre-fusion conformation of the F protein, as "triggering" has not yet occurred. Furthermore, in so-called "competition" experiments in which RSV was incubated with soluble, recombinant nucleolin prior to being added to cell cultures, this state involved exogenous nucleolin saturating F protein binding sites in a pre-fusion state, since there were no cells present during this incubation step.

In our proposed model (Figure 1A), RSV binds cell surface nucleolin via the trimeric pre-fusion form of the F protein. Nucleolin is shown as part of a protein complex which includes either membrane proteins or glycosylphosphatidylinositol (GPI)-linked proteins that tether it to the cell surface. We postulate this binding event triggers the re-folding of the F protein into its extended conformation and once this has occurred, fusion can continue without further need of nucleolin. In this model as many as three molecules of nucleolin can bind one RSV F protein pre-fusion trimer. Refolding of the fusion protein from a pre-fusion to post-fusion conformation is irreversible making the temporal and spatial triggering of this event critical [38]. A fusion receptor like nucleolin helps to ensure that the optimal conditions for viral fusion are met.

Cell surface nucleolin has been found in association with lipid-rich rafts upon anchorage of HIV to permissive cells [40] and efficient RSV infection of human lung epithelial cells requires intact lipid-rich rafts [41]. Nucleolin-mediated trafficking of DNA nanoparticles is lipid raft dependent and nucleolin colocalizes with and co-immunoprecipitates with the raft protein, flotillin [42]. Thus nucleolin may serve to bring RSV in contact to raft domains that may themselves be preferred areas for virus fusion. Alternatively, RSV may be brought into the cell via caveolae or endosomes and triggering/fusion might occur in one of these intracellular compartments. Uptake of virus by bovine dendritic cells has been shown to involve caveolae and RSV colocalizes with caveolin in these cells [43]. However, unlike the case of influenza and Semliki forest virus (SFV) [44], RSV F protein does not appear to be triggered by pH change that occurs during the acidification of lysosomes [45,46]. Interestingly, it has been reported that the internalization of nucleolin on ligand binding is a calcium-dependent process [26] and it has been known for some years that RSV infection is also a calcium-dependent process [47]. On the other hand, there is a body of evidence that supports the idea of clatherin-mediated endocytosis being necessary for RSV infection [48]. Similarly, there are publications that show that nucleolin is internalized after ligand binding (*i.e.*, endostatin) via a clatherin-mediated pathway [49]. It seems possible that RSV and nucleolin may use both types of endosomal pathways in different circumstances however this still remains to be resolved.

Figure 1. (**A**) Model of RSV F-protein binding nucleolin. On the left, the F-protein is shown in its trimeric pre-fusion conformation. The red circles are putative nucleolin binding sites. Nucleolin is shown in orange as part of a protein complex that includes proteins anchored to the membrane by either a transmembrane domain or a GPI anchor. Only one nucleolin molecule is shown binding the F-protein trimer for clarity but in this model as many as three could bind at once. On the right the F-protein is shown in the "extended" conformation with fusion peptides (yellow) inserted into the cell membrane. After this step virus-cell membrane fusion would proceed without nucleolin. (**B**) Diagram of virus binding to the cell surface. Indicated in light yellow are lipid-rich domains/rafts. The virus is shown in a dark magenta covered with F-protein binding to nucleolin that is preferentially located in lipid-rich rafts or caveolae. A caveola is shown covered with caveolin (dark red). This in turn can enter the cell to form a caveozome and join the endosomal or lysosomal pathway. Our proposed model leaves open the possibilities that viral fusion may occur at the cell surface or in a caveozome/endosome/lysosome. Another possibility (not shown) is that virus enters via clathirin-coated pits (see text).

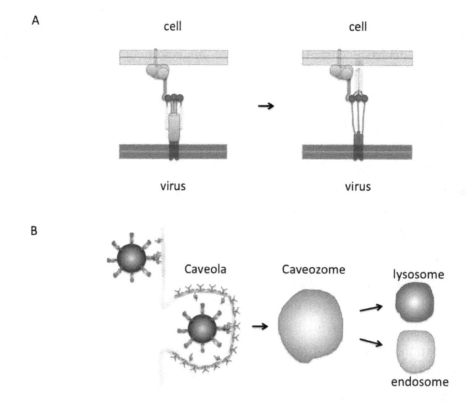

As depicted in Figure 1B, RSV binding to the cell surface is shown incorporating lipid-rich rafts or caveolae. Based on available evidence, including analogies to other pathogens, there exist a number of possibilities by which this can occur and how nucleolin may be involved. For example, nucleolin may either be located within lipid rafts or may become associated with these rafts after binding to the virus. Moreover, lipid raft formation may even be induced by the aggregation of nucleolin around the viral fusion protein. At this point either fusion occurs immediately or the virus is brought into the cell possibly via a caveosome and fusion is triggered later on. Overall, the model we show here, while incomplete, provides a framework with which these various possibilities can be tested experimentally.

6. Future Directions

6.1. Targeting the Host in RSV Prophylaxis and Therapy?

As has been demonstrated for Palivizumab [50], targeting RSV as a strategy for patient management has limitations, since resistant viral strains can arise through random genetic mutation and selective pressure. An alternative strategy is to target the host rather than the virus, the human genome being much more stable. This is not as radical an idea as it may sound if one considers that when immunizing a patient against infection the goal is "conversion" of the host to a virus-resistant state –in effect the host, not the virus, is being targeted. The challenge is to achieve an adequate anti-viral state in the host, and to avoid undesired off-target effects or other toxicity.

6.2. Nucleolin as an Anti-RSV Target

Nucleolin has a rapid half-life on the cell surface: exposure of cells to nucleolin-specific antibody results in rapid internalization of the nucleolin-antibody complex and replacement with "fresh" nucleolin [51]. The rapid turnover of the cell surface nucleolin may be advantageous in the context of designing RSV prophylaxis and/or therapy since it is unlikely there would be any long-lasting disruption of its normal functions. Targeting cell surface nucleolin with the guanine-rich oligonucleotide (GRO), AS1411 [52], is being evaluated in the therapy a variety of cancers in human clinical trials. Other nucleolin-binding compounds (e.g., midkine, pleiotropin, lactoferrin, pseudopeptide HB-19) have been described and in some cases, their safety profiles have already been established in humans. An important practical consideration is that, in contrast to use in chronic diseases such as cancer, nucleolin-binding compounds used for either prophylaxis or therapy of RSV infections (e.g., as a nasal spray formulation) would be administered for relatively short intervals and thus could avoid the development of some of the undesired drug-related effects associated with longer term use.

6.3. RSV-Nucleolin Interaction Domain(s)

Detailed inspection of the primary amino acid sequence of nucleolin does not provide any apparent clues about potential interaction domain(s) with RSV, although one might reasonably exclude the RRMs found in the central portion because these domains are known to be nucleic acid binding motifs [21]. While binding cell surface nucleolin with a specific compound that targets nucleolin and causing it to internalize may be sufficient to make it unavailable for binding to virus, determining the interaction domains of nucleolin and the RSV F protein will be essential for the rational design of small molecule inhibitors. Also, if cell surface nucleolin is part of a larger protein complex [29] that functions to tether it to the cell surface, one could potentially target the other proteins in this complex in order to destabilize it.

One potential site of RSV-F protein interaction with nucleolin may occur with the "head" around amino acids 429–437. This region of the protein binds mAb 19 and mAb 20, both monoclonal antibodies known to inhibit RSV fusion [53–55]. However, such associations based on antibody binding epitopes need to be interpreted cautiously as interference via an antibody may only require that it bind near enough to the interaction domain to be effective at neutralization.

Figure 2. Human airway epithelial cells from bronchial brushings stained with a rabbit polyclonal antibody against human nucleolin (H-250, Santa Cruz Biotechnology Inc., Santa Cruz, CA, USA). Note the positive nucleolin immunostaining (dark brown) at the apical surface of airway epithelial cells (arrows).

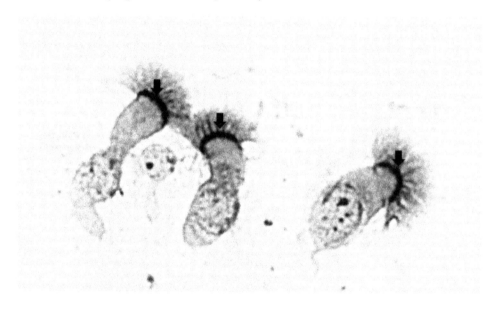

6.4. Nucleolin and RSV Tropism

Because nucleolin is an essential protein found in all cells, it does not by itself account for the apparent restricted tropism of RSV to the respiratory tract and while it is clearly expressed on the cell surface of airway epithelium, the major target for RSV infection, it has not yet been determined if this is the case for other cell types *in vivo* (Figure 2). However, this situation is not unique to RSV, as other viral receptors are widely expressed in various cells and tissues, while tropism is restricted [56]. For example, the cellular receptor of Hepatitis A virus, HAVcr-1, is expressed in various cells within the gastrointestinal tract, salivary glands, kidney, spleen and lymph nodes, yet clinically the virus shows marked tropism to the liver [57]. We speculate that the tropism of RSV for the respiratory tract could involve a combination of the local environment/context and possibly the involvement of more than one receptor/co-receptor, including other molecules postulated to be RSV receptors indicated above. In this context, the viral G protein may be an important determinant of RSV's tropism to the respiratory tract, in terms of the role of RSV G in initial attachment and enabling the virus to recognize nucleolin expressed on the cell surface. Given that the efficiency of RSV infection is markedly decreased in RSVΔG compared to wild-type virus, a role for RSV G as a determinant of tropism is likely.

7. Concluding Remarks

Our discovery of nucleolin as a functional RSV fusion receptor *in vitro* and *in vivo* increases our understanding of the pathobiology of RSV infections, and presents a number of possibilities for novel interventions, including targeting RSV fusion from a "host" perspective. Although the mechanisms of RSV fusion require further study, we present a model of RSV fusion that has a number of testable assumptions and could lead to a deeper understanding of the events underlying RSV fusion and entry into cells.

References

1.   Nair, H.; Nokes, D.J.; Gessner, B.D.; Dherani, M.; Madhi, S.A.; Singleton, R.J.; O'Brien, K.L.; Roca, A.; Wright, P.F.; Bruce, N.; *et al.* Global burden of acute lower respiratory infections due to respiratory syncytial virus in young children: A systematic review and meta-analysis. *Lancet* **2010**, *375*, 1545–1555.

2.   Walsh, E.E. Respiratory syncytial virus infection in adults. *Semin. Respir. Crit. Care Med.* **2011**, *32*, 423–432.

3.   Blount, R.E., Jr.; Morris, J.A.; Savage, R.E. Recovery of cytopathogenic agent from chimpanzees with coryza. *Proc. Soc. Exp. Biol. Med.* **1956**, *92*, 544–549.

4.   Collins, P.L.; Melero, J.A. Progress in understanding and controlling respiratory syncytial virus: Still crazy after all these years. *Virus Res.* **2011**, *162*, 80–99.

5.   Techaarpornkul, S.; Barretto, N.; Peeples, M.E. Functional analysis of recombinant respiratory syncytial virus deletion mutants lacking the small hydrophobic and/or attachment glycoprotein gene. *J. Virol.* **2001**, *75*, 6825–6834.

6.   Behera, A.K.; Matsuse, H.; Kumar, M.; Kong, X.; Lockey, R.F.; Mohapatra, S.S. Blocking intercellular adhesion molecule-1 on human epithelial cells decreases respiratory syncytial virus infection. *Biochem. Biophys. Res. Commun.* **2001**, *280*, 188–195.

7.   Krusat, T.; Streckert, H.J. Heparin-dependent attachment of respiratory syncytial virus (RSV) to host cells. *Arch. Virol.* **1997**, *142*, 1247–1254.

8. Malhotra, R.; Ward, M.; Bright, H.; Priest, R.; Foster, M.R.; Hurle, M.; Blair, E.; Bird, M. Isolation and characterisation of potential respiratory syncytial virus receptor(s) on epithelial cells. *Microbes Infect.* **2003**, *5*, 123–133.

9. Marr, N.; Turvey, S.E. Role of human TLR4 in respiratory syncytial virus-induced NF-kappaB activation, viral entry and replication. *Innate Immun.* **2012**, *18*, 856–865.

10. Harcourt, J.; Alvarez, R.; Jones, L.P.; Henderson, C.; Anderson, L.J.; Tripp, R.A. Respiratory syncytial virus G protein and G protein CX3C motif adversely affect CX3CR1+ T cell responses. *J. Immunol.* **2006**, *176*, 1600–1608.

11. Dimmock, N.J.; Easton, A.J.; Leppard, K. *Introduction to Modern Virology*, 6th ed.; Blackwell Pub.: Malden, MA, USA, 2007; p. 516.

12. Duan, D.; Yue, Y.; Yan, Z.; McCray, P.B., Jr.; Engelhardt, J.F. Polarity influences the efficiency of recombinant adenoassociated virus infection in differentiated airway epithelia. *Hum. Gene Ther.* **1998**, *9*, 2761–2776.

13. Techaarpornkul, S.; Collins, P.L.; Peeples, M.E. Respiratory syncytial virus with the fusion protein as its only viral glycoprotein is less dependent on cellular glycosaminoglycans for attachment than complete virus. *Virology* **2002**, *294*, 296–304.

14. Batonick, M.; Oomens, A.G.; Wertz, G.W. Human respiratory syncytial virus glycoproteins are not required for apical targeting and release from polarized epithelial cells. *J. Virol.* **2008**, *82*, 8664–8672.

15. Tayyari, F.; Marchant, D.; Moraes, T.J.; Duan, W.; Mastrangelo, P.; Hegele, R.G. Identification of nucleolin as a cellular receptor for human respiratory syncytial virus. *Nat. Med.* **2011**, *17*, 1132–1135.

16. Cao, W.; Henry, M.D.; Borrow, P.; Yamada, H.; Elder, J.H.; Ravkov, E.V.; Nichol, S.T.; Compans, R.W.; Campbell, K.P.; Oldstone, M.B. Identification of alpha-dystroglycan as a receptor for lymphocytic choriomeningitis virus and Lassa fever virus. *Science* **1998**, *282*, 2079–2081.

17. Reyes-Reyes, E.M.; Akiyama, S.K. Cell-surface nucleolin is a signal transducing P-selectin binding protein for human colon carcinoma cells. *Exp. Cell Res.* **2008**, *314*, 2212–2223.

18. Losfeld, M.E.; Khoury, D.E.; Mariot, P.; Carpentier, M.; Krust, B.; Briand, J.P.; Mazurier, J.; Hovanessian, A.G.; Legrand, D. The cell surface expressed nucleolin is a glycoprotein that triggers calcium entry into mammalian cells. *Exp. Cell Res.* **2009**, *315*, 357–369.

19. Orrick, L.R.; Olson, M.O.; Busch, H. Comparison of nucleolar proteins of normal rat liver and Novikoff hepatoma ascites cells by two-dimensional polyacrylamide gel electrophoresis. *Proc. Natl. Acad. Sci. USA* **1973**, *70*, 1316–1320.

20. Bugler, B.; Caizergues-Ferrer, M.; Bouche, G.; Bourbon, H.; Amalric, F. Detection and localization of a class of proteins immunologically related to a 100-kDa nucleolar protein. *Eur. J. Biochem.* **1982**, *128*, 475–480.

21. Ginisty, H.; Sicard, H.; Roger, B.; Bouvet, P. Structure and functions of nucleolin. *J. Cell Sci.* **1999**, *112*, 761–772.

22. Bicknell, K.; Brooks, G.; Kaiser, P.; Chen, H.; Dove, B.K.; Hiscox, J.A. Nucleolin is regulated both at the level of transcription and translation. *Biochem. Biophys. Res. Commun.* **2005**, *332*, 817–822.

23. Chen, C.M.; Chiang, S.Y.; Yeh, N.H. Increased stability of nucleolin in proliferating cells by inhibition of its self-cleaving activity. *J. Biol. Chem.* **1991**, *266*, 7754–7758.

24. Srivastava, M.; Pollard, H.B. Molecular dissection of nucleolin's role in growth and cell proliferation: New insights. *FASEB J.* **1999**, *13*, 1911–1922.

25. Tajrishi, M.M.; Tuteja, R.; Tuteja, N. Nucleolin: The most abundant multifunctional phosphoprotein of nucleolus. *Commun. Integr. Biol.* **2011**, *4*, 267–275.

26. Hovanessian, A.G.; Soundaramourty, C.; El Khoury, D.; Nondier, I.; Svab, J.; Krust, B. Surface expressed nucleolin is constantly induced in tumor cells to mediate calcium-dependent ligand internalization. *PLoS One* **2010**, *5*, e15787.

27. Schwab, M.S.; Dreyer, C. Protein phosphorylation sites regulate the function of the bipartite NLS of nucleolin. *EJCB* **1997**, *73*, 287–297.

28. Hovanessian, A.G.; Puvion-Dutilleul, F.; Nisole, S.; Svab, J.; Perret, E.; Deng, J.S.; Krust, B. The cell-surface-expressed nucleolin is associated with the actin cytoskeleton. *Exp. Cell Res.* **2000**, *261*, 312–328.

29. Krust, B.; El Khoury, D.; Nondier, I.; Soundaramourty, C.; Hovanessian, A.G. Targeting surface nucleolin with multivalent HB-19 and related Nucant pseudopeptides results in distinct inhibitory mechanisms depending on the malignant tumor cell type. *BMC Cancer* **2011**, *11*, 333.

30. Chen, X.; Kube, D.M.; Cooper, M.J.; Davis, P.B. Cell surface nucleolin serves as receptor for DNA nanoparticles composed of pegylated polylysine and DNA. *Mol. Ther.* **2008**, *16*, 333–342.

31. Barel, M.; Hovanessian, A.G.; Meibom, K.; Briand, J.P.; Dupuis, M.; Charbit, A. A novel receptor—ligand pathway for entry of Francisella tularensis in monocyte-like THP-1 cells: Interaction between surface nucleolin and bacterial elongation factor Tu. *BMC Microbiol.* **2008**, *8*, 145.

32. Sinclair, J.F.; Dean-Nystrom, E.A.; O'Brien, A.D. The established intimin receptor Tir and the putative eucaryotic intimin receptors nucleolin and beta1 integrin localize at or near the site of enterohemorrhagic Escherichia coli O157:H7 adherence to enterocytes *in vivo*. *Infect. Immun.* **2006**, *74*, 1255–1265.

33. Calle, A.; Ugrinova, I.; Epstein, A.L.; Bouvet, P.; Diaz, J.J.; Greco, A. Nucleolin is required for an efficient herpes simplex virus type 1 infection. *J. Virol.* **2008**, *82*, 4762–4773.

34. Greco, A.; Arata, L.; Soler, E.; Gaume, X.; Coute, Y.; Hacot, S.; Calle, A.; Monier, K.; Epstein, A.L.; Sanchez, J.C.; *et al.* Nucleolin interacts with US11 protein of herpes simplex virus 1 and is involved in its trafficking. *J. Virol.* **2012**, *86*, 1449–1457.

35. Kusakawa, T.; Shimakami, T.; Kaneko, S.; Yoshioka, K.; Murakami, S. Functional interaction of hepatitis C Virus NS5B with Nucleolin GAR domain. *J. Biochem.* **2007**, *141*, 917–927.

36. Strang, B.L.; Boulant, S.; Kirchhausen, T.; Coen, D.M. Host cell nucleolin is required to maintain the architecture of human cytomegalovirus replication compartments. *mBio* **2012**, *3*, e00301–11.

37. Cancio-Lonches, C.; Yocupicio-Monroy, M.; Sandoval-Jaime, C.; Galvan-Mendoza, I.; Urena, L.; Vashist, S.; Goodfellow, I.; Salas-Benito, J.; Gutierrez-Escolano, A.L. Nucleolin interacts with the feline calicivirus 3' untranslated region and the protease-polymerase NS6 and NS7 proteins, playing a role in virus replication. *J. Virol.* **2011**, *85*, 8056–8068.

38. Chang, A.; Dutch, R.E. Paramyxovirus fusion and entry: Multiple paths to a common end. *Viruses* **2012**, *4*, 613–636.

39. Harrison, S.C. Viral membrane fusion. *Nat. Struct. Mol. Biol.* **2008**, *15*, 690–698.

40. Nisole, S.; Krust, B.; Hovanessian, A.G. Anchorage of HIV on permissive cells leads to coaggregation of viral particles with surface nucleolin at membrane raft microdomains. *Exp. Cell. Res.* **2002**, *276*, 155–173.

41. Chang, T.H.; Segovia, J.; Sabbah, A.; Mgbemena, V.; Bose, S. Cholesterol-rich lipid rafts are required for release of infectious human respiratory syncytial virus particles. *Virology* **2012**, *422*, 205–213.

42. Chen, X.; Shank, S.; Davis, P.B.; Ziady, A.G. Nucleolin-mediated cellular trafficking of DNA nanoparticle is lipid raft and microtubule dependent and can be modulated by glucocorticoid. *Mol. Ther.* **2011**, *19*, 93–102.

43. Werling, D.; Hope, J.C.; Chaplin, P.; Collins, R.A.; Taylor, G.; Howard, C.J. Involvement of caveolae in the uptake of respiratory syncytial virus antigen by dendritic cells. *J. Leukoc. Biol.* **1999**, *66*, 50–58.

44. White, J.M.; Delos, S.E.; Brecher, M.; Schornberg, K. Structures and mechanisms of viral membrane fusion proteins: Multiple variations on a common theme. *Crit. Rev. Biochem. Mol. Biol.* **2008**, *43*, 189–219.

45. Kahn, J.S.; Schnell, M.J.; Buonocore, L.; Rose, J.K. Recombinant vesicular stomatitis virus expressing respiratory syncytial virus (RSV) glycoproteins: RSV fusion protein can mediate infection and cell fusion. *Virology* **1999**, *254*, 81–91.

46. Srinivasakumar, N.; Ogra, P.L.; Flanagan, T.D. Characteristics of fusion of respiratory syncytial virus with HEp-2 cells as measured by R18 fluorescence dequenching assay. *J. Virol.* **1991**, *65*, 4063–4069.

47. Shahrabadi, M.S.; Lee, P.W. Calcium requirement for syncytium formation in HEp-2 cells by respiratory syncytial virus. *J. Clin. Microbiol.* **1988**, *26*, 139–141.

48. Kolokoltsov, A.A.; Deniger, D.; Fleming, E.H.; Roberts, N.J., Jr.; Karpilow, J.M.; Davey, R.A. Small interfering RNA profiling reveals key role of clathrin-mediated endocytosis and early endosome formation for infection by respiratory syncytial virus. *J. Virol.* **2007**, *81*, 7786–7800.

49. Song, N.; Ding, Y.; Zhuo, W.; He, T.; Fu, Z.; Chen, Y.; Song, X.; Fu, Y.; Luo, Y. The nuclear translocation of endostatin is mediated by its receptor nucleolin in endothelial cells. *Angiogenesis* **2012**, *15*, 697–711.

50. Adams, O.; Bonzel, L.; Kovacevic, A.; Mayatepek, E.; Hoehn, T.; Vogel, M. Palivizumab-resistant human respiratory syncytial virus infection in infancy. *Clin. Infect. Dis.* **2010**, *51*, 185–188.

51. Deng, J.S.; Ballou, B.; Hofmeister, J.K. Internalization of anti-nucleolin antibody into viable HEp-2 cells. *Mol. Biol. Rep.* **1996**, *23*, 191–195.

52. Bates, P.J.; Laber, D.A.; Miller, D.M.; Thomas, S.D.; Trent, J.O. Discovery and development of the G-rich oligonucleotide AS1411 as a novel treatment for cancer. *Exp. Mol. Pathol.* **2009**, *86*, 151–164.

53. Taylor, G.; Stott, E.J.; Furze, J.; Ford, J.; Sopp, P. Protective epitopes on the fusion protein of respiratory syncytial virus recognized by murine and bovine monoclonal antibodies. *J. Gen. Virol.* **1992**, *73*, 2217–2223.

54. Arbiza, J.; Taylor, G.; Lopez, J.A.; Furze, J.; Wyld, S.; Whyte, P.; Stott, E.J.; Wertz, G.; Sullender, W.; Trudel, M.; *et al.* Characterization of two antigenic sites recognized by neutralizing monoclonal antibodies directed against the fusion glycoprotein of human respiratory syncytial virus. *J. Gen. Virol.* **1992**, *73*, 2225–2234.

55. McLellan, J.S.; Yang, Y.; Graham, B.S.; Kwong, P.D. Structure of respiratory syncytial virus fusion glycoprotein in the postfusion conformation reveals preservation of neutralizing epitopes. *J. Virol.* **2011**, *85*, 7788–7796.

56. Schneider-Schaulies, J. Cellular receptors for viruses: Links to tropism and pathogenesis. *J. Gen. Virol.* **2000**, *81*, 1413–1429.

57. Asher, L.V.; Binn, L.N.; Mensing, T.L.; Marchwicki, R.H.; Vassell, R.A.; Young, G.D. Pathogenesis of hepatitis A in orally inoculated owl monkeys (Aotus trivirgatus). *J. Med. Virol.* **1995**, *47*, 260–268.

9

Breaking In: Human Metapneumovirus Fusion and Entry

Reagan G. Cox [1] and John V. Williams [2],*

[1] Department of Pathology, Microbiology and Immunology, Vanderbilt University School of Medicine, 1161 21st Ave. S., Nashville, TN 37232, USA; E-Mail: reagan.j.cox@vanderbilt.edu

[2] Departments of Pediatrics and Pathology, Microbiology, and Immunology, Vanderbilt University School of Medicine, 1161 21st Ave. S., Nashville, TN 37232, USA

* Author to whom correspondence should be addressed; E-Mail: john.williams@vanderbilt.edu

Abstract: Human metapneumovirus (HMPV) is a leading cause of respiratory infection that causes upper airway and severe lower respiratory tract infections. HMPV infection is initiated by viral surface glycoproteins that attach to cellular receptors and mediate virus membrane fusion with cellular membranes. Most paramyxoviruses use two viral glycoproteins to facilitate virus entry—an attachment protein and a fusion (F) protein. However, membrane fusion for the human paramyxoviruses in the *Pneumovirus* subfamily, HMPV and respiratory syncytial virus (hRSV), is unique in that the F protein drives fusion in the absence of a separate viral attachment protein. Thus, pneumovirus F proteins can perform the necessary functions for virus entry, *i.e.*, attachment and fusion. In this review, we discuss recent advances in the understanding of how HMPV F mediates both attachment and fusion. We review the requirements for HMPV viral surface glycoproteins during entry and infection, and review the identification of cellular receptors for HMPV F. We also review our current understanding of how HMPV F mediates fusion, concentrating on structural regions of the protein that appear to be critical for membrane fusion activity. Finally, we illuminate key unanswered questions and suggest how further studies can elucidate how this clinically important paramyxovirus fusion protein may have evolved to initiate infection by a unique mechanism.

Keywords: metapneumovirus; fusion protein; paramyxovirus; integrin

1. Introduction

Human metapneumovirus (HMPV) was first isolated in 2001 in the Netherlands [1]. Dutch investigators discovered an unknown virus in respiratory secretions collected from young children with lower respiratory illness. Virus-infected cell supernatants were examined by electron microscopy and found to contain pleomorphic virus particles measuring 150 to 600 nm, with spike-like envelope projections of 13 to 17 nm [2]. PCR and sequence analysis revealed a single-stranded, negative-sense RNA genome with close resemblance to avian metapneumovirus (AMPV), an avian virus that causes serious respiratory disease in chickens and turkeys [3]. Based upon virion morphology and genome organization, HMPV was classified as the first human member of the *Metapneumovirus* genus, in the subfamily *Pneumovirinae* of the paramyxovirus family [1,4].

HMPV is a ubiquitous respiratory pathogen that has been circulating in human populations undetected for decades. The original report detected HMPV-specific antibodies in archived human sera from the 1950s [1] and HMPV has been detected by RT-PCR in specimens from 1976 [5]. Phylogenetic analysis of multiple HMPV gene sequences suggests that HMPV diverged from AMPV between 200–300 years ago [6,7]. HMPV is a leading cause of lower respiratory infection in infants and children worldwide [5,8–18]. HMPV is also associated with severe disease in immunocompromized hosts or persons with underlying conditions [19–25]. HMPV causes a clinical spectrum of illness from upper airway infection to severe lower respiratory tract infections (e.g., bronchiolitis and pneumonia) [5,26]. HMPV pathogenesis is similar to hRSV and causes inflammation, sloughing and necrosis of the bronchiolar epithelium [27]. Experimental studies in nonhuman primates and small animal models (hamsters, cotton rats, and mice) indicate that HMPV replicates in the upper and lower respiratory tract epithelium and demonstrate no evidence of viral dissemination, indicating a distinct tissue tropism for HMPV which is consistent with clinical illness observed during human infection [28–30].

2. HMPV F: A Dual Function Fusion Protein

The HMPV virion is similar to other paramyxoviruses. The viral lipid bilayer is likely derived from the plasma membrane of infected cells during virus egress, as virions are thought to bud from the infected cell surface. The closely related pneumovirus, hRSV forms filaments at and buds from the apical surface of polarized epithelial cells [31,32]. Similar to hRSV [32], the HMPV matrix (M) protein has been shown to assemble into filaments on the surface of HMPV-infected cells [33]. The HMPV M protein lines the inner leaflet of the viral lipid bilayer, and virions contain three integral membrane surface glycoproteins, the fusion (F), glycoprotein (G) and short hydrophobic (SH) proteins (Figure 1). The envelope contains a helical ribonucleoprotein (RNAP) complex consisting of nucleoprotein (N), phosphoprotein (P), matrix 2 protein (M2), large polymerase protein (L), and the single-stranded, negative-sense RNA genome.

Figure 1. Schematic representation of a human metapneumovirus (HMPV) virion.
The fusion (orange), attachment (red), and short hydrophobic (black) glycoproteins are
depicted at the virion surface. The matrix protein (gray ovals) lines the inner leaflet of the
virus membrane. Encapsidated within the viral envelope is the ribonucleoprotein (RNAP)
complex consisting of the helical, genomic RNA wrapped by the nucleoprotein (N), the
viral RNA-dependent, RNA polymerase (L), phosphoprotein (P), and matrix 2 protein (M2).

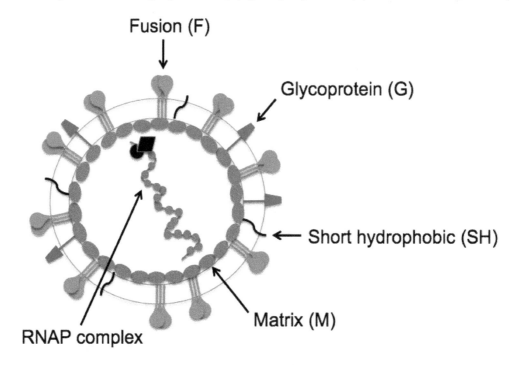

HMPV infection is initiated by viral surface glycoproteins that attach to cellular receptors and
mediate virus membrane fusion with cellular membranes. Most paramyxoviruses use two viral
glycoproteins to facilitate virus entry—an attachment protein, called HN, H or G (depending on
the virus), and a fusion (F) protein. Indeed, elegant studies on paramyxoviruses in the subfamily
Paramyxovirinae have demonstrated that viral attachment and fusion are mediated by two individual
viral proteins that act in concert during virus entry (reviewed in [34]). For the *Paramyxovirinae*, F is
capable of catalyzing membrane fusion only in the presence of the attachment protein. The proposed
model for paramyxovirus entry is a stepwise process where: (1) the attachment protein binds to cellular
receptors; (2) the bound attachment protein directly interacts with and transmits a signal to the F
protein; (3) the F protein becomes activated to undergo structural changes; (4) F refolds from a
prefusion to postfusion structural conformation, resulting in the merging of the viral membrane with
the plasma membrane; and (5) the genome is delivered into the cytoplasm from a fusion pore created
at the cell surface.

However, membrane fusion for paramyxoviruses in the *Pneumovirus* subfamily is unique in that F
drives fusion in the absence of a separate viral attachment protein. The pneumoviruses incorporate
three surface glycoproteins that could potentially facilitate entry: F, SH, and G (termed the attachment
protein based upon homology to other paramyxoviruses). The first indication that pneumovirus

entry may not absolutely depend upon all surface glycoproteins was the identification of a live, cold-passaged hRSV strain (cp-52) that had a large deletion spanning most of the SH and G coding sequences but replicated efficiently in Vero cells [35]. Thus, in the absence of SH and G, hRSV was infectious and capable of replicating to high titer *in vitro*, although cp-52 replication was severely attenuated *in vivo* in both animals and humans [35]. Subsequent studies with hRSV engineered without the SH and G genes have confirmed that hRSV F is sufficient for virus entry in cell culture, but replication is attenuated in animal models of infection [36–42]. The invention of reverse genetics for HMPV has enabled researchers to rescue viruses engineered to express the F protein in the absence of G and/or SH, and define the individual contributions of each protein for virus entry. Deletion of the SH gene from HMPV did not alter viral growth in cell culture or animal models of infection [43,44], confirming that the SH protein does not serve a role in virus entry. HMPV lacking both G and SH replicated efficiently in cell culture [44] and in both the upper and lower respiratory tracts of hamsters after intranasal inoculation [44]. HMPV lacking G (HMPVΔG) infected and was shed from both the upper and lower respiratory tracts of African green monkeys, a permissive nonhuman primate host. However, HMPVΔG replication was attenuated compared to wild type infection (viral titers were reduced six-fold in the upper respiratory tract and 3200-fold in the lower respiratory tract) [43].

The fact that both hRSV and HMPV viruses lacking the G and SH genes are infectious indicates that the F proteins from these pneumoviruses can perform the necessary functions for virus entry, *i.e.*, attachment and fusion. However, the G protein is clearly important for virus fitness *in vivo*. Despite the fact that hRSV and HMPV G proteins share no homology and are very different in size [4], the G proteins are thought to serve similar functions in the pneumovirus lifecycle. Current evidence suggests that pneumovirus G proteins help tether virus particles to the cell surface, and are likely important for strengthening particle adhesion and concentrating virions on the cell surface. Techaarpornkul *et al.* demonstrated that hRSV G is required for optimal virus attachment to the cell surface, but not for virus fusion and entry as the F protein alone is sufficient for efficient virus fusion with cultured cells [39]. HRSV and HMPV G have been shown to bind adhesion molecules on the cell surface such as heparan sulfate or glycosaminoglycans (GAGs) [45–47]. Pretreatment of HMPV with soluble heparin inhibits infection, and recombinant G protein binds to heparin-agarose columns and cells in a GAG-dependent manner [47]. Thus, HMPV G is capable of binding cell surface GAGs and may contribute to virus attachment; however, because G is dispensable for viral entry, it is not absolutely required for the membrane fusion activity of F during the virus entry process.

Thus, HMPV F is necessary and sufficient for membrane fusion and capable of mediating entry without an additional attachment protein, in contrast to the firmly established model for most paramyxoviruses that absolutely require two viral proteins. To be sufficient for virus entry, HMPV F must be able to attach to cellular receptors and this attachment should activate F-mediated membrane fusion. How HMPV F mediates both attachment to cellular receptors and membrane fusion has been the focus of several recent studies and will be the topic of this review.

3. HMPV F: The Key to Intrusion

All paramyxovirus F proteins are class I fusion proteins that due to the conservation of structural domains are thought to mediate fusion via the same global mechanism (reviewed in [48]). HMPV F is a trimeric, type I membrane glycoprotein. A schematic of the HMPV F protein structure is shown in Figure 2. Each F monomer is translated as an inactive precursor, F0, which is proteolytically cleaved at a monobasic consensus site by host cell proteases into two disulfide-linked subunits, F1 and F2. This cleavage reveals a hydrophobic fusion peptide (FP) at the N-terminus of the larger F1 subunit, which inserts into target cell membranes to initiate membrane fusion. Two heptad repeat (HR) regions are located in the F1 subunit; HRA is adjacent to the FP and HRB is adjacent to the transmembrane (TM) domain. During fusion a metastable, prefusion conformation of F refolds into a highly stable postfusion conformation. During the prefusion-to-postfusion transition, the HRA and HRB form trimeric coiled-coils that rearrange to fold into a highly stable six-helix bundle that drives the formation of a fusion pore between the virus and cell membranes. Formation of the six-helix bundle is essentially irreversible and is directly linked to membrane merging, as peptides mimicking the heptad repeats are capable of blocking membrane fusion [49–51].

Figure 2. Schematic representation of the cleaved HMPV fusion protein. The mature, proteolytically cleaved HMPV F protein contains 522 amino acids (without signal sequence), with 82 residues in the F2 subunit and 440 residues in the F1 subunit, which includes a large extracellular domain, an ~23-amino acid transmembrane domain and a cytoplasmic tail of 25 residues. FP = fusion peptide; HRA = heptad repeat A; HRB = heptad repeat B; TM = transmembrane domain; CT = cytoplasmic tail. The approximate location of a conserved RGD motif (residues 329–331) is indicated as a magenta box. Arrows indicate the three N-linked glycosylation sites. The location of two disulfide bonds that connect the F1 and F2 protein subunits are shown. (Scale bar, amino acids.)

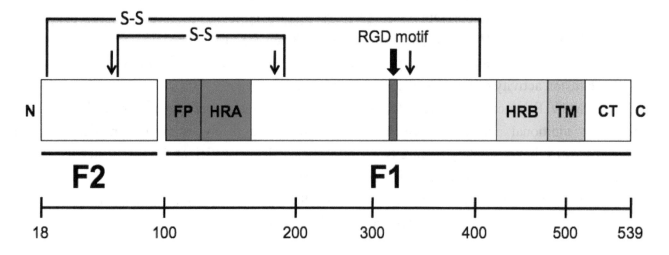

Figure 3. Structures of paramyxovirus F proteins. (**A**) The prefusion conformation of the PIV5 F trimer and the postfusion conformation of the hRSV F trimer. A schematic of the F protein color-coded to identify structural domains is shown below the structures. The DI domain is shown in orange, the DII domain is shown in red, and the DIII domain is shown in blue. HRA is shown in light blue, HRB is shown in cyan and the HRB linker domain is shown in gray. The fusion peptide is shown in green for prefusion PIV5 F, but was not solved in the hRSV F structure. The GCNt domain (shown in yellow) was added to the PIV5 F trimer for crystallization. (**B**) HMPV F in complex with a neutralizing antibody (DS7 Fab, shown as gray surface). DI, DII, and DIII coloring is as for the F trimers shown in (A). The conserved RGD motif is shown as magenta spheres. Residue 294 (Glu) is shown as green spheres. Conserved charged residues in DIII that impact fusion activity are indicated as spheres (yellow, acidic residues; brown, basic residues). (**C**) Side and top views of the prefusion PIV5 F trimer are shown with the homologous residues to HMPV F-RGD shown as magenta spheres. Each monomer is shown in blue, yellow, or green. (**D**) Side and top views of the postfusion hRSV F trimer are shown with the homologous residues to HMPV F-RGD shown as magenta spheres. Coloring is as for PIV5 F in (C). Structural coordinates were obtained from the Protein Data Bank [52] and figure constructed with PyMOL. PIV5 F, PDB ID: 2B9B [53]; hRSV F, PDB ID: 3RKI [54]; HMPV F complex, PDB ID: 4DAG [55].

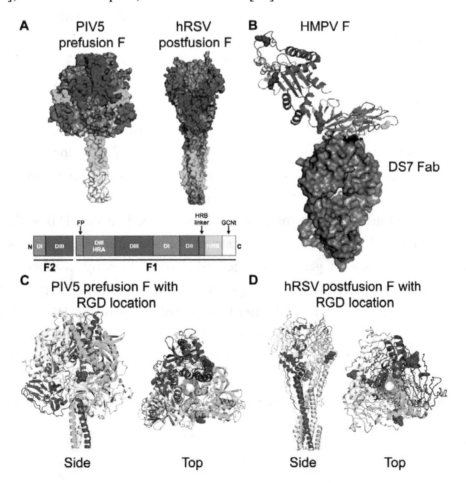

Crystal structures for the PIV5 prefusion F [53] and the hRSV postfusion F [54] have been determined and are shown in Figure 3A. Three discrete domains, DI (orange), DII (red) and DIII (blue), have been colored to indicate how the linear sequence of amino acids is arranged in the tertiary structure of the prefusion and postfusion F proteins. The HRA domain (light blue) changes significantly in both secondary structure and location, and the F head domain becomes more compact, during the prefusion-to-postfusion F transition (reviewed in [48]). A crystal structure of HMPV F in complex with a neutralizing antibody (DS7 Fab) has recently been described [55]. The HMPV F structure was solved as a monomer, and is depicted in Figure 3B. The HMPV F DIII domain is similar to the prefusion PIV5 F protein but overall the HMPV F structure resembled the hRSV postfusion F [55].

HMPV F amino acid sequences are highly conserved, falling into two major lineages (A and B), each with two subgroups (1 and 2), which exhibit a mean of ~96% identity [7,56]. A study in 2004 comparing 64 partial F gene sequences from the United States, Canada, Peru, France, Israel, Republic of South Africa, Australia and the Netherlands confirmed that HMPV isolates circulating around the world encode F proteins from the A1, A2, B1 and B2 genetic lineages [57]. Distinct canonical amino acid differences are present between major subgroups, and polymorphic variations tend to cluster in discrete regions [7,57]. Amino acid identity within and between subgroups is higher than nucleotide identity, suggesting structural or functional constraints on F protein diversity. A study comparing 85 full-length F gene sequences collected over a 20-year period from the United States (all isolated in Tennessee), Canada, Japan and the Netherlands suggested that there was no progressive genetic drift over time, and the genetic lineages were stable over time in circulating viruses in a population of children with respiratory illnesses [7].

The HMPV F protein is glycosylated at three Asn residues (residues 57, 172 and 353) [58,59]. Mutating the F2 subunit glycosylation site at N_{57} results in an F protein that is expressed and processed at near wild type levels, and efficiently mediates both cell-cell fusion [58] and virus growth in a mouse model of infection [59]. Glycosylation of N_{172} appears to be critical for proper F protein folding, fusion activity, and virus growth in mice [58,59]. Glycosylation of N_{353} appears to be critical for proper F folding and cleavage [58], which results in the inability to recover viruses with an N353Q mutation [59].

An arginine-glycine-aspartate (RGD) motif at residues 329–331 in the HMPV F1 subunit, along with 5 N- and 16 C-terminal flanking residues, is strictly conserved in all gene sequences that have been studied to date, regardless of genetic lineage and despite diversity in other regions of the F gene [60]. This motif is unique to HMPV F among human paramyxovirus fusion proteins and absent in all published HRSV F sequences. The RGD motif is located in DI of the HMPV F protein and is shown in Figure 3B as magenta spheres. Based upon homology, the predicted location of the RGD motif is also shown on the PIV5 prefusion (Figure 3C, magenta spheres) and the hRSV postfusion (Figure 3D, magenta spheres) F structures. The presence of the invariant RGD motif led to the speculation that integrins function as receptors for HMPV, discussed in more detail in the next section.

4. HMPV Binding: Identifying the Door

As noted, HMPV diverged from an avian pneumovirus (AMPV-C) between 200–300 years ago [6,7]. HMPV does not replicate in birds and evidence of AMPV infection has not been detected in humans [1]. The switch in virus tropism appears to be due to the attachment function of the F protein. In cell culture, HMPV expressing only F (HMPVΔGΔSH) binds to the cell surface with the same efficiency as wild type virus [61]. Moreover, HMPV F confers species specificity of infection, as F was found to be primarily responsible for the difference in the ability of AMPV-C and HMPV to infect quail fibroblast (QT6) cells [62]. Further, the F2 subunit (and not the G protein) of both hRSV [38] and HMPV [62] has been shown to confer species-specific infection of cells. This evidence strongly indicated that HMPV F interacts with cell surface receptors, and both protein and carbohydrate receptors for HMPV F have been discovered.

We identified a conserved RGD motif in the HMPV F1 subunit, and speculated that integrins might serve as receptors for HMPV. Integrins are heterodimeric integral membrane proteins composed of one α and one β subunit. A subset of integrins (αVβ1, αVβ3, αVβ5, αVβ6, αVβ8, α5β1, α8β1 and αIIbβ3) bind proteins with RGD motifs, such as fibronectin and vitronectin. Integrins are adhesion receptors that bind extracellular proteins to modulate cell behavior and survival. Integrins associate with cytoskeletal proteins, adaptors, and kinases via the cytoplasmic tails of the α and β subunits, allowing them to transduce bidirectional signals between the intra- and extra-cellular environments [63]. The intimate link between integrins and cell signaling cascades, as well as endosomal sorting pathways, makes them a desirable receptor for mammalian viruses. Several viruses, including adenovirus, hantavirus, herpesvirus, picornavirus, and reovirus, utilize integrins during entry, either as attachment or internalization receptors (reviewed in [64]).

Initial experiments in our laboratory found that the RGD-binding integrin αVβ1 promoted HMPV infection [60,65]. EDTA, which chelates divalent cations required for integrin function, exhibited a dose-dependent inhibition of HMPV infection. Synthetic RGD peptides blocked HMPV infection, while RGE peptides did not. Function-blocking monoclonal antibodies (mAbs) directed against RGD-binding integrins inhibited HMPV infection, with mAbs against αV and β1 exhibiting the most potent effect. Similarly, reduction of αV and β1 expression by siRNA reduced HMPV infection. Importantly, none of these loss-of-function experiments inhibited hRSV, which has a very similar F protein but lacks an RGD motif. Transfection of poorly permissive cells with αV or β1 cDNAs conferred HMPV infectivity. These data suggested that αVβ1 integrin is a receptor for HMPV.

Subsequent studies using both virus and virus-like particles showed that HMPV F is capable of binding multiple RGD-binding integrins in addition to αVβ1, specifically α5β1 and other αV-integrin heterodimers that may differ depending upon target cells [65]. Furthermore, recent data suggest that HMPV F utilizes RGD-binding integrins as attachment and entry receptors. HMPV F binds RGD-binding integrins during attachment, and this interaction is necessary for virus attachment and subsequent productive infection [65]. Blockade of integrin function with mAbs inhibits approximately half of virus binding, but >90% of virus infectivity. Thus, while HMPV can bind to other cell surface molecules, integrin binding is required for efficient entry. Furthermore, mutating the conserved RGD motif significantly attenuated HMPV growth *in vitro* and altered the extent of virus-infected cell-cell fusion, suggesting a key role for the integrin-binding motif during F-mediated entry and fusion [65]. In addition to being necessary for efficient HMPV F-mediated attachment, our experiments suggest that integrin engagement is also required for postbinding events during HMPV entry, because blocking RGD-binding integrin attachment results in significantly lower levels of viral transcripts at eight hours post infection [65]. Thus, in the absence of integrin-mediated entry, virus transcription is impaired. These data suggest that RGD-binding integrin engagement is necessary but not sufficient for HMPV attachment (40%–50% of HMPV F-specific binding is mediated by integrins), and that integrin engagement is important for post-binding events that occur during HMPV entry [65].

Chang *et al.* recently identified heparan sulfate as a receptor for HMPV F, and suggested that the carbohydrate moiety was the first binding partner for HMPV F during virus attachment [61]. Experiments with Chinese hamster ovary (CHO-K1) cells and mutant CHO-K1-derived cell lines unable to synthesize GAGs demonstrated that heparan sulfate proteoglycans were required for HMPV binding and infection [61]. These authors concluded that β1 integrin was not a direct cellular receptor for HMPV because virus still bound β1 integrin-deficient murine embryonic fibroblasts [61]. However, when β1-null fibroblasts were complemented with human β1 integrin, HMPV infection was significantly enhanced, supporting a role for β1 integrin in promoting HMPV infection [61]. In light of our recent findings that HMPV F binds multiple integrins during attachment, HMPV F would be expected to bind to other RGD-binding integrins such as αVβ5, αVβ6 and/or αVβ8 on the β1-null cell surface. The β1-null fibroblasts express several αV heterodimers, including αVβ3 and αVβ5 [66,67]. These data show that an HMPV F interaction with heparan sulfate moieties on the cell surface contributes to HMPV attachment and infection, and heparan sulfate may be the first cell surface receptor that HMPV engages during virus attachment.

Interestingly, recent findings by Chang *et al.* suggest that efficient HMPV infection depends upon the expression of a proteinaceous receptor that is trypsin- and proteinase K-sensitive (integrins are reported to be resistant to both types of protease treatment) [61]. Thus, HMPV entry appears to involve more than one cell surface receptor: heparan sulfate, RGD-binding integrins, and other protease-sensitive surface proteins. However, further studies are needed to identify other putative proteinaceous receptors for HMPV.

Together, recent studies on the receptors involved in HMPV entry suggest that HMPV F interacts with multiple binding partners during attachment. We propose a multi-step model of HMPV attachment where F first binds heparan sulfate before engaging specific proteinaceous receptors including RGD-binding integrins, which mediate post-binding events that lead to productive HMPV infection.

5. HMPV Fusion: Entering the Premises

The mature HMPV F protein must be proteolytically cleaved to convert the F0 precursor into the fusion-competent, disulfide-linked F1/F2 heterodimer. The monobasic, consensus cleavage site (PRQSR) is a trypsin-like cleavage motif, which is cleaved after the final Arg residue. For most cell types, cell surface HMPV F is expressed in the F0 precursor form. In cell culture, F protein cleavage occurs when trypsin is added to the cell medium. Indeed, HMPV grows poorly (or not at all) unless trypsin is added to virus growth medium during virus propagation in cell culture [1,44,68]. Trypsin treatment of HMPV F-expressing cells is also required for cell-cell fusion activity [58]. *In vivo*, cleavage is likely mediated by extracellular proteases such as TMPRSS2 [69] or mini-plasmin [70] expressed in the respiratory tract of infected humans. HMPV F cleavage activates the protein by creating a new F1 N-terminus, the fusion peptide, which is inserted into target cell membranes during the fusion process.

Most paramyxovirus F proteins require an attachment protein to drive membrane fusion, both during entry (virus-cell fusion) and to induce syncytia (cell-cell fusion). Transient transfection of HMPV F is sufficient to induce cell-cell fusion, and co-expression of the G protein does not significantly enhance fusion [58]. Moreover, using virus-like particles containing only F or F+G, we have demonstrated that the G protein does not alter particle-cell hemifusion kinetics or the extent of fusion [65]. This evidence coupled with the observation that HMPV lacking the G protein is infectious suggests that the G protein is not a critical component of the HMPV fusion machinery.

To better understand how the HMPV F protein functions alone to mediate fusion, recent studies have explored the requirements for fusion and investigated the importance of specific residues within the extracellular domain of the protein for fusion activity. Paramyxovirus fusion proteins mediate fusion in a pH-independent manner [71], and commonly induce fusion of cultured cells at neutral pH resulting in syncytium formation during virus infection. Surprisingly, the first report of HMPV F-mediated cell-cell fusion activity suggested that HMPV F required low pH for activation [58]. Schowalter *et al.* determined that HMPV F required both trypsin treatment, to mediate proteolytic processing, and low pH pulses for fusion activity of the A2 genotype strain CAN97-83 [58]. A follow-up study suggested that the low-pH-induced fusion phenotype of HMPV CAN97-83 may be strain-specific [72]. Herfst *et al.* used prototype F proteins from the four HMPV genetic lineages to demonstrate that fusion for lineage B strains was pH-independent, but fusion for some lineage A strains (one A1 and one of two A2 strains tested) was enhanced by pH 5 pulses [72]. Mutagenesis studies determined that a Gly residue at position 294 was a key determinant of the low-pH-induced fusion phenotype for HMPV A strains, but inserting the Gly_{294} residue into HMPV B F proteins did not confer pH sensitivity [72]. We compared the sequences of more than 1000 published full-length and partial HMPV F sequences from around the world to determine the frequency of the residue present at position 294 (see Figure 3B, green spheres). Most HMPV strains encode a Glu residue at position 294, 6% encode a Gly (59 of 1005), and rarely a Lys residue is found at this position in the sequence (15 of 1005). The lack of HMPV F proteins with the low-pH sensitive Gly_{294} suggests that exposure to low pH is not a general requirement for fusion activity. Thus, the general trigger that activates HMPV F to drive the membrane fusion process is still not known.

The finding that some HMPV F strains may require low pH for fusogenicity has led to follow-up studies that have elucidated the importance of other residues in the HMPV F protein that serve a role in protein stability and fusion triggering. Mutagenesis studies of CAN97-83 suggest that protonation of a conserved His residue at position 435 in the HRB linker domain serves a critical role in the low pH activation of the F protein [73,74]. A predicted cluster of basic residues Lys_{295}, Arg_{396}, and Arg_{438} are also important for the low pH fusion phenotype [73]. Interestingly, a predicted cluster of positively charged residues in this same region of the AMPV-A F protein (a distantly related pneumovirus) are important for fusion activity at neutral pH [75]. These studies suggest that the His residue at position 435 may serve as a low-pH sensor, and one model proposed that protonation of the His residue at low pH induces localized electrostatic repulsion that leads to the destabilization of F and fusion triggering [73,76]. Alternatively, electrostatic repulsion among the basic residues induced by receptor binding could destabilize the HRB linker domain and trigger fusion [75]. In any case, mutational analyses suggest that specific residues in domain II of HMPV F (Figure 3B, red residues) impact the initiation of membrane fusion. It is interesting that the cluster of basic residues is located in close proximity to a recently identified epitope that is recognized by a potently neutralizing mAb [55,77]. Thus, structural and functional studies support a significant role for domain II in the fusion activity of HMPV F.

Another charged region in the HMPV F extracellular head domain has recently been implicated in the low-pH sensitive fusion phenotype. Acidic residues Glu_{51}, Asp_{54}, and Glu_{56} (Figure 3B, yellow spheres) are important for low-pH triggered F-mediated cell-cell fusion, but also appear to be critical for protein stability [76]. These residues are clustered in a charged region present in the F2 subunit of F in close proximity to two basic residues (Figure 3B, brown spheres) [76]. The specific acidic residues in the F2 subunit and basic residues in the HRA domain are highly conserved in all HMPV strains; therefore, others have predicted that salt bridges and/or electrostatic interactions in this region may contribute to F triggering during HMPV fusion [76]. This hypothesis is supported by another study that indicated that the F2 subunit from AMPV-C could confer a hyperfusogenic phenotype to HMPV F1 [62].

Taking these studies together, it is clear that multiple regions in the HMPV F head domain are critical for fusion activity. Interestingly, two distal regions with predicted charged residue clusters have been implicated in fusion triggering (located in domains II and III). The idea that electrostatic repulsions can trigger the HMPV F prefusion protein to spring into the postfusion conformation during the fusion process is logical. The HRA region of F must undergo a significant structural rearrangement during fusion, extending to form a long coiled-coil and moving a long distance to refold into a six-helix bundle with HRB coils near the TM domain [48]. This structural change must also occur at the right time and place, as refolding of class I fusion proteins is irreversible under physiological conditions. Thus, sensor residues could act as molecular switches that modulate electrostatic interactions, leading to repulsive forces that drive movement of structural elements within the F protein. While histidine protonation at residue 435 appears to serve as one sensor in HMPV strains that exhibit enhanced fusogenicity at low pH, it remains unclear how pH-independent HMPV F fusion is triggered. Perhaps receptor interactions serve to augment local protein structure, driving the same electrostatic repulsion that can be triggered by exposure to low pH in some HMPV strains.

It is tempting to speculate that a direct interaction between HMPV F and RGD-binding integrins serves to initiate F-mediated fusion. However, current evidence does not support this hypothesis. We recently found that blocking HMPV F interaction with RGD-binding integrins did not alter virus-cell hemifusion kinetics, and virus-like particles bearing an F-RAE mutation fused with the same hemifusion kinetics as wild type F particles [65]. Moreover, Chang *et al.* showed that an HMPV F-RGA mutant promoted cell-cell fusion at levels approximately 80% of the wild type F protein [61], indicating that the RGD motif was not absolutely required for fusion activity. However, our results support a post-binding role for RGD-binding integrins during HMPV entry, as integrin blockade reduced HMPV transcription at 8 hours by 50%, in addition to a 40–50% block during virus attachment [65]. Further, when we introduced the F-RAE mutation into a virus, the F-RAE virus was severely attenuated and exhibited a small plaque phenotype that lacked the characteristic syncytia (indicative of F-mediated cell-cell fusion) of wild type virus [65]. Thus, while it appears that an F-integrin interaction is not required for efficient HMPV hemifusion, it remains possible that this interaction promotes fusion pore opening during virus-cell fusion.

6. HMPV Entry: Unlocking the Mystery

The solved crystal structures of postfusion PIV3, NDV, and hRSV F proteins are similar [54,78,79], supporting the model that all paramyxovirus F proteins mediate fusion via a highly conserved mechanism. Only one paramyxovirus F protein, PIV5, has been crystallized in the prefusion structural conformation (shown in Figure 3A, [53]). Comparison of this structure to the postfusion conformation has facilitated our understanding of the paramyxovirus fusion process (reviewed in [48]). The unique activity of pneumovirus fusion proteins to mediate fusion in the absence of an attachment protein suggests that hRSV and HMPV F may have unique prefusion structures compared to the *Paramyxovirinae* subfamily F proteins. Unfortunately, crystal structures of hRSV and HMPV prefusion trimers have not been published. The recently described structure of HMPV F in complex with a neutralizing antibody [55] provides insight into the structure of the protein, but HMPV F may trimerize slightly differently than PIV5 F [53]. Furthermore, while the HMPV F DIII domain had a similar fold to the PIV5 prefusion protein, the overall structural fold more closely resembled the postfusion hRSV F protein [55]. Thus, a crystal structure of a prefusion pneumovirus F trimer will be required to understand how these proteins have evolved to mediate fusion in the absence of an attachment protein. Further, because hRSV and HMPV F proteins utilize distinct proteinaceous cellular receptors [65,80], these proteins may also have unique prefusion structures. Such structures could provide insight into how pneumovirus F proteins couple receptor-binding and fusion activities.

The proverbial "black box" with respect to paramyxovirus entry is a lack of understanding of the fusion protein triggering process. For all paramyxoviruses, the process by which receptor binding triggers conformational changes in F remains unclear. HMPV F interacts with at least two different cell surface receptors during entry, heparan sulfate and RGD-binding integrins. How binding to receptor(s) results in structural changes in F that drive fusion is not clear. Furthermore, whether HMPV binds receptors simultaneously or sequentially is not known. Simultaneously binding to multiple receptors may induce conformational changes in multiple sites of the HMPV F extracellular domain, thereby promoting destabilization, protein refolding, and fusion. Alternatively, HMPV F binding to one receptor may expose the receptor binding site for another co-receptor, similar to the strategy utilized by HIV gp120/gp41 during fusion [81]. Our understanding of HMPV F triggering is further complicated by observations that some F proteins are more fusogenic at low pH. Typically, enveloped viruses either fuse at neutral pH or require exposure to low pH for fusion activity. We speculate that low pH treatment could result in histidine protonation events that serve to destabilize HMPV F in a similar manner to receptor engagement, although this hypothesis requires further investigation. This could explain why not all strains require low-pH exposure, but highly conserved charged regions of F are critical for function of all HMPV strains.

The role of low pH in HMPV entry is still unclear. Inhibitors of endosomal acidification such as bafilomycin A1 and concanamycin A have been shown to partially reduce HMPV infection of the low-pH sensitive CAN97-83 virus strain [73]. Intriguingly, bafilomycin A1 and concanamycin A also partially inhibit infection by the pH-independent NL199 (B1) strain of HMPV, but not the NL1-00 (A1) strain which has been shown to be triggered by low pH exposure in syncytium assays [74]. Because the low-pH-sensitive phenotype observed in cell-cell fusion assays does not necessarily correlate with inhibition of HMPV infection by endosomal acidification inhibitors, it is not clear that the ability to enhance fusogenicity with low pH pulses is correlated with a requirement for endosomal acidification during entry. Furthermore, whether particle-cell fusion requires exposure to low pH requires further investigation to determine whether low pH is an absolute requirement for triggering of F proteins from some HMPV strains. The site of HMPV fusion also requires further investigation. Schowalter et al. reported that infection by the low-pH sensitive HMPV strain CAN97-83 was significantly impaired by chemical inhibitors of endocytosis pathways, e.g., chlorpromazine and dynasore [73]. Thus, one study suggests that HMPV entry may involve virus internalization, although this speculation requires further studies with other HMPV lineage strains and more specific inhibitors of various endocytosis pathways.

7. Conclusions

HMPV is a leading cause of lower respiratory illness in adults and children. Although the virus was only discovered in 2001, remarkable progress has been made in elucidating the biology of HMPV. The F protein serves both to bind cellular receptors and to mediate fusion, although G protein is required for full virulence. HMPV F binds to heparan sulfate, and uniquely among human paramyxoviruses uses multiple RGD-binding integrins as attachment and entry receptors. Some HMPV F molecules exhibit sensitivity to low pH, though the function of this low pH triggering during the context of infection is not clear. While HMPV F shares many features of other paramyxovirus fusion proteins, there are distinct aspects of the attachment, entry, and fusion mechanisms of this recently discovered virus.

Acknowledgments

This work was supported by Public Health Service grants AI-73697 and AI-85062 (JVW) and T32 AI-7611 (RGC), from the National Institute of Allergy and Infectious Diseases. We thank current and past members of the Williams laboratory for helpful discussion.

References

1. Van den Hoogen, B.G.; de Jong, J.C.; Groen, J.; Kuiken, T.; de Groot, R.; Fouchier, R.A.; Osterhaus, A.D. A newly discovered human pneumovirus isolated from young children with respiratory tract disease. *Nat. Med.* **2001**, *7*, 719–724.

2. Schildgen, V.; van den Hoogen, B.; Fouchier, R.; Tripp, R.A.; Alvarez, R.; Manoha, C.; Williams, J.; Schildgen, O. Human metapneumovirus: Lessons learned over the first decade. *Clin. Microbiol. Rev.* **2011**, *24*, 734–754.

3. Cook, J.K. Avian pneumovirus infections of turkeys and chickens. *Vet. J.* **2000**, *160*, 118–125.

4. Van den Hoogen, B.G.; Bestebroer, T.M.; Osterhaus, A.D.; Fouchier, R.A. Analysis of the genomic sequence of a human metapneumovirus. *Virology* **2002**, *295*, 119–132.

5. Williams, J.V.; Harris, P.A.; Tollefson, S.J.; Halburnt-Rush, L.L.; Pingsterhaus, J.M.; Edwards, K.M.; Wright, P.F.; Crowe, J.E., Jr. Human metapneumovirus and lower respiratory tract disease in otherwise healthy infants and children. *N. Engl. J. Med.* **2004**, *350*, 443–450.

6. De Graaf, M.; Osterhaus, A.D.; Fouchier, R.A.; Holmes, E.C. Evolutionary dynamics of human and avian metapneumoviruses. *J. Gen. Virol.* **2008**, *89*, 2933–2942.

7. Yang, C.F.; Wang, C.K.; Tollefson, S.J.; Piyaratna, R.; Lintao, L.D.; Chu, M.; Liem, A.; Mark, M.; Spaete, R.R.; Crowe, J.E., Jr.; *et al.* Genetic diversity and evolution of human metapneumovirus fusion protein over twenty years. *Virol. J.* **2009**, *6*, 138.

8. Williams, J.V.; Wang, C.K.; Yang, C.F.; Tollefson, S.J.; House, F.S.; Heck, J.M.; Chu, M.; Brown, J.B.; Lintao, L.D.; Quinto, J.D.; *et al.* The role of human metapneumovirus in upper respiratory tract infections in children: A 20-year experience. *J. Infect. Dis.* **2006**, *193*, 387–395.

9. Van den Hoogen, B.G.; van Doornum, G.J.; Fockens, J.C.; Cornelissen, J.J.; Beyer, W.E.; de Groot, R.; Osterhaus, A.D.; Fouchier, R.A. Prevalence and clinical symptoms of human metapneumovirus infection in hospitalized patients. *J. Infect. Dis.* **2003**, *188*, 1571–1577.

10. Peiris, J.S.; Tang, W.H.; Chan, K.H.; Khong, P.L.; Guan, Y.; Lau, Y.L.; Chiu, S.S. Children with respiratory disease associated with metapneumovirus in hong kong. *Emerg. Infect. Dis.* **2003**, *9*, 628–633.

11. Mullins, J.A.; Erdman, D.D.; Weinberg, G.A.; Edwards, K.; Hall, C.B.; Walker, F.J.; Iwane, M.; Anderson, L.J. Human metapneumovirus infection among children hospitalized with acute respiratory illness. *Emerg. Infect. Dis.* **2004**, *10*, 700–705.

12. McAdam, A.J.; Hasenbein, M.E.; Feldman, H.A.; Cole, S.E.; Offermann, J.T.; Riley, A.M.; Lieu, T.A. Human metapneumovirus in children tested at a tertiary-care hospital. *J. Infect. Dis.* **2004**, *190*, 20–26.

13. Mackay, I.M.; Bialasiewicz, S.; Jacob, K.C.; McQueen, E.; Arden, K.E.; Nissen, M.D.; Sloots, T.P. Genetic diversity of human metapneumovirus over 4 consecutive years in australia. *J. Infect. Dis.* **2006**, *193*, 1630–1633.

14. Foulongne, V.; Guyon, G.; Rodiere, M.; Segondy, M. Human metapneumovirus infection in young children hospitalized with respiratory tract disease. *Pediatr. Infect. Dis. J.* **2006**, *25*, 354–359.

15. Esper, F.; Martinello, R.A.; Boucher, D.; Weibel, C.; Ferguson, D.; Landry, M.L.; Kahn, J.S. A 1-year experience with human metapneumovirus in children aged <5 years. *J. Infect. Dis.* **2004**, *189*, 1388–1396.

16. Ebihara, T.; Endo, R.; Kikuta, H.; Ishiguro, N.; Ishiko, H.; Hara, M.; Takahashi, Y.; Kobayashi, K. Human metapneumovirus infection in japanese children. *J. Clin. Microbiol.* **2004**, *42*, 126–132.

17. Dollner, H.; Risnes, K.; Radtke, A.; Nordbo, S.A. Outbreak of human metapneumovirus infection in norwegian children. *Pediatr. Infect. Dis. J.* **2004**, *23*, 436–440.

18. Boivin, G.; de Serres, G.; Cote, S.; Gilca, R.; Abed, Y.; Rochette, L.; Bergeron, M.G.; Dery, P. Human metapneumovirus infections in hospitalized children. *Emerg. Infect. Dis.* **2003**, *9*, 634–640.

19. Williams, J.V.; Martino, R.; Rabella, N.; Otegui, M.; Parody, R.; Heck, J.M.; Crowe, J.E., Jr. A prospective study comparing human metapneumovirus with other respiratory viruses in adults with hematologic malignancies and respiratory tract infections. *J. Infect. Dis.* **2005**, *192*, 1061–1065.

20. Williams, J.V.; Crowe, J.E., Jr.; Enriquez, R.; Minton, P.; Peebles, R.S., Jr.; Hamilton, R.G.; Higgins, S.; Griffin, M.; Hartert, T.V. Human metapneumovirus infection plays an etiologic role in acute asthma exacerbations requiring hospitalization in adults. *J. Infect. Dis.* **2005**, *192*, 1149–1153.

21. Vicente, D.; Montes, M.; Cilla, G.; Perez-Trallero, E. Human metapneumovirus and chronic obstructive pulmonary disease. *Emerg. Infect. Dis.* **2004**, *10*, 1338–1339.

22. Pelletier, G.; Dery, P.; Abed, Y.; Boivin, G. Respiratory tract reinfections by the new human metapneumovirus in an immunocompromised child. *Emerg. Infect. Dis.* **2002**, *8*, 976–978.

23. Madhi, S.A.; Ludewick, H.; Abed, Y.; Klugman, K.P.; Boivin, G. Human metapneumovirus-associated lower respiratory tract infections among hospitalized human immunodeficiency virus type 1 (hiv-1)-infected and hiv-1-uninfected african infants. *Clin. Infect. Dis.* **2003**, *37*, 1705–1710.

24. Larcher, C.; Geltner, C.; Fischer, H.; Nachbaur, D.; Muller, L.C.; Huemer, H.P. Human metapneumovirus infection in lung transplant recipients: Clinical presentation and epidemiology. *J. Heart Lung Transplant.* **2005**, *24*, 1891–1901.

25. Englund, J.A.; Boeckh, M.; Kuypers, J.; Nichols, W.G.; Hackman, R.C.; Morrow, R.A.; Fredricks, D.N.; Corey, L. Brief communication: Fatal human metapneumovirus infection in stem-cell transplant recipients. *Ann. Intern. Med.* **2006**, *144*, 344–349.

26. Brodzinski, H.; Ruddy, R.M. Review of new and newly discovered respiratory tract viruses in children. *Pediatr. Emerg. Care* **2009**, *25*, 352–360.

27. Loughlin, G.M.; Moscona, A. The cell biology of acute childhood respiratory disease: Therapeutic implications. *Pediatr. Clin. North Am.* **2006**, *53*, 929–959.

28. Kuiken, T.; van den Hoogen, B.G.; van Riel, D.A.; Laman, J.D.; van Amerongen, G.; Sprong, L.; Fouchier, R.A.; Osterhaus, A.D. Experimental human metapneumovirus infection of cynomolgus macaques (macaca fascicularis) results in virus replication in ciliated epithelial cells and pneumocytes with associated lesions throughout the respiratory tract. *Am. J. Pathol.* **2004**, *164*, 1893–1900.

29. Williams, J.V.; Tollefson, S.J.; Johnson, J.E.; Crowe, J.E., Jr. The cotton rat (sigmodon hispidus) is a permissive small animal model of human metapneumovirus infection, pathogenesis, and protective immunity. *J. Virol.* **2005**, *79*, 10944–10951.

30. Hamelin, M.E.; Prince, G.A.; Gomez, A.M.; Kinkead, R.; Boivin, G. Human metapneumovirus infection induces long-term pulmonary inflammation associated with airway obstruction and hyperresponsiveness in mice. *J. Infect. Dis.* **2006**, *193*, 1634–1642.

31. Roberts, S.R.; Compans, R.W.; Wertz, G.W. Respiratory syncytial virus matures at the apical surfaces of polarized epithelial cells. *J. Virol.* **1995**, *69*, 2667–2673.

32. Shaikh, F.Y.; Cox, R.G.; Lifland, A.W.; Hotard, A.L.; Williams, J.V.; Moore, M.L.; Santangelo, P.J.; Crowe, J.E., Jr. A critical phenylalanine residue in the respiratory syncytial virus fusion protein cytoplasmic tail mediates assembly of internal viral proteins into viral filaments and particles. *MBio* **2012**, *3*, doi: 10.1128/mBio.00270-11.

33. Sabo, Y.; Ehrlich, M.; Bacharach, E. The conserved yagl motif in human metapneumovirus is required for higher-order cellular assemblies of the matrix protein and for virion production. *J. Virol.* **2011**, *85*, 6594–6609.

34. Lamb, R.A. Paramyxovirus fusion: A hypothesis for changes. *Virology* **1993**, *197*, 1–11.

35. Karron, R.A.; Buonagurio, D.A.; Georgiu, A.F.; Whitehead, S.S.; Adamus, J.E.; Clements-Mann, M.L.; Harris, D.O.; Randolph, V.B.; Udem, S.A.; Murphy, B.R.; *et al.* Respiratory syncytial virus (rsv) sh and g proteins are not essential for viral replication *in vitro*: Clinical evaluation and molecular characterization of a cold-passaged, attenuated rsv subgroup b mutant. *Proc. Natl. Acad. Sci. USA* **1997**, *94*, 13961–13966.

36. Feldman, S.A.; Audet, S.; Beeler, J.A. The fusion glycoprotein of human respiratory syncytial virus facilitates virus attachment and infectivity via an interaction with cellular heparan sulfate. *J. Virol.* **2000**, *74*, 6442–6447.

37. Kahn, J.S.; Schnell, M.J.; Buonocore, L.; Rose, J.K. Recombinant vesicular stomatitis virus expressing respiratory syncytial virus (rsv) glycoproteins: Rsv fusion protein can mediate infection and cell fusion. *Virology* **1999**, *254*, 81–91.

38. Schlender, J.; Zimmer, G.; Herrler, G.; Conzelmann, K.K. Respiratory syncytial virus (rsv) fusion protein subunit f2, not attachment protein g, determines the specificity of rsv infection. *J. Virol.* **2003**, *77*, 4609–4616.

39. Techaarpornkul, S.; Barretto, N.; Peeples, M.E. Functional analysis of recombinant respiratory syncytial virus deletion mutants lacking the small hydrophobic and/or attachment glycoprotein gene. *J. Virol.* **2001**, *75*, 6825–6834.

40. Techaarpornkul, S.; Collins, P.L.; Peeples, M.E. Respiratory syncytial virus with the fusion protein as its only viral glycoprotein is less dependent on cellular glycosaminoglycans for attachment than complete virus. *Virology* **2002**, *294*, 296–304.

41. Widjojoatmodjo, M.N.; Boes, J.; van Bers, M.; van Remmerden, Y.; Roholl, P.J.; Luytjes, W. A highly attenuated recombinant human respiratory syncytial virus lacking the g protein induces long-lasting protection in cotton rats. *Virol. J.* **2010**, *7*, 114.

42. Teng, M.N.; Whitehead, S.S.; Collins, P.L. Contribution of the respiratory syncytial virus g glycoprotein and its secreted and membrane-bound forms to virus replication *in vitro* and *in vivo*. *Virology* **2001**, *289*, 283–296.

43. Biacchesi, S.; Pham, Q.N.; Skiadopoulos, M.H.; Murphy, B.R.; Collins, P.L.; Buchholz, U.J. Infection of nonhuman primates with recombinant human metapneumovirus lacking the sh, g, or m2-2 protein categorizes each as a nonessential accessory protein and identifies vaccine candidates. *J. Virol.* **2005**, *79*, 12608–12613.

44. Biacchesi, S.; Skiadopoulos, M.H.; Yang, L.; Lamirande, E.W.; Tran, K.C.; Murphy, B.R.; Collins, P.L.; Buchholz, U.J. Recombinant human metapneumovirus lacking the small hydrophobic sh and/or attachment g glycoprotein: Deletion of g yields a promising vaccine candidate. *J. Virol.* **2004**, *78*, 12877–12887.

45. Hallak, L.K.; Collins, P.L.; Knudson, W.; Peeples, M.E. Iduronic acid-containing glycosaminoglycans on target cells are required for efficient respiratory syncytial virus infection. *Virology* **2000**, *271*, 264–275.

46. Krusat, T.; Streckert, H.J. Heparin-dependent attachment of respiratory syncytial virus (rsv) to host cells. *Arch. Virol.* **1997**, *142*, 1247–1254.

47. Thammawat, S.; Sadlon, T.A.; Hallsworth, P.G.; Gordon, D.L. Role of cellular glycosaminoglycans and charged regions of viral g protein in human metapneumovirus infection. *J. Virol.* **2008**, *82*, 11767–11774.

48. Lamb, R.A.; Jardetzky, T.S. Structural basis of viral invasion: Lessons from paramyxovirus f. *Curr. Opin. Struct. Biol.* **2007**, *17*, 427–436.

49. Russell, C.J.; Jardetzky, T.S.; Lamb, R.A. Membrane fusion machines of paramyxoviruses: Capture of intermediates of fusion. *EMBO J.* **2001**, *20*, 4024–4034.

50. Miller, S.A.; Tollefson, S.; Crowe, J.E., Jr.; Williams, J.V.; Wright, D.W. Examination of a fusogenic hexameric core from human metapneumovirus and identification of a potent synthetic peptide inhibitor from the heptad repeat 1 region. *J. Virol.* **2007**, *81*, 141–149.

51. Deffrasnes, C.; Hamelin, M.E.; Prince, G.A.; Boivin, G. Identification and evaluation of a highly effective fusion inhibitor for human metapneumovirus. *Antimicrob. Agents Chemother.* **2008**, *52*, 279–287.

52. Berman, H.M.; Westbrook, J.; Feng, Z.; Gilliland, G.; Bhat, T.N.; Weissig, H.; Shindyalov, I.N.; Bourne, P.E. The protein data bank. *Nucleic Acids Res.* **2000**, *28*, 235–242.

53. Yin, H.S.; Wen, X.; Paterson, R.G.; Lamb, R.A.; Jardetzky, T.S. Structure of the parainfluenza virus 5 f protein in its metastable, prefusion conformation. *Nature* **2006**, *439*, 38–44.

54. Swanson, K.A.; Settembre, E.C.; Shaw, C.A.; Dey, A.K.; Rappuoli, R.; Mandl, C.W.; Dormitzer, P.R.; Carfi, A. Structural basis for immunization with postfusion respiratory syncytial virus fusion f glycoprotein (rsv f) to elicit high neutralizing antibody titers. *Proc. Natl. Acad. Sci. USA* **2011**, *108*, 9619–9624.

55. Wen, X.; Krause, J.C.; Leser, G.P.; Cox, R.G.; Lamb, R.A.; Williams, J.V.; Crowe, J.E., Jr.; Jardetzky, T.S. Structure of the human metapneumovirus fusion protein with neutralizing antibody identifies a pneumovirus antigenic site. *Nat. Struct. Mol. Biol.* **2012**, *19*, 461–463.

56. Van den Hoogen, B.G.; Herfst, S.; Sprong, L.; Cane, P.A.; Forleo-Neto, E.; de Swart, R.L.; Osterhaus, A.D.; Fouchier, R.A. Antigenic and genetic variability of human metapneumoviruses. *Emerg. Infect. Dis.* **2004**, *10*, 658–666.

57. Boivin, G.; Mackay, I.; Sloots, T.P.; Madhi, S.; Freymuth, F.; Wolf, D.; Shemer-Avni, Y.; Ludewick, H.; Gray, G.C.; LeBlanc, E. Global genetic diversity of human metapneumovirus fusion gene. *Emerg. Infect. Dis.* **2004**, *10*, 1154–1157.

58. Schowalter, R.M.; Smith, S.E.; Dutch, R.E. Characterization of human metapneumovirus f protein-promoted membrane fusion: Critical roles for proteolytic processing and low ph. *J. Virol.* **2006**, *80*, 10931–10941.

59. Zhang, J.; Dou, Y.; Wu, J.; She, W.; Luo, L.; Zhao, Y.; Liu, P.; Zhao, X. Effects of n-linked glycosylation of the fusion protein on replication of human metapneumovirus *in vitro* and in mouse lungs. *J. Gen. Virol.* **2011**, *92*, 1666–1675.

60. Cseke, G.; Maginnis, M.S.; Cox, R.G.; Tollefson, S.J.; Podsiad, A.B.; Wright, D.W.; Dermody, T.S.; Williams, J.V. Integrin alphavbeta1 promotes infection by human metapneumovirus. *Proc. Natl. Acad. Sci. USA* **2009**, *106*, 1566–1571.

61. Chang, A.; Masante, C.; Buchholz, U.J.; Dutch, R.E. Human metapneumovirus (hmpv) binding and infection are mediated by interactions between the hmpv fusion protein and heparan sulfate. *J. Virol.* **2012**, *86*, 3230–3243.

62. De Graaf, M.; Schrauwen, E.J.; Herfst, S.; van Amerongen, G.; Osterhaus, A.D.; Fouchier, R.A. Fusion protein is the main determinant of metapneumovirus host tropism. *J. Gen. Virol.* **2009**, *90*, 1408–1416.

63. Hynes, R.O. Integrins: Bidirectional, allosteric signaling machines. *Cell* **2002**, *110*, 673–687.

64. Stewart, P.L.; Nemerow, G.R. Cell integrins: Commonly used receptors for diverse viral pathogens. *Trends Microbiol.* **2007**, *15*, 500–507.

65. Cox, R.G.; Livesay, S.B.; Johnson, M.; Ohi, M.D.; Williams, J.V. The human metapneumovirus fusion protein mediates entry via an interaction with rgd-binding integrins. *J. Virol.* **2012**, *86*, 12148–12160.

66. Wennerberg, K.; Lohikangas, L.; Gullberg, D.; Pfaff, M.; Johansson, S.; Fassler, R. Beta 1 integrin-dependent and -independent polymerization of fibronectin. *J. Cell. Biol.* **1996**, *132*, 227–238.

67. Fassler, R.; Pfaff, M.; Murphy, J.; Noegel, A.A.; Johansson, S.; Timpl, R.; Albrecht, R. Lack of beta 1 integrin gene in embryonic stem cells affects morphology, adhesion, and migration but not integration into the inner cell mass of blastocysts. *J. Cell. Biol.* **1995**, *128*, 979–988.

68. Tollefson, S.J.; Cox, R.G.; Williams, J.V. Studies of culture conditions and environmental stability of human metapneumovirus. *Virus Res.* **2010**, *151*, 54–59.

69. Shirogane, Y.; Takeda, M.; Iwasaki, M.; Ishiguro, N.; Takeuchi, H.; Nakatsu, Y.; Tahara, M.; Kikuta, H.; Yanagi, Y. Efficient multiplication of human metapneumovirus in vero cells expressing the transmembrane serine protease tmprss2. *J. Virol.* **2008**, *82*, 8942–8946.

70. Murakami, M.; Towatari, T.; Ohuchi, M.; Shiota, M.; Akao, M.; Okumura, Y.; Parry, M.A.; Kido, H. Mini-plasmin found in the epithelial cells of bronchioles triggers infection by broad-spectrum influenza a viruses and sendai virus. *Eur. J. Biochem.* **2001**, *268*, 2847–2855.

71. Lamb, R.A.; Parks, G.D. Paramyxoviridae: The Viruses and their Replication. In *Fields virology*, 5th ed.; Knipe, D.M., Howley, P.M., Eds.; Lippincott Williams & Wilkins: Philadelphia, PA, USA, 2007; Volume 1, pp. 1449–1646.

72. Herfst, S.; Mas, V.; Ver, L.S.; Wierda, R.J.; Osterhaus, A.D.; Fouchier, R.A.; Melero, J.A. Low-ph-induced membrane fusion mediated by human metapneumovirus f protein is a rare, strain-dependent phenomenon. *J. Virol.* **2008**, *82*, 8891–8895.

73. Schowalter, R.M.; Chang, A.; Robach, J.G.; Buchholz, U.J.; Dutch, R.E. Low-ph triggering of human metapneumovirus fusion: Essential residues and importance in entry. *J. Virol.* **2009**, *83*, 1511–1522.

74. Mas, V.; Herfst, S.; Osterhaus, A.D.; Fouchier, R.A.; Melero, J.A. Residues of the human metapneumovirus fusion (f) protein critical for its strain-related fusion phenotype: Implications for the virus replication cycle. *J. Virol.* **2011**, *85*, 12650–12661.

75. Wei, Y.; Feng, K.; Yao, X.; Cai, H.; Li, J.; Mirza, A.M.; Iorio, R.M. Localization of a region in the fusion protein of avian metapneumovirus that modulates cell-cell fusion. *J. Virol.* **2012**, *86*, 11800–11814.

76. Chang, A.; Hackett, B.; Winter, C.C.; Buchholz, U.J.; Dutch, R.E. Potential electrostatic interactions in multiple regions affect hmpv f-mediated membrane fusion. *J. Virol.* **2012**, *86*, 9843–9853.

77. Williams, J.V.; Chen, Z.; Cseke, G.; Wright, D.W.; Keefer, C.J.; Tollefson, S.J.; Hessell, A.; Podsiad, A.; Shepherd, B.E.; Sanna, P.P.; *et al.* A recombinant human monoclonal antibody to human metapneumovirus fusion protein that neutralizes virus *in vitro* and is effective therapeutically *in vivo. J. Virol.* **2007**, *81*, 8315–8324.

78. Swanson, K.; Wen, X.; Leser, G.P.; Paterson, R.G.; Lamb, R.A.; Jardetzky, T.S. Structure of the newcastle disease virus f protein in the post-fusion conformation. *Virology* **2010**, *402*, 372–379.

79. Yin, H.S.; Paterson, R.G.; Wen, X.; Lamb, R.A.; Jardetzky, T.S. Structure of the uncleaved ectodomain of the paramyxovirus (hpiv3) fusion protein. *Proc. Natl. Acad. Sci. USA* **2005**, *102*, 9288–9293.

80. Tayyari, F.; Marchant, D.; Moraes, T.J.; Duan, W.; Mastrangelo, P.; Hegele, R.G. Identification of nucleolin as a cellular receptor for human respiratory syncytial virus. *Nat. Med.* **2011**, *17*, 1132–1135.

81. Wilen, C.B.; Tilton, J.C.; Doms, R.W. Molecular mechanisms of hiv entry. *Adv. Exp. Med. Biol.* **2012**, *726*, 223–242.

10

The Pneumonia Virus of Mice (PVM) Model of Acute Respiratory Infection

Kimberly D. Dyer [1],*, Katia E. Garcia-Crespo [1], Stephanie Glineur [1], Joseph B. Domachowske [2] and Helene F. Rosenberg [1]

[1] Laboratory of Allergic Diseases, National Institute of Allergy and Infectious Diseases, National Institutes of Health, Bethesda, MD 20892, USA;
E-Mails: garciacrespoke@niaid.nih.gov (K.E.G.-C.); stephanie.glineur@nih.gov (S.G.); hrosenberg@niaid.nih.gov (H.F.R.)

[2] Department of Pediatrics, SUNY Upstate Medical University, Syracuse, NY 13210, USA;
E-Mail: domachoj@upstate.edu

*   Author to whom correspondence should be addressed; E-Mail: kdyer@niaid.nih.gov

Abstract: Pneumonia Virus of Mice (PVM) is related to the human and bovine respiratory syncytial virus (RSV) pathogens, and has been used to study respiratory virus replication and the ensuing inflammatory response as a component of a natural host—pathogen relationship. As such, PVM infection in mice reproduces many of the clinical and pathologic features of the more severe forms of RSV infection in human infants. Here we review some of the most recent findings on the basic biology of PVM infection and its use as a model of disease, most notably for explorations of virus infection and allergic airways disease, for vaccine evaluation, and for the development of immunomodulatory strategies for acute respiratory virus infection.

Keywords: PVM; inflammation; leukocytes; eosinophils; respiratory syncytial virus; RSV; TLR; IFN; heterologous immunity; MIP-1α

1. Introduction

Pneumonia virus of mice (PVM), human respiratory syncytial virus (hRSV) and bovine respiratory syncytial virus (bRSV) are enveloped, negative sense, single-stranded RNA viruses of the family *Paramyxoviridae*, subfamily Pneumovirinae, genus Pneumovirus [1]. PVM was originally discovered in 1939 by researchers Horsfall and Hahn at The Rockefeller University as part of an attempt to identify pathogens from human clinical samples that would replicate in lung tissues of inbred mice. PVM was isolated from lung tissue of what had been presumed to be healthy control mice that had been subjected to serial mouse-to-mouse passage [2]. PVM virions are polymorphic and found in diverse shapes, from spheres of 80–120 μm in diameter to filaments up to 3 μm in length. The virus replicates over a period of 24–30 h in mouse lung tissue, with virus amplification proceeding at 16-fold per cycle [2].

PVM is one of the many virus pathogens that are monitored in commercial and research rodent colonies [3,4]. In a study covering the years 2004–2007, Liang and colleagues [5] reported that 0.2%–1.0% of isolates from mouse colonies and 6.4%–25.8% of isolates from rat colonies tested positive for PVM. Information on wild rodents is somewhat limited. However, an extensive three-year study performed by Kaplan and colleagues [6] documented over 40% seropositivity for PVM in nearly 300 small wild rodents tested at 11 field sites in the United Kingdom. In contrast, Smith and colleagues [7] found no seropositivity for PVM among wild house mice in Southern Australia.

It is not yet clear how or if PVM replicates and induces pathology in non-rodent hosts. In a study carried out in 1986, Pringle and Eglin [8] found that more than 75% of adult sera had PVM-neutralizing activity that did not correlate with hRSV or parainfluenza virus (PIV)-3 neutralizing activity. More recently, Brock and colleagues [9] explored this question further, and determined that PVM did not replicate *in situ* when administered to the respiratory tracts of non-human primates, and that the PVM-neutralizing factor(s) in human sera did not interact specifically with virion components. In another recent development, Dubovi and colleagues [10,11] reported the isolation of canine pneumovirus (CnPnV) from the respiratory tracts of shelter-confined dogs with apparent respiratory illness. CnPnV is very similar overall to PVM (Figure 1), replicates in the lungs of BALB/c mice and induces inflammatory pathology, morbidity and mortality similar to that elicited by PVM [12] but a much higher initial inoculum is required to elicit these effects. The specific virulence attributable to this virus in canine species remains to be explored.

There are two characterized strains of PVM, strain 15 (two variants) and strain J3666 in current use in the research community. The original studies by Horsfall and co-workers [2,13–15] were performed on an isolate named strain 15, which was reported to be highly pathogenic in mice. Since that time, this strain had reportedly undergone tissue-culture passage, resulting in loss of its pathogenicity *in vivo*. Strain 15/Warwick is highly attenuated and elicits minimal inflammatory response [16] while strain 15/ATCC (American Tissue Culture Collection VR-25), in our hands, elicits inflammatory pathology in BALB/c mice but substantially less disease pathology in C57BL/6 mice [17]. Strain J3666 has reportedly been maintained via mouse passage [18] and thus retains full pathogenicity. The molecular organization of the PVM genome was elucidated by Easton and colleagues [19–22] and Krempl and colleagues [23,24]. The most significant differences between strains 15 and J3666 are in the G attachment protein. Anh and colleagues [25] documented the susceptibility of various strains of mice to strain J3666 as follows: 129/Sv > DBA > C3H/HeJ > BALB/c > C57BL/6 > SJL. Glineur and colleagues [26] have recently explored PVM infection in crosses between 129/Sv and SJL mice and have documented the polygenic nature of resistance and susceptibility to severe virus infection. A third strain, PVM strain Y, originally derived from a spontaneous infection in athymic mice [27] and featured in an early study of disease exacerbation in mice with severe combined immunodeficiency disease [28] has recently been sequenced (Figure 1; [29]).

Figure 1. (**A**) Although there is little direct amino acid sequence homology between PVM and hRSV, the two viruses share the same gene order. (**B**) Neighbor-joining tree featuring the amino acid sequences of the G glycoproteins of selected pneumoviruses; Genbank accession numbers include FJ614813.1; NC_001989.1; NC_006579; AY729016.1; JQ899033.1; HQ734815; AY743910.1. Panel A reprinted with permission from [1].

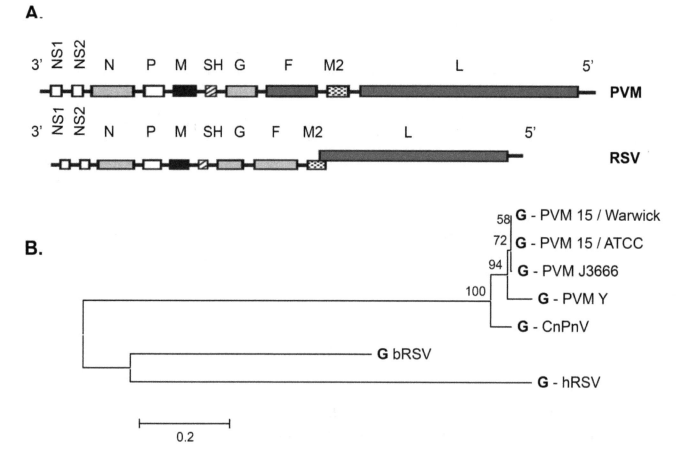

Horsfall and Ginsberg [14] recognized the potential of PVM for the exploration of acute respiratory virus infection in an evolutionarily relevant host. These authors were also the first to relate the development of lung lesions to ongoing virus replication and to evaluate altered morbidity and mortality in response to immunomodulatory therapy, specifically in response to administration of bacterial capsular polysaccharide [13–15]. We, and others, are using the PVM infection model to study the importance of virus-induced inflammatory responses in the development of severe respiratory virus disease and as a platform for the development of novel immunomodulatory strategies (see section on PVM and Disease, Heterologous Immunity).

2. The PVM Model of Acute Respiratory Infection

Our initial studies on PVM focused on the inflammatory responses to respiratory virus infection in a natural, evolutionarily relevant host [30,31]. We reproduced the findings of Horsfall and colleagues and reported robust virus replication *in situ* (to titers $>10^8$ pfu/gm lung tissue), progressing to marked morbidity (hunching, fur ruffling), weight loss, and mortality in response to a minimal virus inoculum of the highly pathogenic strain PVM J3666 [32,33]. We have localized immunoreactive PVM to the bronchiolar epithelium [34], in a distribution similar to what has been observed for RSV in human post-mortem specimens [35]. Profound inflammation of the lungs is evident and especially noteworthy is the recruitment of granulocytes and severe pulmonary edema. PVM replication in the mouse lung tissue is associated with local production of proinflammatory mediators including MIP-1α, MIP-2, and MCP-1 [34], consistent with those detected in lung and nasal washings in association with the more severe forms of RSV disease in human infants [1,36]. Although some features of the PVM model clearly conform to human pathophysiology, others do not. For example, neonatal mice exhibit little to no overt inflammation in response to PVM infection [37], nor can we establish a distinct pattern of infection in aged mice [38]. Similarly, it is crucial to recognize that PVM has no direct cross-reactivity with the human RSV pathogen, thus one's ability to perform studies of antigen-specific acquired immunity are limited.

3. Host Immune Response to PVM Infection

3.1. Neutrophils and Eosinophils

Microscopic examination of bronchoalveolar lavage fluid and lung tissue from morbid mice reveals profound inflammation, most notable for recruitment of granulocytes and progression to pulmonary edema (Figure 2). Similar to findings from the mouse model of influenza virus [39], MIP-1α signaling through CC chemokine receptor (CCR)-1, its major receptor on neutrophils and eosinophils, is crucial for granulocyte recruitment in response to PVM infection [33]. We have built on this observation to explore immunomodulatory therapies for pneumovirus infection directed at limiting uncontrolled neutrophil influx [40,41] as discussed below.

The role of eosinophils in respiratory virus infection is controversial and somewhat of a "double-edged sword" (reviewed in [42–44]). Eosinophils are among the granulocytes recruited at the earliest time points in response to PVM infection [32]. We and others have shown that eosinophils have antiviral properties against RSV [32,45,46]; recent findings from our laboratory demonstrate that activated eosinophils promote survival against lethal PVM infection [47]. PVM replicates in mouse eosinophils and promotes cytokine release [48].

3.2. T Lymphocytes

Although T cells have no apparent impact on the outcome of acute lethal PVM infection, both CD4$^+$ and CD8$^+$ T cells are required for virus clearance in response to sublethal infection [49]. Claassen and colleagues [50] documented influx of activated CD8$^+$ T cells into the lungs of infected mice and characterized PVM-specific responses against epitopes in the virus M (matrix; M_{43-51}), F (fusion; $F_{304-312}$) and P (phosphoprotein; $P_{261-269}$) virion proteins. The relatively limited frequency of functional virus-specific CD8$^+$ T cells suggested that PVM infection resulted in inactivation of effector T cells, similar to what has been reported in acute RSV infections [51]. Claassen and colleagues [52] have also identified a CD4$^+$ T cell epitope in the G attachment protein, $G_{381-385}$ and demonstrated protective immunity against lethal PVM challenge when mice were immunized simultaneously with both the CD4$^+$ $G_{381-385}$ and the $P_{261-269}$ CD8$^+$ T cell epitope peptides.

While CD4$^+$ and CD8$^+$ T cells have been reported to promote virus clearance, IL-21, a type I cytokine produced primarily by activated CD4$^+$T cells, promotes pathology in response to PVM infection [53]. Mice devoid of the unique receptor for IL-21 (IL21R$^{-/-}$) have diminished levels of the proinflammatory chemokine KC, and recruit fewer neutrophils, CD4$^+$, CD8$^+$ and gamma-delta T cells to the lungs, and survive longer in response to PVM infection than their PVM-infected wild-type counterparts.

Figure 2. (A) Detection of PVM in bronchiolar epithelial cells, original magnification 63×; **(B,C)** Histology of lung tissue from PVM-infected wild-type C57BL/6 mice, featuring multifocal acute alveolitis with intra-alveolar edema with scattered hemorrhage and moderate granulocytic infiltrates throughout; original magnifications 63× and 20×, respectively; **(D)** Flow cytometric profiles of Gr1$^+$ granulocytes in single cell suspensions from lung tissue of naïve and PVM-infected BALB/c mice. Reprinted with permission from (A) [34]; (B) and (C) [54].

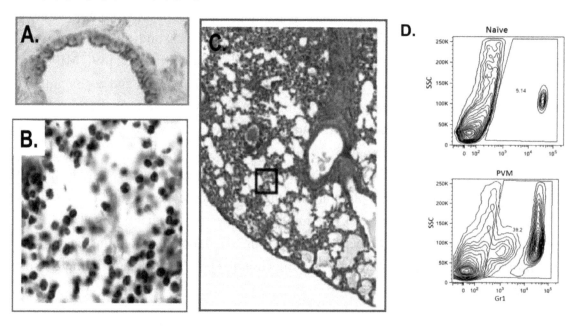

3.3. Macrophages

Macrophages are the main resident phagocytes in the lung and, working together with intact muco-ciliary to clear unwelcome debris including pathogens. Rigaux and colleagues [55] showed that depletion of alveolar macrophage prior to PVM infection resulted in a small increase in virus recovery and paradoxically prolonged survival. Macrophage depleted PVM-infected mice exhibited enhanced NK cell recruitment to the lungs accompanied by increased production of IFNγ by recruited NK cells, CD4$^+$ and CD8$^+$ T cells. Interestingly, in similar studies featuring RSV challenge, Pribul and colleagues [56] found that macrophage depletion had no impact on virus-mediated T cell recruitment, weight loss or lung function, while Reed and colleagues [57] found that macrophage depletion prior to RSV challenge resulted in prominent airway occlusion in association with ongoing disease.

3.4. Toll-Like Receptors

Several studies have elucidated the nature and function of pattern recognition receptors (PRRs) that are involved in initiating the immune response to hRSV [58–60]. Despite findings that focused on hRSV signaling via TLR4, Faisca and colleagues [61] found that the sequelae of PVM infection—specifically, virus recovery, histopathology, body weight, and pulmonary function—were indistinguishable from one another when examined in wild-type and TLR4 gene-deleted mice. The results with the PVM model are consistent with recent findings from Marr and Turvey [62] who found that NF-kB activation mediated by infectious RSV particles in cell culture does not require the presence of a functional human TLR4/MD-2/CD14 complex.

Davidson and colleagues [63] utilized the PVM model to explore the role of TLR7 in promoting host defense against acute pneumovirus infection. Among their findings, PVM infection in TLR7 gene-deleted mice was associated with delayed induction of interferons and diminished recruitment of NK cells and neutrophils; adoptive transfer of TLR7-sufficient plasmacytoid dendritic cells restored innate antiviral responses and promoted virus clearance. Interestingly, TLR7-sufficient eosinophils also promote virus clearance in mouse models of RSV challenge [46].

3.5. Type I Interferons

Pneumoviruses have developed an efficient strategy to circumvent the host IFN response (reviewed in [64]). Among the most prominent of these findings, the non-structural NS1 and NS2 proteins of both human and bovine RSV inhibit the IFN alpha and beta (type I IFN) signaling pathways via several independent mechanisms [65–68], including degradation of the STAT2 signaling intermediate and blockade of activation and nuclear translocation of the transcription factor, interferon-regulatory factor 3.

Garvey and colleagues [54] were the first to evaluate the interactions of PVM and type I interferons in their study of the sequelae of virus infection in mice devoid of the receptor for type I interferons (IFNαβR$^{-/-}$ mice). PVM infection clearly elicited preferential expression of a wide spectrum of interferon-regulated and interferon-response genes, and virus replication *in vivo* was relatively suppressed in wild-type *vs.* IFNαβR$^{-/-}$ mice. However, paradoxically prolonged survival was observed among the IFNαβR$^{-/-}$ mice, which may be attributed to the overriding impact of differential inflammatory pathology. Among the most striking differences, the IFNαβR$^{-/-}$ mice developed tertiary mucosal associated lymphoid tissue (MALT, or B (bronchus) ALT) which has been associated with protection against virus pathogens in other settings (reviewed in [69]).

There are two studies that have directly addressed the role of PVM NS1 and NS2 using the recombinant virus (rPVM). In the first, Buchholz and colleagues [70] identified both NS1 and NS2 as virulence factors, as rPVMΔNS1 (*i.e.*, with the NS1 gene-deletion), and more notably, rPVMΔNS2, and rPVMΔNS1ΔNS2 replicate less efficiently in BALB/c mice than the parent wild-type rPVM, and resulted in fewer clinical symptoms. Interestingly, the ΔNS1 elicited production of both IFNα and IFNβ was indistinguishable from that of the parent rPVM; ΔNS2 and ΔNS1ΔNS2 gene-deleted viruses elicited higher levels of both IFNα and IFNβ than the parent rPVM at early time points during infection. In the second study, Heinze and colleagues [71] found that all three of the aforementioned deletion mutants replicated more effectively in IFNαβR$^{-/-}$ mice than they did in wild type mice; replication of the mutant viruses was further enhanced in mice devoid of both IFNαβR and IL28Rα, the receptor for the type III interferon, IFNλ.

4. Using the PVM Model to Explore Human Disease

4.1. Inflammation and Acute Infection

Among the primary reasons to explore respiratory virus infection using the PVM model is to improve our understanding of the molecular basis of severe disease so as to design novel therapeutic strategies. As a natural rodent pathogen, PVM undergoes robust virus replication in lung tissue [31]. However, we have found that even highly effective antiviral therapy—strategies such as systemic ribavirin that result in immediate cessation of all further virus replication—do not provide tangible benefits when one is evaluating morbidity and mortality as endpoints (reviewed in [72]). Indeed, our experience with the PVM model mirrors the human clinical observations with ribavirin use for RSV infection. Ribavirin was once administered routinely to infants hospitalized with RSV disease; and although it was quite effective as an antiviral, clinical benefits were not observed [73,74]. As such, the PVM model has provided the impetus to explore several specific immunomodulatory strategies. Among the most promising directions are combined antivirals and immunomodulatory blockade of the proinflammatory cytokine, MIP-1α [40,41]. Specifically, we have shown that antibody-mediated blockade of the actions of MIP-1α resulted in improved survival, from 20% in response to ribavirin alone to 60% in response to ribavirin together with anti-MIP-1α monoclonal antibody. Survival in response to acute PVM infection was also enhanced in response to increasing concentrations of metRANTES, which blocks MIP-1α signaling via its primary receptor, CCR1.

A similar study documented the effectiveness of ribavirin in PVM infection in conjunction with montelukast a cysteinyl-leukotriene inhibitor [75]. Neither agent was effective at reducing morbidity or mortality when administered alone. However, significant improvements in long-term survival were observed when provided as combined therapy. Interestingly, montelukast had little impact on neutrophil recruitment, suggesting that the presence of neutrophils alone does not indicate inevitable progression to intractable disease.

The chemerin/ChemR23 (also known as CMKLR1) pathway is another potential therapeutic target [76]. pDCs preferentially express chemerin and prochemerin is processed by neutrophil proteases. Given that pDCs and neutrophils play an important role in the physiopathology of viral infections of the lung, the role of chemerin/ChemR23 in PVM was investigated. PVM-infected ChemR23$^{-/-}$ mice responded with augmented neutrophil recruitment, delayed virus clearance, and higher rates of morbidity and mortality than wild type counterparts, a response suggesting the therapeutic value of supplementation with the activated adipokine, chemerin, during acute virus infection.

Glucocorticoids are in general use as potent and non-specific anti-inflammatory agents but have only limited benefit for the treatment of severe hRSV-associated inflammation [77–80]. We have shown that hydrocortisone therapy has no effect on the production of MIP-1α or on the influx of neutrophils during acute severe PVM infection. In fact, PVM-infected mice responded to hydrocortisone with enhanced viral replication and slightly accelerated mortality [81] suggesting that the added immunosupression of glucocortcoids in this context contributed to illness severity.

Bem and colleagues [82] explored the impact of mechanical ventilation on the acute inflammatory response in mice infected with PVM. In addition to increased levels of cytokines in the airways, mechanical ventilation activated caspase-dependent cell death pathways leading to acute lung injury in PVM-infected mice. In a subsequent study, van den Berg and colleagues [83] found that inflammatory injuries associated with mechanical ventilation were less severe in *lpr* (Fas-deficient) mice although all mice ultimately succumbed to infection.

4.2. Asthma and Allergic Airway Disease

The role of respiratory virus infection in promoting and exacerbating asthma and existing respiratory allergies is an area of significant medical concern [84,85]. Siegle and colleagues [86,87] have used PVM to determine how recovery from a respiratory virus infection early in life might alter subsequent responses to an unrelated allergen. Mice that recovered from a sublethal PVM infection displayed an exaggerated Th2 response to a chronic intranasal ovalbumin sensitization followed by a moderate challenge, with elevated levels of serum IgE and augmented expression of IL-4, IL-5 and IL-13; these responses were suppressed by a combination of neutralizing antibodies against both IL-4 and IL-25. Similarly, Barends and colleagues [88] found that PVM could exacerbate an ongoing allergic response. When PVM was administered to sensitized mice together with an intranasal antigen challenge, the virions elicited augmented eosinophil recruitment together with local elevation of Th2 cytokines.

4.3. Vaccines

The first RSV vaccination trial, performed in the early 1960s with a formalin-inactivated preparation (FI-RSV, lot 100) resulted in an aberrant deleterious response following natural hRSV infection. Numerous vaccinated infants developed severe respiratory complications from subsequent natural RSV infection including two deaths, a phenomenon later referred to as "enhanced disease" [89]. Enhanced disease has been studied extensively, and has been modeled in BALB/c mice inoculated with formalin-inactivated RSV and RSV virion components (reviewed in [90,91]). PVM antigens, when prepared and administered in a manner analogous to the hRSV lot 100 vaccine also induces the enhanced disease response, likewise characterized by elevated levels of Th2 cytokines and eosinophil recruitment to airways and lung tissue [92]. Interestingly, the eosinophils, long perceived to be the cells promoting respiratory pathology in this setting, had no impact on virus recovery or weight loss in this experimental model.

Enhanced disease observed during the FI-RSV lot 100 study was among the issues that constrained further progress in the development of an RSV vaccine. Now, several decades later, a small number of human infant RSV vaccine trials are underway. Among the current vaccines under study, recent success with recombinant rodent Sendai virus (SeV) used to deliver RSV antigens [93,94] suggests that a similar approach may be feasible utilizing recombinant PVM [9,71]. Most recently, van Helden and colleagues [95] used the PVM model to explore the role of antigen-specific CD8$^+$ T cells as a useful vaccine strategy. Among their findings, adoptive transfer of PVM-specific CD8$^+$ T cells do provide at least partial protection against acute pneumovirus disease, and do not appear to contribute to immunopathology.

4.4. Heterologous Immunity

As part of an exploration of the immunomodulatory potential of probiotic *Lactobacillus* strains, we found that wild-type mice primed via intranasal inoculation with *Lactobacillus plantarum* or *Lactobacillus reuteri* were fully protected against lethal sequelae of a subsequent PVM infection ([96], Figure 3). These findings are a particularly robust example of heterologous immunity, a concept recently introduced into the literature that explains observations such as this, in which increased resistance (or susceptibility) to an unrelated (*i.e.*, not cross-reactive) pathogen can be observed upon recovery from an inflammatory insult [97–99]. There are a number of examples in which PVM has been featured as a target pathogen in studies of heterologous immunity. One such study is that of Wiley and colleagues [100] who elicited protection against PVM (within a larger series of respiratory viruses) via instillation of protein cage nanoparticles, which are multi-subunit homopolymers of unique heat shock proteins from the thermophilic bacterium, *Methanocaldococcus jannaschii*). Likewise, Easton and colleagues [101] found that inoculation of mice with the defective interfering (DI) deletion mutant influenza 244/PR8 protects against subsequent infection with PVM. Interestingly, although each of these initial priming events—*Lactobacillus*, nanoparticles or defective interfering virus—all lead to a shared outcome, specifically, protection from the lethal sequelae of PVM infection, the cellular and biochemical mechanisms promoting these responses are unique and stimulus-specific [102].

Figure 3. (**A**) Mice primed via intranasal inoculation with *L. plantarum* or *L. reuteri* are fully (100%) protected from the lethal sequelae of PVM infection. (**B**) Prolonged survival and significant long-term protection results even when virus challenge was delayed until 91 days (3 months) after initial *Lactobacillus*-mediated priming. Reprinted with permission from [96].

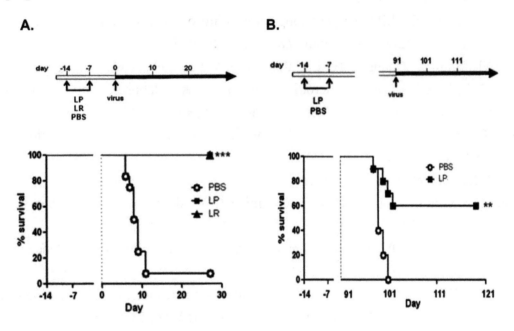

5. Conclusions

The PVM model holds great promise for the elucidation of inflammatory mechanisms associated with pneumovirus infection. Studies carried out to date have provided a rationale for the use of chemokine and/or chemokine receptor blockade alone and/or in conjunction with appropriate antiviral therapy as a means to reduce the inflammatory pathology in severe pneumovirus disease. Likewise, PVM is an excellent system in which to explore the molecular mechanisms of heterologous immunity to pneumovirus infection, information that may assist in the development of vaccines and other novel prevention strategies.

Acknowledgments

Funding for this work was provided by the NIAID Division of Intramural Research (AI000943 to HFR) and from the Children's Miracle Network of NY (to JBD).

References

1. Easton, A.J.; Domachowske, J.B.; Rosenberg, H.F. Animal pneumoviruses: Molecular genetics and pathogenesis. *Clin. Microbiol. Rev.* **2004**, *17*, 390–412.

2. Horsfall, F.L.; Hahn, R.G. A latent virus in normal mice capable of producing pneumonia in its natural host. *J. Exp. Med.* **1940**, *71*, 391–408.

3. Miyata, H.; Kishikawa, M.; Kondo, H.; Kai, C.; Watanabe, Y.; Ohsawa, K.; Sato, H. New isolates of pneumonia virus of mice (PVM) from Japanese rat colonies and their characterization. *Exp. Anim.* **1995**, *44*, 95–104.

4. Zenner, L.; Regnault, J.P. Ten-year long monitoring of laboratory mouse and rat colonies in French facilities: A retrospective study. *Lab. Anim.* **2000**, *34*, 76–83.

5. Liang, C.T.; Shih, A.; Chang, Y.H.; Liu, C.W.; Lee, Y.T.; Hsieh, W.C.; Huang, Y.L.; Huang, W.T.; Kuang, C.H.; Lee, K.H.; *et al.* Microbial contaminations of laboratory mice and rats in Taiwan from 2004 to 2007. *J. Am. Assoc. Lab. Anim. Sci.* **2009**, *48*, 381–386.

6. Kaplan, C.; Healing, T.D.; Evans, N.; Healing, L.; Prior, A. Evidence of infection by viruses in small British field rodents. *J. Hyg.* **1980**, *84*, 285–294.

7. Smith, A.L.; Singleton, G.R.; Hansen, G.M.; Shellam, G. A serologic survey for viruses and Mycoplasma pulmonis among wild house mice (Mus domesticus) in southeastern Australia. *J. Wildl. Dis.* **1993**, *29*, 219–229.

8. Pringle, C.R.; Eglin, R.P. Murine pneumonia virus: Seroepidemiological evidence of widespread human infection. *J. Gen. Virol.* **1986**, *67*, 975–982.

9. Brock, L.G.; Karron, R.A.; Krempl, C.D.; Collins, P.L.; Buchholz, U.J. Evaluation of pneumonia virus of mice as a possible human pathogen. *J. Virol.* **2012**, *86*, 5829–5843.

10. Renshaw, R.; Laverack, M.; Zylich, N.; Glaser, A.; Dubovi, E. Genomic analysis of a pneumovirus isolated from dogs with acute respiratory disease. *Vet. Microbiol.* **2011**, *150*, 88–95.

11. Renshaw, R.W.; Zylich, N.C.; Laverack, M.A.; Glaser, A.L.; Dubovi, E.J. Pneumovirus in dogs with acute respiratory disease. *Emerg. Infect. Dis.* **2010**, *16*, 993–995.

12. Percopo, C.M.; Dubovi, E.J.; Renshaw, R.W.; Dyer, K.D.; Domachowske, J.B.; Rosenberg, H.F. Canine pneumovirus replicates in mouse lung tissue and elicits inflammatory pathology. *Virology* **2011**, *416*, 26–31.

13. Ginsberg, H.S.; Horsfall, F.L., Jr. Concurrent infection with influenza virus and mumps virus or pneumonia virus of mice as bearing on the inhibition of virus multiplication by bacterial polysaccharides. *J. Exp. Med.* **1949**, *89*, 37–52.

14. Ginsberg, H.S.; Horsfall, F.L., Jr. Therapy of infection with pneumonia virus of mice (PVM); effect of a polysaccharide on the multiplication cycles of the virus and on the course of the viral pneumonia. *J. Exp. Med.* **1951**, *93*, 161–171.

15. Horsfall, F.L., Jr.; Ginsberg, H.S. The dependence of the pathological lesion upon the multiplication of pneumonia virus of mice (PVM); kinetic relation between the degree of viral multiplication and the extent of pneumonia. *J. Exp. Med.* **1951**, *93*, 139–150.

16. Thorpe, L.C.; Easton, A.J. Genome sequence of the non-pathogenic strain 15 of pneumonia virus of mice and comparison with the genome of the pathogenic strain J3666. *J. Gen. Virol.* **2005**, *86*, 159–169.

17. Ellis, J.A.; Martin, B.V.; Waldner, C.; Dyer, K.D.; Domachowske, J.B.; Rosenberg, H.F. Mucosal inoculation with an attenuated mouse pneumovirus strain protects against virulent challenge in wild type and interferon-gamma receptor deficient mice. *Vaccine* **2007**, *25*, 1085–1095.

18. Easton, A.J. University of Warwick, Coventry, UK. Personal communication, 1997.

19. Ahmadian, G.; Chambers, P.; Easton, A.J. Detection and characterization of proteins encoded by the second ORF of the M2 gene of pneumoviruses. *J. Gen. Virol.* **1999**, *80*, 2011–2016.

20. Barr, J.; Easton, A.J. Characterisation of the interaction between the nucleoprotein and phosphoprotein of pneumonia virus of mice. *Virus Res.* **1995**, *39*, 221–235.

21. Chambers, P.; Pringle, C.R.; Easton, A.J. Sequence analysis of the gene encoding the fusion glycoprotein of pneumonia virus of mice suggests possible conserved secondary structure elements in paramyxovirus fusion glycoproteins. *J. Gen. Virol.* **1992**, *73*, 1717–1724.

22. Easton, A.J.; Chambers, P. Nucleotide sequence of the genes encoding the matrix and small hydrophobic proteins of pneumonia virus of mice. *Virus Res.* **1997**, *48*, 27–33.

23. Krempl, C.D.; Collins, P.L. Reevaluation of the virulence of prototypic strain 15 of pneumonia virus of mice. *J. Virol.* **2004**, *78*, 13362–13365.

24. Krempl, C.D.; Wnekowicz, A.; Lamirande, E.W.; Nayebagha, G.; Collins, P.L.; Buchholz, U.J. Identification of a novel virulence factor in recombinant pneumonia virus of mice. *J. Virol.* **2007**, *81*, 9490–9501.

25. Anh, D.B.; Faisca, P.; Desmecht, D.J. Differential resistance/susceptibility patterns to pneumovirus infection among inbred mouse strains. *Am. J. Physiol. Lung Cell Mol. Physiol.* **2006**, *291*, L426–L435.

26. Glineur, S.; Tran Anh, D.B.; Sarlet, M.; Michaux, C.; Desmecht, D. Characterization of the resistance of SJL/J mice to pneumonia virus of mice, a model for infantile bronchiolitis due to a respiratory syncytial virus. *PLoS One* **2012**, *7*, e44581.

27. Weir, E.C.; Brownstein, D.G.; Smith, A.L.; Johnson, E.A. Respiratory disease and wasting in athymic mice infected with pneumonia virus of mice. *Lab. Anim. Sci.* **1988**, *38*, 133–137.

28. Roths, J.B.; Smith, A.L.; Sidman, C.L. Lethal exacerbation of Pneumocystis carinii pneumonia in severe combined immunodeficiency mice after infection by pneumonia virus of mice. *J. Exp. Med.* **1993**, *177*, 1193–1198.

29. Compton, C. Yale University, New Haven, CT, USA. Personal communication, 2012.

30. Bem, R.A.; Domachowske, J.B.; Rosenberg, H.F. Animal models of human respiratory syncytial virus disease. *Am. J. Physiol. Lung Cell Mol. Physiol.* **2011**, *301*, L148–L156.

31. Rosenberg, H.F.; Domachowske, J.B. Pneumonia virus of mice: Severe respiratory infection in a natural host. *Immunol. Lett.* **2008**, *118*, 6–12.

32. Domachowske, J.B.; Bonville, C.A.; Dyer, K.D.; Easton, A.J.; Rosenberg, H.F. Pulmonary eosinophilia and production of MIP-1alpha are prominent responses to infection with pneumonia virus of mice. *Cell Immunol.* **2000**, *200*, 98–104.

33. Domachowske, J.B.; Bonville, C.A.; Gao, J.L.; Murphy, P.M.; Easton, A.J.; Rosenberg, H.F. The chemokine macrophage-inflammatory protein-1 alpha and its receptor CCR1 control pulmonary inflammation and antiviral host defense in paramyxovirus infection. *J. Immunol.* **2000**, *165*, 2677–2682.

34. Bonville, C.A.; Bennett, N.J.; Koehnlein, M.; Haines, D.M.; Ellis, J.A.; DelVecchio, A.M.; Rosenberg, H.F.; Domachowske, J.B. Respiratory dysfunction and proinflammatory chemokines in the pneumonia virus of mice (PVM) model of viral bronchiolitis. *Virology* **2006**, *349*, 87–95.

35. Welliver, T.P.; Garofalo, R.P.; Hosakote, Y.; Hintz, K.H.; Avendano, L.; Sanchez, K.; Velozo, L.; Jafri, H.; Chavez-Bueno, S.; Ogra, P.L.; *et al.* Severe human lower respiratory tract illness caused by respiratory syncytial virus and influenza virus is characterized by the absence of pulmonary cytotoxic lymphocyte responses. *J. Infect. Dis.* **2007**, *195*, 1126–1136.

36. Domachowske, J.B.; Bonville, C.A.; Rosenberg, H.F. Animal models for studying respiratory syncytial virus infection and its long term effects on lung function. *Pediatr. Infect. Dis. J.* **2004**, *23*, S228–S234.

37. Bonville, C.A.; Bennett, N.J.; Percopo, C.M.; Branigan, P.J.; Del Vecchio, A.M.; Rosenberg, H.F.; Domachowske, J.B. Diminished inflammatory responses to natural pneumovirus infection among older mice. *Virology* **2007**, *368*, 182–190.

38. Bonville, C.A.; Ptaschinski, C.; Percopo, C.M.; Rosenberg, H.F.; Domachowske, J.B. Inflammatory responses to acute pneumovirus infection in neonatal mice. *Virol. J.* **2010**, *7*, 320.

39. Cook, D.N.; Beck, M.A.; Coffman, T.M.; Kirby, S.L.; Sheridan, J.F.; Pragnell, I.B.; Smithies, O. Requirement of MIP-1 alpha for an inflammatory response to viral infection. *Science* **1995**, *269*, 1583–1585.

40. Bonville, C.A.; Easton, A.J.; Rosenberg, H.F.; Domachowske, J.B. Altered pathogenesis of severe pneumovirus infection in response to combined antiviral and specific immunomodulatory agents. *J. Virol.* **2003**, *77*, 1237–1244.

41. Bonville, C.A.; Lau, V.K.; DeLeon, J.M.; Gao, J.L.; Easton, A.J.; Rosenberg, H.F.; Domachowske, J.B. Functional antagonism of chemokine receptor CCR1 reduces mortality in acute pneumovirus infection *in vivo. J. Virol.* **2004**, *78*, 7984–7989.

42. Rosenberg, H.F.; Dyer, K.D.; Domachowske, J.B. Eosinophils and their interactions with respiratory virus pathogens. *Immunol. Res.* **2009**, *43*, 128–137.

43. Rosenberg, H.F.; Dyer, K.D.; Domachowske, J.B. Respiratory viruses and eosinophils: Exploring the connections. *Antivir. Res.* **2009**, *83*, 1–9.

44. Rosenberg, H.F.; Dyer, K.D.; Foster, P.S. Eosinophils: Changing perspectives in health and disease. *Nat. Rev. Immunol.* **2013**, *13*, 9–22.

45. Adamko, D.J.; Yost, B.L.; Gleich, G.J.; Fryer, A.D.; Jacoby, D.B. Ovalbumin sensitization changes the inflammatory response to subsequent parainfluenza infection. Eosinophils mediate airway hyperresponsiveness, m(2) muscarinic receptor dysfunction, and antiviral effects. *J. Exp. Med.* **1999**, *190*, 1465–1478.

46. Phipps, S.; Lam, C.E.; Mahalingam, S.; Newhouse, M.; Ramirez, R.; Rosenberg, H.F.; Foster, P.S.; Matthaei, K.I. Eosinophils contribute to innate antiviral immunity and promote clearance of respiratory syncytial virus. *Blood* **2007**, *110*, 1578–1586.

47. Percopo, C.M.; Dyer, K.D.; Ochkur, S.I.; Lee, J.J.; Domachowske, J.B.; Rosenberg, H.F. Activated eosinophils protect against lethal respiratory virus infection. *J. Immunol.* **2013**, to be submitted for publication.

48. Dyer, K.D.; Percopo, C.M.; Fischer, E.R.; Gabryszewski, S.J.; Rosenberg, H.F. Pneumoviruses infect eosinophils and elicit MyD88-dependent release of chemoattractant cytokines and interleukin-6. *Blood* **2009**, *114*, 2649–2656.

49. Frey, S.; Krempl, C.D.; Schmitt-Graff, A.; Ehl, S. Role of T cells in virus control and disease after infection with pneumonia virus of mice. *J. Virol.* **2008**, *82*, 11619–11627.

50. Claassen, E.A.; van der Kant, P.A.; Rychnavska, Z.S.; van Bleek, G.M.; Easton, A.J.; van der Most, R.G. Activation and inactivation of antiviral CD8 T cell responses during murine pneumovirus infection. *J. Immunol.* **2005**, *175*, 6597–6604.

51. Chang, J.; Braciale, T.J. Respiratory syncytial virus infection suppresses lung CD8+ T-cell effector activity and peripheral CD8+ T-cell memory in the respiratory tract. *Nat. Med.* **2002**, *8*, 54–60.

52. Claassen, E.A.; van Bleek, G.M.; Rychnavska, Z.S.; de Groot, R.J.; Hensen, E.J.; Tijhaar, E.J.; van Eden, W.; van der Most, R.G. Identification of a CD4 T cell epitope in the pneumonia virus of mice glycoprotein and characterization of its role in protective immunity. *Virology* **2007**, *368*, 17–25.

53. Spolski, R.; Wang, L.; Wan, C.K.; Bonville, C.A.; Domachowske, J.B.; Kim, H.P.; Yu, Z.; Leonard, W.J. IL-21 promotes the pathologic immune response to pneumovirus infection. *J. Immunol.* **2012**, *188*, 1924–1932.

54. Garvey, T.L.; Dyer, K.D.; Ellis, J.A.; Bonville, C.A.; Foster, B.; Prussin, C.; Easton, A.J.; Domachowske, J.B.; Rosenberg, H.F. Inflammatory responses to pneumovirus infection in IFN-alpha beta R gene-deleted mice. *J. Immunol.* **2005**, *175*, 4735–4744.

55. Rigaux, P.; Killoran, K.E.; Qiu, Z.; Rosenberg, H.F. Depletion of alveolar macrophages prolongs survival in response to acute pneumovirus infection. *Virology* **2012**, *422*, 338–345.

56. Pribul, P.K.; Harker, J.; Wang, B.; Wang, H.; Tregoning, J.S.; Schwarze, J.; Openshaw, P.J. Alveolar macrophages are a major determinant of early responses to viral lung infection but do not influence subsequent disease development. *J. Virol.* **2008**, *82*, 4441–4448.

57. Reed, J.L.; Brewah, Y.A.; Delaney, T.; Welliver, T.; Burwell, T.; Benjamin, E.; Kuta, E.; Kozhich, A.; McKinney, L.; Suzich, J.; *et al.* Macrophage impairment underlies airway occlusion in primary respiratory syncytial virus bronchiolitis. *J. Infect. Dis.* **2008**, *198*, 1783–1793.

58. Klein Klouwenberg, P.; Tan, L.; Werkman, W.; van Bleek, G.M.; Coenjaerts, F. The role of Toll-like receptors in regulating the immune response against respiratory syncytial virus. *Crit. Rev. Immunol.* **2009**, *29*, 531–550.

59. Kurt-Jones, E.A.; Popova, L.; Kwinn, L.; Haynes, L.M.; Jones, L.P.; Tripp, R.A.; Walsh, E.E.; Freeman, M.W.; Golenbock, D.T.; Anderson, L.J.; *et al.* Pattern recognition receptors TLR4 and CD14 mediate response to respiratory syncytial virus. *Nat. Immunol.* **2000**, *1*, 398–401.

60. Ehl, S.; Bischoff, R.; Ostler, T.; Vallbracht, S.; Schulte-Monting, J.; Poltorak, A.; Freudenberg, M. The role of Toll-like receptor 4 *versus* interleukin-12 in immunity to respiratory syncytial virus. *Eur. J. Immunol.* **2004**, *34*, 1146–1153.

61. Faisca, P.; Tran Anh, D.B.; Thomas, A.; Desmecht, D. Suppression of pattern-recognition receptor TLR4 sensing does not alter lung responses to pneumovirus infection. *Microbes Infect.* **2006**, *8*, 621–627.

62. Marr, N.; Turvey, S.E. Role of human TLR4 in respiratory syncytial virus-induced NF-kappaB activation, viral entry and replication. *Innate Immun.* **2012**, *18*, 856–865.

63. Davidson, S.; Kaiko, G.; Loh, Z.; Lalwani, A.; Zhang, V.; Spann, K.; Foo, S.Y.; Hansbro, N.; Uematsu, S.; Akira, S.; *et al.* Plasmacytoid dendritic cells promote host defense against acute pneumovirus infection via the TLR7-MyD88-dependent signaling pathway. *J. Immunol.* **2011**, *186*, 5938–5948.

64. Fontana, J.M.; Bankamp, B.; Rota, P.A. Inhibition of interferon induction and signaling by paramyxoviruses. *Immunol. Rev.* **2008**, *225*, 46–67.

65. Bossert, B.; Conzelmann, K.K. Respiratory syncytial virus (RSV) nonstructural (NS) proteins as host range determinants: A chimeric bovine RSV with NS genes from human RSV is attenuated in interferon-competent bovine cells. *J. Virol.* **2002**, *76*, 4287–4293.

66. Ramaswamy, M.; Shi, L.; Monick, M.M.; Hunninghake, G.W.; Look, D.C. Specific inhibition of type I interferon signal transduction by respiratory syncytial virus. *Am. J. Respir. Cell Mol. Biol.* **2004**, *30*, 893–900.

67. Schlender, J.; Hornung, V.; Finke, S.; Gunthner-Biller, M.; Marozin, S.; Brzozka, K.; Moghim, S.; Endres, S.; Hartmann, G.; Conzelmann, K.K. Inhibition of toll-like receptor 7- and 9-mediated alpha/beta interferon production in human plasmacytoid dendritic cells by respiratory syncytial virus and measles virus. *J. Virol.* **2005**, *79*, 5507–5515.

68. Spann, K.M.; Tran, K.C.; Chi, B.; Rabin, R.L.; Collins, P.L. Suppression of the induction of alpha, beta, and lambda interferons by the NS1 and NS2 proteins of human respiratory syncytial virus in human epithelial cells and macrophages [corrected]. *J. Virol.* **2004**, *78*, 4363–4369.

69. Randall, T.D. Bronchus-associated lymphoid tissue (BALT) structure and function. *Adv. Immunol.* **2010**, *107*, 187–241.

70. Buchholz, U.J.; Ward, J.M.; Lamirande, E.W.; Heinze, B.; Krempl, C.D.; Collins, P.L. Deletion of nonstructural proteins NS1 and NS2 from pneumonia virus of mice attenuates viral replication and reduces pulmonary cytokine expression and disease. *J. Virol.* **2009**, *83*, 1969–1980.

71. Heinze, B.; Frey, S.; Mordstein, M.; Schmitt-Graff, A.; Ehl, S.; Buchholz, U.J.; Collins, P.L.; Staeheli, P.; Krempl, C.D. Both nonstructural proteins NS1 and NS2 of pneumonia virus of mice are inhibitors of the interferon type I and type III responses *in vivo*. *J. Virol.* **2011**, *85*, 4071–4084.

72. Rosenberg, H.F.; Domachowske, J.B. Inflammatory responses to respiratory syncytial virus (RSV) infection and the development of immunomodulatory pharmacotherapeutics. *Curr. Med. Chem.* **2012**, *19*, 1424–1431.

73. Reassessment of the indications for ribavirin therapy in respiratory syncytial virus infections. American Academy of Pediatrics Committee on Infectious Diseases. *Pediatrics* **1996**, *97*, 137–140.

74. Van Woensel, J.B.; Kimpen, J.L.; Brand, P.L. Respiratory tract infections caused by respiratory syncytial virus in children. Diagnosis and treatment. *Minerva Pediatr.* **2001**, *53*, 99–106.

75. Bonville, C.A.; Rosenberg, H.F.; Domachowske, J.B. Ribavirin and cysteinyl leukotriene-1 receptor blockade as treatment for severe bronchiolitis. *Antivir. Res.* **2006**, *69*, 53–59.

76. Bondue, B.; Vosters, O.; de Nadai, P.; Glineur, S.; de Henau, O.; Luangsay, S.; van Gool, F.; Communi, D.; de Vuyst, P.; Desmecht, D.; *et al.* ChemR23 dampens lung inflammation and enhances anti-viral immunity in a mouse model of acute viral pneumonia. *PLoS Pathog.* **2011**, *7*, e1002358.

77. Buckingham, S.C.; Jafri, H.S.; Bush, A.J.; Carubelli, C.M.; Sheeran, P.; Hardy, R.D.; Ottolini, M.G.; Ramilo, O.; DeVincenzo, J.P. A randomized, double-blind, placebo-controlled trial of dexamethasone in severe respiratory syncytial virus (RSV) infection: Effects on RSV quantity and clinical outcome. *J. Infect. Dis.* **2002**, *185*, 1222–1228.

78. Patel, H.; Platt, R.; Lozano, J.M.; Wang, E.E. Glucocorticoids for acute viral bronchiolitis in infants and young children. *Cochrane Database Syst. Rev.* **2004**, CD004878.

79. Van Woensel, J.B.; Lutter, R.; Biezeveld, M.H.; Dekker, T.; Nijhuis, M.; van Aalderen, W.M.; Kuijpers, T.W. Effect of dexamethasone on tracheal viral load and interleukin-8 tracheal concentration in children with respiratory syncytial virus infection. *Pediatr. Infect. Dis. J.* **2003**, *22*, 721–726.

80. Van Woensel, J.B.; van Aalderen, W.M.; de Weerd, W.; Jansen, N.J.; van Gestel, J.P.; Markhorst, D.G.; van Vught, A.J.; Bos, A.P.; Kimpen, J.L. Dexamethasone for treatment of patients mechanically ventilated for lower respiratory tract infection caused by respiratory syncytial virus. *Thorax* **2003**, *58*, 383–387.

81. Domachowske, J.B.; Bonville, C.A.; Ali-Ahmad, D.; Dyer, K.D.; Easton, A.J.; Rosenberg, H.F. Glucocorticoid administration accelerates mortality of pneumovirus-infected mice. *J. Infect. Dis.* **2001**, *184*, 1518–1523.

82. Bem, R.A.; van Woensel, J.B.; Bos, A.P.; Koski, A.; Farnand, A.W.; Domachowske, J.B.; Rosenberg, H.F.; Martin, T.R.; Matute-Bello, G. Mechanical ventilation enhances lung inflammation and caspase activity in a model of mouse pneumovirus infection. *Am. J. Physiol. Lung Cell Mol. Physiol.* **2009**, *296*, L46–56.

83. Van den Berg, E.; van Woensel, J.B.; Bos, A.P.; Bem, R.A.; Altemeier, W.A.; Gill, S.E.; Martin, T.R.; Matute-Bello, G. Role of the Fas/FasL system in a model of RSV infection in mechanically ventilated mice. *Am. J. Physiol. Lung Cell Mol. Physiol.* **2011**, *301*, L451–L460.

84. Lukacs, N.W.; Smit, J.; Lindell, D.; Schaller, M. Respiratory syncytial virus-induced pulmonary disease and exacerbation of allergic asthma. *Contrib. Microbiol.* **2007**, *14*, 68–82.

85. Xepapadaki, P.; Papadopoulos, N.G. Viral infections and allergies. *Immunobiology* **2007**, *212*, 453–459.

86. Siegle, J.S.; Hansbro, N.; Dong, C.; Angkasekwinai, P.; Foster, P.S.; Kumar, R.K. Blocking induction of T helper type 2 responses prevents development of disease in a model of childhood asthma. *Clin. Exp. Immunol.* **2011**, *165*, 19–28.

87. Siegle, J.S.; Hansbro, N.; Herbert, C.; Rosenberg, H.F.; Domachowske, J.B.; Asquith, K.L.; Foster, P.S.; Kumar, R.K. Early-life viral infection and allergen exposure interact to induce an asthmatic phenotype in mice. *Respir. Res.* **2010**, *11*, 14.

88. Barends, M.; de Rond, L.G.; Dormans, J.; van Oosten, M.; Boelen, A.; Neijens, H.J.; Osterhaus, A.D.; Kimman, T.G. Respiratory syncytial virus, pneumonia virus of mice, and influenza A virus differently affect respiratory allergy in mice. *Clin. Exp. Allergy* **2004**, *34*, 488–496.

89. Kapikian, A.Z.; Mitchell, R.H.; Chanock, R.M.; Shvedoff, R.A.; Stewart, C.E. An epidemiologic study of altered clinical reactivity to respiratory syncytial (RS) virus infection in children previously vaccinated with an inactivated RS virus vaccine. *Am. J. Epidemiol.* **1969**, *89*, 405–421.

90. Castilow, E.M.; Olson, M.R.; Meyerholz, D.K.; Varga, S.M. Differential role of gamma interferon in inhibiting pulmonary eosinophilia and exacerbating systemic disease in fusion protein-immunized mice undergoing challenge infection with respiratory syncytial virus. *J. Virol.* **2008**, *82*, 2196–2207.

91. Castilow, E.M.; Olson, M.R.; Varga, S.M. Understanding respiratory syncytial virus (RSV) vaccine-enhanced disease. *Immunol. Res.* **2007**, *39*, 225–239.

92. Percopo, C.M.; Qiu, Z.J.; Phipps, S.; Foster, P.S.; Domachowske, J.B.; Rosenberg, H.F. Pulmonary eosinophils and their role in immunopathologic responses to formalin-inactivated pneumonia virus of mice. *J. Immunol.* **2009**, *183*, 604–612.

93. Hurwitz, J.L. Respiratory syncytial virus vaccine development. *Expert Rev. Vaccines.* **2011**, *10*, 1415–1433.

94. Jones, B.G.; Sealy, R.E.; Rudraraju, R.; Traina-Dorge, V.L.; Finneyfrock, B.; Cook, A.; Takimoto, T.; Portner, A.; Hurwitz, J.L. Sendai virus-based RSV vaccine protects African green monkeys from RSV infection. *Vaccine* **2012**, *30*, 959–968.

95. Van Helden, M.J.; van Kooten, P.J.; Bekker, C.P.; Grone, A.; Topham, D.J.; Easton, A.J.; Boog, C.J.; Busch, D.H.; Zaiss, D.M.; Sijts, A.J. Pre-existing virus-specific CD8(+) T-cells provide protection against pneumovirus-induced disease in mice. *Vaccine* **2012**, *30*, 6382–6388.

96. Gabryszewski, S.J.; Bachar, O.; Dyer, K.D.; Percopo, C.M.; Killoran, K.E.; Domachowske, J.B.; Rosenberg, H.F. Lactobacillus-mediated priming of the respiratory mucosa protects against lethal pneumovirus infection. *J. Immunol.* **2011**, *186*, 1151–1161.

97. Didierlaurent, A.; Goulding, J.; Hussell, T. The impact of successive infections on the lung microenvironment. *Immunology* **2007**, *122*, 457–465.

98. Goulding, J.; Snelgrove, R.; Saldana, J.; Didierlaurent, A.; Cavanagh, M.; Gwyer, E.; Wales, J.; Wissinger, E.L.; Hussell, T. Respiratory infections: Do we ever recover? *Proc. Am. Thorac. Soc.* **2007**, *4*, 618–625.

99. Hussell, T.; Cavanagh, M.M. The innate immune rheostat: Influence on lung inflammatory disease and secondary bacterial pneumonia. *Biochem. Soc. Trans.* **2009**, *37*, 811–813.

100. Wiley, J.A.; Richert, L.E.; Swain, S.D.; Harmsen, A.; Barnard, D.L.; Randall, T.D.; Jutila, M.; Douglas, T.; Broomell, C.; Young, M. Inducible Bronchus-associated lymphoid tissue elicited by a protein cage nanoparticle enhances protection in mice against diverse respiratory viruses. *PLoS One* **2009**, *4*, e7142.

101. Easton, A.J.; Scott, P.D.; Edworthy, N.L.; Meng, B.; Marriott, A.C.; Dimmock, N.J. A novel broad-spectrum treatment for respiratory virus infections: Influenza-based defective interfering virus provides protection against pneumovirus infection *in vivo*. *Vaccine* **2011**, *29*, 2777–2784.

102. Garcia-Crespo, K.E.; Chan, C.C.; Gabryszewski, S.J.; Percopo, C.M.; Rigaux, P.; Dyer, K.D.; Domachowske, J.B.; Rosenberg, H.F. Lactobacillus priming of the respiratory tract: Heterologous immunity and protection against lethal pneumovirus infection. *Antivir. Res.* **2013**, *97*, 270–279.

11

Human Metapneumovirus in Adults

Lenneke E. M. Haas [1],*, **Steven F. T. Thijsen** [2], **Leontine van Elden** [3] **and Karen A. Heemstra** [2]

[1] Department of Intensive Care Medicine, Diakonessenhuis, Utrecht, 3582 KE, The Netherlands
[2] Department of Microbiology, Diakonessenhuis, Utrecht, 3582 KE, The Netherlands;
     E-Mails: sthijsen@diakhuis.nl (S.F.T.T.); K.A.Heemstra@umcutrecht.nl (K.A.H.)
[3] Department of Pulmonary Diseases, Diakonessenhuis, Utrecht, 3582 KE, The Netherlands;
     E-Mail: lvelden@diakhuis.nl

* Author to whom correspondence should be addressed; E-Mail: lvlelyveld@diakhuis.nl

Abstract: Human metapneumovirus (HMPV) is a relative newly described virus. It was first isolated in 2001 and currently appears to be one of the most significant and common human viral infections. Retrospective serologic studies demonstrated the presence of HMPV antibodies in humans more than 50 years earlier. Although the virus was primarily known as causative agent of respiratory tract infections in children, HMPV is an important cause of respiratory infections in adults as well. Almost all children are infected by HMPV below the age of five; the repeated infections throughout life indicate transient immunity. HMPV infections usually are mild and self-limiting, but in the frail elderly and the immunocompromised patients, the clinical course can be complicated. Since culturing the virus is relatively difficult, diagnosis is mostly based on a nucleic acid amplification test, such as reverse transcriptase polymerase chain reaction. To date, no vaccine is available and treatment is supportive. However, ongoing research shows encouraging results. The aim of this paper is to review the current literature concerning HMPV infections in adults, and discuss recent development in treatment and vaccination.

Keywords: human metapneumovirus; HMPV; respiratory tract infection; adults; intensive care; diagnosis; treatment; vaccination

Abbreviations

HMPV	human metapneumovirus
RTI	respiratory tract infection
NAAT	nucleic acid amplification test
HRSV	human respiratory syncytial virus
COPD	chronic obstructive pulmonary disease
RT-PCR	reverse transcriptase polymerase chain reaction assay
CE	Conformité Européenne
FDA	Food and Drug Administration
EIA	enzyme immuno-assay
ELISA	enzyme-linked immunosorbent assay
IFA	direct immunofluorescent-antibody test
ICU	intensive care unit
RNAi	RNA interference
miRNA	microRNA
siRNA	small interfering RNA
HSCT	hematopoietic stem cell transplant
CAP	community acquired pneumonia

1. Introduction

The most common illness experienced by people of all ages worldwide is an acute respiratory tract infection (RTI). It is a leading cause of mortality and morbidity worldwide. Viruses are responsible for a large proportion of RTI's [1]. A significant portion of the infections with viral etiology can be attributed to the human metapneumovirus (HMPV), also in adults [2–9].

HMPV was first identified in the Netherlands in 2001, but serologic studies of antibodies against HMPV indicate that the virus is not new and circulated in humans for at least 50 years [4].

The aim of this paper is to review the current literature concerning HMPV infections in adults, and discuss recent development in treatment and vaccination.

2. Virology

HMPV is classified as the first human member of the *Metapneumovirus* genus in the *Pneumovirinae* subfamily within the *Paramyxoviridae* family. It is an enveloped negative-sense single-stranded RNA virus. The RNA genome includes 8 genes coding for 9 different proteins. HMPV is identical in gene order to the avian pneumovirus (AMPV), which also belongs to the *Metapneumovirus* genus [10].

Phylogenetic analysis has identified two genotypes of HMPV, namely A and B [4]. Both genotypes may co-circulate simultaneously, but during an epidemic, one genotype usually dominates [11,12]. Within each of these subgroups two clades are designated (designated A1, A2, B1 and B2 [12,13].

This classification is mainly based on the sequence variability of the attachment (G) and fusion (F) surface glycoproteins [4]. The highly conserved F protein constitutes an antigenic determinant that mediates cross-lineage neutralization and protection [14]. In 2006, two further subgroups, A2a and A2b, were described, but this further splitting was based on limited data and has not been confirmed by other groups [15]. In addition, no clinical significance of these subgroups has yet been shown.

3. Pathogenesis and Susceptibility

For extensive explanation about pathogenesis of HMPV and animal models, we refer to the review of Schildgen et al. [16]. The pathogenesis of HMPV infections in adults seems to be similar to that in children.

HMPV is associated with severe infection in patients with pulmonary disease and chronic obstructive pulmonary disease (COPD). Studies on HMPV in BALB/c in mice and cotton rats show airway obstruction and hyperresponsiveness after infection. Initially HMPV infection in the lung is characterized by interstitial inflammation with alveolitis starting on day 3 with a peak on day 5 and subsequently decreasing inflammation [17]. However, after 2–3 weeks this develops in a more prominent peribronchiolar and perivascular infiltrate. Hamelin et al. also show airway obstruction in BALB/c mice after a single HMPV challenge with a peak on day 5, but still present until day 70 [18]. In addition, significant hyperresponsiveness after methacholine challenge was also shown until day 70, indicating long-term pulmonary inflammation after HMPV infection.

Darniot and colleagues demonstrated in a mice model that susceptibility to HMPV infection is age related with aged mice showing severer illness and mortality compared to young mice. Aged mice showed greater virus replication in the lung; however, viral clearance was not delayed. In addition, lower levels of virus specific antibodies, neutralizing antibodies and interferon gamma with a significant increase in IL4 and CD4$^+$ lymphocytes were observed in aged mice after HMPV infection. This suggests an important role for the cellular immune response in controlling HMPV infection [19]. This hypothesis is partially confirmed by Ditt et al., who found that HMPV infection in aged mice results in a diminished TNF-alfa expression resulting in low levels of NF-Kb compared to young mice [20].

Lüsebrink et al. demonstrated that neutralizing antibodies seem to be present in all age groups in humans and that neutralizing capacities remain high, with a minor decrease for individuals over 69 years of age. Therefore, they hypothesized that the cellular response has a more important role in the clearing of HMPV infection than the neutralizing humoral immune response [21].

Sastre et al. used a recombinant fusion protein-based enzyme linked immunosorbent assay (F-ELISA) in the same set of sera. Their results support the hypothesis that it appears likely that neutralizing antibodies play a minor role in the control of HMPV infections in humans [22]. In addition, Falsey et al. found higher serum antibodies at baseline, a greater response in binding antibody and a trend towards greater neutralizing antibody responses in older adults compared to younger adults with HMPV illness of the same severity suggesting immune dysregulation in aged patients with an HMPV infection [23].

Overall, neutralizing antibodies seem to play a minor role in controlling HMPV infections. Cellular immune responses seem to be more important for the susceptibility of HMPV infections in aged patients.

4. Epidemiology

HMPV is distributed worldwide and has a seasonal distribution comparable to that of influenza viruses and RSV. It tends to strike in the late winter and early spring [11,24,25]. In young children, HMPV is the second most common cause of lower RTI after RSV, with children less than one year of age showing the highest rates of infection [26,27]. Seroprevalence at the age of 5 is almost 100% [4,25–36].

However, due to incompletely protective immune responses or infection with a new genotype reinfection occurs, especially in elderly and high risk patients [9,37]. Van den Hoogen *et al.* demonstrated that experimental HMPV infection induces transient protective immunity in cynomolgus macaques [38].

Walsh *et al.* found that the proportion of HMPV infections in adults varied between 3%–7.1% in four consecutive winters [9]. This is similar to the annual average infection rate for RSV (5.5%) and greater than that of influenza A (2.4%) in the same cohorts during the same time frame [39].

HMPV was identified in 2.2% of patients who visited a general practitioner because of community-acquired acute RTI who were negative for RSV and influenza virus [5].

HMPV infection is associated with hospitalization for acute RTI in adults in the study of Walsh *et al.* [9]. The incidence of HMPV infection in this hospitalized adults varied from year to year ranging from 4.3%–13.2%. This is in accordance with the rates for RSV and influenza A. Average annual infection rates for RSV and influenza A were 9.6% and 10.5% in the same cohorts [39]. Two-third of these hospitalized patients had underlying disease. Twenty-tree percent of these patients had a co-infection with another respiratory virus.

Widmer *et al.* found that HMPV accounted for 4.5% of hospitalizations for acute RTI in adults older then 50 years during the winter season in 3 consecutive years [8]. Rates for RSV and influenza A were 6.1% and 6.5% respectively. Average annual rates of hospitalization for HMPV were 1.8/10,000 residents in adults from 50–65 years and 22.1/10,000 residents in adults >65 years. Patients with HMPV infections were older, had more cardiovascular disease and were more likely to be vaccinated with influenza vaccination compared to patients with influenza.

Boivin *et al.* found HMPV in 2.3% of respiratory samples during the winter season 2000–2001 [29]. Of the 26 HMPV infected hospitalized patient 35% was aged <5 years and 46% aged >65 years. One third of the hospitalized children aged <5 years, two-third of the patients aged 15–65 years and all patients aged >65 years had an underlying disease.

Data from our hospital suggest a comparable incidence in adult patients and pediatric patients. We analyzed all polymerase chain reaction (PCR) tests for respiratory viruses of the last 19 months in our hospital. A total of 283 adults were tested for HMPV because of symptoms of RTI and almost five percent of the patients (14 of 283 patients) tested positive for HMPV.

5. Transmission

HMPV is thought to be transmitted by direct or close contact with contaminated secretions, which may involve saliva, droplets or large particle aerosols [40–42]. HMPV RNA is found in excretions five days to two weeks after initiation of symptoms [43]. However, the extent of contagiousness is unknown since detection of HMPV RNA in respiratory samples from patients recovering from infection does not per se indicate viable contagious viral particles.

Based on two single cases of nosocomial HMPV infections the incubation period of HMPV is estimated to be 4 to 6 days [44]. Another nosocomial HMPV infection study in a pediatric hemato-oncology ward found an estimated incubation period of 7–9 days. In a retrospective study HMPV transmission in households in Japan was studied. Of the 15 studied families all index-patients were children attending primary school, childcare or nursery homes. Contact cases developed symptoms with a median of five days (range 3–7 days) after the index case developed symptoms [40]. As this was a retrospective study including only symptomatic patients, no reliable exact number of transmissions in households could be determined. Two studies found HMPV carriage in 4.1% of asymptomatic adults, which suggests that asymptomatic adults might be a neglected source of HMPV transmission [3,45]. However, other studies found that the presence of HMPV RNA in excretions of asymptomatic persons is uncommon [4,24,27,29,46].

6. Clinical Manifestations

In general, HMPV infection can not be distinguished from other respiratory viruses on clinical grounds only [5]. Adult patients with an HMPV infection might be asymptomatic or might have symptoms ranging from mild upper RTI symptoms to severe pneumonia [9]. Most patients present with cough, nasal congestion and dyspnoea. Purulent cough, wheezing, sore throat, fever, pneumonia, bronchi(oli)tis, conjunctivitis and otitis media are other reported symptoms [47]. Li *et al.* described a HMPV infection in an immunocompetent adult presenting as a mononucleosis-like illness [48]. Adults with HMPV infection were less likely to report fever in contrast to adults with RSV or influenza infection [8,49,50]. In addition, adults with an HMPV infection presented more often with wheezing compared to adults with RSV or influenza [9]. Falsey *et al.* showed that this is mainly in the elderly population (>65 years) [49]. Elder patients also showed more dyspnoea compared to younger adults [49]. Young adults with HMPV infection had greater complaints of hoarseness [44]. In the frail elderly patients, the patients with pulmonary or cardiovascular disease and immunocompromised patients, infections can be severe [51–55].

Laboratory examination may show lymphopenia, neutropenia and elevated transaminases. Studies on imaging with chest X-ray and computed tomotography (CT) show initially signs of acute interstitial pneumonia (ground glass opacity and air-space consolidation) turning into signs of bronchiolitis/bronchitis (bronchial(ar) wall thickening or impaction) [56–58].

Compared to RSV and influenza, similar rates of intensive care unit (ICU) admission, mechanical ventilation, length of stay for hospitalization and length of stay in ICU were seen for HMPV infection in adults [8,9].

7. Diagnosis

The diagnosis of HMPV infection can be made by several techniques, including culture, nucleic acid amplification tests (NAAT), antigen detection and serologic testing.

Virus culture is relatively difficult, because HMPV grows slowly in conventional cell culture and has mild cytopathic effects. The rapid culture technique is known as shell vial amplification [59].

Detection of viral RNA by NAAT such as reverse transcriptase-PCR (RT-PCR) assay is the most sensitive method for diagnosis of HMPV infection [53,60,61].

Methods for detection of HMPV antigens, such as enzyme immuno-assay (EIA) and enzyme-linked immunosorbent assay (ELISA) are not commonly used. No commercial immunochromatographic assays are available. A direct immunofluorescent-antibody (IFA) test—which is a rapid test in which labeled antibodies to detect specific viral antigens in direct patients materials are used—could be useful for the diagnosis of HMPV infections in outbreaks. The test results are known within two hours. However, the sensitivity of IFA is lower than that of RT-PCR and needs to be validated before use.

Detection of the immune response against the virus by serologic testing is only used for epidemiologic studies. One of the disadvantages of serology is the fact that the interval between virus spreading and detection of HMPV-specific IgM and IgG antibodies is relatively long. However, a combined approach of serology and RT-PCR has added diagnostic value in the diagnosis of HMPV infections in the case of investigating the magnitude of an outbreak for instance in long term care facilities [43,61].

8. Treatment and Prevention

8.1. Treatment

To date, treatment of HMPV infection is mainly supportive. Several treatment regimes have been investigated. Most of these therapeutic options, like innovative approaches based on fusion inhibitors and on RNA interference, seemed effective *in vitro* and in animal studies.

Ribavirin is a nucleoside with broad spectrum inhibitory activity against a variety of RNA and DNA viruses, including HMPV. Ribavirin has demonstrated *in vitro* inhibition of tumor necrosis factor-alfa, interferon-gamma and interleukin (IL)-10, suggesting a down regulation in Th1 and Th2 cytokine production and an increase of IL-2 production by peripheral blood mononuclear cells [43,62]. Ribavirin may terminate T-cell immune-mediated damage caused by viral infections. It limits viral transcription and showed to have immunomodulatory effects [63]. The *in vitro* results are confirmed by an *in vivo* study in BALB/c mouse [64–69].

Immunoglobulins for therapeutical goals can be divided in specific and non specific.

Palivizumab (Synagis®) contains humanized monoclonal antibodies that can recognize a highly conserved neutralizing epitope on the fusion protein of RSV. It showed to have preventive effects in infants at high risk of severe hRSV infections; monthly palivizumab injections reduced RSV hospitalizations by 50% compared with placebo [70–73]. Motavizumab is another RSV specific monoclonal antibody preparation, which is developed after the success of palivizumab. It showed to be non-inferior to palivizumab for prevention of RSV hospitalization in high-risk children [74]. These data of effectiveness of humanized monoclonal Abs against RSV infection has prompted a similar approach for protection against HMPV.

MAb 338 is one of the antibodies that was developed to target the HMPV fusion protein. It appeared effective in animal models in which it neutralized the prototypic strains of the four subgroups of HMPV, significantly reduced the pulmonary viral titer, limited severe acute manifestations and limited bronchial hyper-reactivity. In mice, it appears to have both prophylactic and therapeutic benefits [75]. Hamelin *et al.* also showed that it could be useful after infection and not only as preventive measure [76].

Williams *et al.* tested a fully human monoclonal antibody fragment (Human Fab DS7) with biological activity against HMPV *in vivo* and *in vitro* and demonstrated a prophylactic and therapeutic potential against severe HMPV infection. When Fab DS7 was given intranasally to cotton rats, a >1,500-fold reduction in viral titer in the lungs and a modest 4-fold reduction in the nasal tissues was found. A dose-response relationship between the dose of DS7 and virus titer was seen [77,78].

Wyde *et al.* showed that standard immune globulin preparations (thus without selection for antibodies to a particular microorganism or its toxin), initially used as preventive measure against hRSV, also inhibit replication of HMPV *in vitro* [64].

The combination of oral and aerosolized ribavirin with polyclonal intravenous immune globulin (IVIG) seems an effective treatment for severe HMPV infections, but no randomized controlled trials in humans have been performed. Despite this lack of good trials in human, a lot of experience has been gained meanwhile in individual cases and small case series [69,79,80].

Both ribavirin and IVIG are expensive and have disadvantages. Ribavirin is potential teratogen and administration by nebulization must be carried out via a small particle aerosol generator [81]. Therefore, in daily practice ribavirin nebulization is seldom used for HMPV infection. In addition, health care providers who are pregnant or attempting to become pregnant should avoid contact with patients receiving treatment with aerosolized ribavirin. Furthermore, IVIG requires large fluid volumes infusions, generates a high protein load and is associated with adverse side effects in children with congenital heart disease [82].

Fusion inhibitors target the first steps of the viral replication cycle. Deffrasnes and colleagues tested nine inhibitory peptides with sequences homology with the HRA en HRB domains of the HMPV fusion protein and demonstrated potent viral inhibitory activity *in vitro* of five of these peptides. One peptide, HRA2, displayed very potent activity against all four HMPV subgroups. BALB/c mice that received the HRA2 peptide and a lethal HMPV intranasal challenge simultaneously were completely protected from clinical symptoms and mortality [83]. The study of Miller and colleagues demonstrated that individual HR-1 peptides could lead to effective viral inhibition [84]. These peptides could be used in the prevention of severe infection in vulnerable patients after exposure, but the clinical role post-infection has to be investigated.

RNA interference (RNAi) is a recently discovered interesting approach for treatment of RNA virus infections. RNAi is a naturally occurring intracellular inhibitory process that regulates gene expression through the silencing of specific mRNAs. The small RNAs, the microRNA (miRNA) and small interfering RNA (siRNA), can down-regulate protein production by inhibiting targeted mRNA in a sequence-specific manner. RNAi therapeutics have been shown to be active *in vitro* and *in vivo* against respiratory syncytial virus, parainfluenza and influenza [85–87]. Deffrasnes *et al.* successfully identified two highly efficient siRNAs against HMPV *in vitro*, targeting essential components of the HMPV replication complex [88]. Very recently, Preston and colleagues designed and validate a siRNA molecule that is effective against the G gene of hMPV *in vitro*. Although, a significant reduction in G mRNA did not reduce viral growth *in vitro* or induce a significant type I interferon (IFN) response, hMPV G might still be a valid target for RNAi as G is required for viral replication *in vivo* [89].

Wyde *et al.* have also demonstrated that both the sulfated sialyl lipid (NMSO3) and heparin have antiviral activity against HMPV *in vitro*. NMSO3 acts most likely by inhibiting attachment and penetration of the virus and may inhibit cell-to-cell spread [90].

8.2. Vaccination

Several *in vitro* and animal studies have been performed investigating the development of an HMPV vaccine. However, no human studies have been performed yet and no vaccine is available up till now.

Results of studies performed in rodent and non-human primate models look promising, but very little research is performed in human volunteers. A variety of live attenuated, virus vectored, inactivated virus and subunit vaccines have been tested in animal models and showed to have immunogenicity and protective efficacy [91].

HMPV expresses the major surface glycoproteins F and G. Two main genetic virus lineages exist worldwide which have a similar highly conserved F (fusion) protein. Immunization strategies have been targeted against these surface proteins. Immunization with monoclonal antibodies against the F protein shows a prophylactic effect [77,78,92,93]. Several animal studies investigating the immunization with a chimeric virus vector using a bovine parainfluenza virus 3 expressing the HMPV F protein, adjuvanted soluble F protein or F protein DNA show protective immunity after a HMPV challenge [92–96].

Immunization with the HMPV attachment (G) glycoproteins did not show any production of antibodies or protection [97]. Ryder *et al.* also demonstrated that HMPV G is not a protective antigen. They evaluated the protective efficacy of immunization with a recombinant form of G ectodomain (GDeltaTM) in cotton rats. Although immunized animals developed high levels of serum antibodies to both recombinant and native G protein, they did not develop neutralizing antibodies and were not protected against virus challenge [98].

Studies investigating immunization with inactivated HMPV show an enhanced immune response with even lethal outcome following HMPV infection in animals [99–101]. Use of live-attenuated viruses generated by reverse genetics or recombinant proteins, tested in animals, showed encouraging results. Live vaccines are mimicking natural infection; however natural infection does only lead to transient protective immunity [38]. This makes an extra challenge for vaccine development.

The primary strategy is to develop a live-attenuated virus for intranasal immunization. Reverse genetics provides a means of developing highly characterized 'designer' attenuated vaccine candidates. To date, several promising vaccine candidates have been developed, each using a different mode of attenuation. The first candidate involves deletion of the G glycoprotein, providing attenuation that is probably based on reduced efficiency of attachment. The second candidate involves deletion of the M2-2 protein, which participates in regulating RNA synthesis and whose deletion has the advantageous property of up-regulating transcription and increasing antigen synthesis. A third candidate involves replacing the P protein gene of HMPV with its counterpart from the related avian metapneumovirus, thereby introducing attenuation owing to its chimeric nature and host range restriction. Another live vaccine strategy involves using an attenuated parainfluenza virus as a vector to express HMPV protective antigens, providing a bivalent pediatric vaccine [102].

8.3. Infection Control Measures

As outbreaks with HMPV are frequently described, control measures to prevent HMPV transmission in hospitals and long-term care facilities seem justifiable [43,103–105]. When patients with HMPV infection are hospitalized, infection control measures similar to those taken in case of RSV infection should be taken including droplet isolation until clinical recovery. The Dutch working party on infection prevention advises to apply droplet isolation to all patients hospitalized with bronchiolitis until clinical recovery [106]. No specific advice is formulated for HMPV infections. The CDC advises contact and droplet precautions for infants and young children with respiratory infections; however no advice for adults is given [107]. In our hospitals (Diakonessenhuis Utrecht and the University Medical Centre Utrecht, Utrecht, The Netherlands), droplet isolation is applied to all patients with HMPV infection until clinical recovery. We do not routinely perform control RT-PCR on nasopharyngeal swabs after clinical recovery.

9. Risk Groups

HMPV infections may be more severe in older patients or patients with underlying medical conditions. It is a significant cause of acute respiratory diseases in adults over 65 years and adults with comorbid diseases, such as COPD, asthma, cancer, immunocompromised status, including HIV or post transplantation.

9.1. Adults with Pulmonary Disease or Congestive Heart Disease

Respiratory viruses are a common trigger for exacerbations of COPD, and have been associated with respiratory failure in patients with cardiopulmonary disease such as COPD and congestive heart failure [108,109]. Walsh *et al.* performed a cohort-study during four winters to investigate the clinical outcome and incidence of HMPV infections [110]. Serum samples were taken before and after the observation period (November 15 to April 15) each year. In case of respiratory symptoms a nasopharyngeal swab for HMPV RNA analysis and serum were sampled. They showed that 71% of infections with HMPV were asymptomatic in the healthy young adults (19–40 years) in contrast to 39% in the high risk adults (patients with symptomatic lung disease, COPD, congestive heart failure). These patients were also more likely to use medical care service. Patients were ill for a mean of 10 days in the young adults *versus* 16 days in the high risk group. Johnstone *et al.* investigated the potential role of respiratory viruses in the natural history of community-acquired pneumonia (CAP). In 39% of the 193 patients who were admitted because of CAP, a pathogen was identified. Of these pathogens, 39% were viruses and the easily transmissible viruses such as influenza, HMPV, and RSV were the most common (respectively 24, 24 and 17%). There were few clinically meaningful differences in presentation and no differences in outcomes according to the presence or absence of viral infection. The patients with viral infection were, compared with bacterial infection, significant older, more likely to have cardiac disease and more frail [111].

This is in accordance with the results of Hamelin *et al.* who found HMPV in 4.1% of patients with CAP or exacerbation of chronic obstructive pulmonary disease [112]. Martinello *et al.* also showed that HMPV was frequently identified in patients hospitalized because of an exacerbation of COPD [113]. HMPV (both genotype A and B) was identified in nasopharyngeal specimens (by RT-PCR) in 12% of these patients (6/50). RSV, influenza A and parainfluenza type 3 were identified in respectively 8%, 4% and 2%.

Along with these results, Williams and colleagues showed that HMPV was detected (by RT-PCR of nasal wash specimens) in almost 7% (7/101) of the adults hospitalized for an acute asthma exacerbation, compared to 1.3% in follow-up patients ($p = 0.03$). While none of these patients tested positive for HMPV three months after discharge, a direct etiologic role of the virus seems very likely [114,115].

Recently, we reported a case series of adult patients, including two patients known with COPD, with severe HMPV infections with respiratory insufficiency and the need of ICU admission [116].

9.2. Healthy Elderly Patients over 65 Years

Since adults are not routinely screened for HMPV in the hospital and clinical course can be asymptomatic or mild, infections in the elderly are likely to be underreported. The reported yearly incidence in adults is between 4 and 11% and in adults aged over 50 years; hospitalization rates for HMPV were similar to those associated with influenza and RSV [8].

Walsh *et al.* showed that the risk for symptomatic severe HMPV infection was higher in the elderly. HMPV infection was asymptomatic in 44% of the healthy elderly in contrast to 71% of the healthy young adults. Thirty-eight % of the elderly with HMPV infection used medical care in contrast to 9% in the young adults [23]. Rates for hospitalization in elderly patients over 65 years were also significantly higher for HMPV infection (22.1/10,000 residents) compared to influenza virus (12.3/10,000 residents), but similar to those of RSV infection (25.4/10,000 residents) [8,23]. Antibody levels prior to infection were higher in elderly, suggesting possible immune dysregulation associated with decreased viral clearance in elderly [117].

9.3. Outbreaks in Long Term Care Facilities

Several studies have reported outbreaks in long-term care facilities for elderly. Boivin et al. studied a large outbreak in a long term care facility in Canada in which 96 (27%) op the 364 residents had respiratory symptoms. Six out of 13 tested residents were HMPV positive by RT-PCR. Nine patients died, of which three residents tested HMPV positive [103]. In a 23-bed ward in a hospital for older people in Japan, all 8 residents with respiratory symptoms were HMPV positive by RT-PCR [118]. None of these residents died. Tu et al. found 10 of 13 tested residents of a 53-bed psychiatric ward of an armed forces general hospital in Taiwan HMPV positive by RT-PCR [41]. In a summer outbreak in a long term care facility in California 26 (18%) of residents developed respiratory symptoms. Five of the 13 tested residents were HMPV positive [105]. In an outbreak that the authors of this review described, the attack rate was 13% in a long term care facility [43]. Three patients died, however these were only possible cases. Osbourn et al. found an attack rate of 16.4% in HMPV outbreak in a long-term care facility in Australia, in which two residents died [104]. Sixteen (36%) of 44 residents in a long-term care facility in Oregon had respiratory symptoms of which 6 of 10 tested residents were HMPV positive by RT-PCR [119]. Another study in a community hospital in England reported an attack rate of 29.4%. The different settings (residential care facilities for elderly versus hospital settings) and different case definitions might partly explain the difference in attack rate and mortality.

9.4. Immunocompromised

Several case reports and case series concerning HMPV infections in immunocompromised patients have been published reporting varying morbidity and mortality [67,120–124]. While immunocompromised patients, including patients with haematological malignancies and solid organ and hematopoietic stem cell transplant (HSCT) patients appear to acquire HMPV infection at the same frequency as immunocompetent individuals, they seem to be at risk for severe infections, probably due to poor viral clearance [125–127]. Clinical course is prolonged and respiratory failure may develop [121]. However, Debiaggi showed that HSCT recipients may frequently develop symptomless HMPV infection [128].

Sumino et al. examined a cohort of 688 patients who underwent a bronchoscopy. Of these patients, 72% were immunocompromised (mainly lung transplant patients) and 30% were patients without acute illness who underwent routine bronchoscopy for surveillance after lung transplantation or follow-up of rejection. Six cases of HMPV infection were identified using RT-PCR; four of these were immunocompromised hosts. In the asymptomatic individuals, no cases were identified [129].

Kamboj *et al.* showed that HMPV is detected in 2.7% of cancer patients with respiratory disease. However, HMPV was associated with mild respiratory disease and RSV and influenza were more often found. In patients with hematologic malignancies HMPV was found more often [58].

Debur *et al.* showed that HMPV was present in 2.5% of hematologic stem cell transplant recipients with respiratory disease. Most patients presented with upper RTI, while 27% had a lower RTA. No patients died [130].

Englund *et al.* performed a retrospective survey to demonstrate the importance of HMPV in hematopoietic stem-cell transplant recipients [131]. In 3% of these patients who underwent a BAL because of LRTI was HMPV detected (by RT-PCR). Clinical course in this group was severe and 80% died with acute respiratory failure.

Williams *et al.* showed that HMPV is found in the same frequency as RSV, influenza and parainfluenzavirus in hematologic malignancy patients with acute respiratory disease. All patients presented with an upper RTI, but 41% progressed to a lower RTI. One third (three patients) of these patients died, however in two of these patients potential bacterial pathogens were also found in their BAL fluid [125].

Cane *et al.* published a case report about a HSCT recipient who succumbed to progressive respiratory failure following an upper respiratory prodrome and where HMPV was detected as the sole pathogen in the nasopharyngeal aspirate [132].

In lung transplant patients, HMPV was found in 6% of adults with RTI. This was significantly lower then the most frequently found viral cause, namely parainfluenza virus (17%) [133]. RSV and influenza were found in 12% and 14% respectively. The rate of required hospitalization and length of stay of hospitalization were not different between HMPV and other respiratory viruses. In this study, viral RTI was associated with acute graft rejection. However, this rate was significantly higher for RSV infection compared to HMPV infection.

Larcher *et al.* found HMPV in 25% of BAL fluids from lung transplant patients. Not al of them had respiratory symptoms at the time of the lavage. In this study, HMPV infection seems associated with acute graft rejection, but not with the development of bronchiolitis obliterans [134]. However, other studies suggest that viral RTI is associated with the risk of the development of bronchiolitis obliterans [135,136].

10. Complications

Bacterial and fungal superinfections might complicate viral respiratory infections. To our knowledge no studies specific addressing this issue have been executed, although some studies report the presence of potential bacterial pathogens in the BAL fluid, sputum or blood cultures in those patients with sometimes lethal outcome [9,50,114,125].

In a mouse model that HMPV infection predisposes to severe bacterial infections [137]. Higher levels of airway obstruction, pneumococcal replication and inflammatory cytokines and chemokines were observed in the lungs of superinfected mice, which were challenged with *Streptococcus pneumoniae* (*S. pneumoniae*) five days after HMPV infection. Inactivated HMPV did not result in these changes after a pneumococcal challenge, suggesting that HMPV replication rather than the host response to HMPV may be responsible for these effects. Mice infected with influenza A show long-term impairment of *S. pneumoniae* lung clearance, but the mechanism producing these effects might be different. In contrast to these findings, Ludewick *et al.* showed that BALB/c mice infected with HMPV had a normal bacterial lung clearance when they were challenged with *S. pneumoniae* 14 days after HMPV infection [138].

11. Discussion

The last years more knowledge is obtained about the significance of HMPV infection in adult patients.

Thanks to more sensitive diagnostic tools, like PCR, the proportion of known viral etiologies has increased and HMPV is recognized as a major cause of respiratory disease in patients of all ages. Reported yearly incidences in adults are up to 11%, but the real incidence of HMPV infections is difficult to measure or estimate. First, because a great part of the HMPV infections is asymptomatic or mild and these patients do not present to the hospital. Secondly, the majority of the patients with respiratory symptoms presenting to our hospital are not tested for viral infections.

Epidemiological studies show that elderly over 65 years, patients with cardiac or pulmonary diseases and immunocompromised patients are at high risk for an HMPV infection presenting with severer disease than younger adults without co-morbidity [8,9,114,125]. As serious outbreaks of HMPV with mortality have been reported in long-term care facilities and among immunocompromised patients, infection control measures should be taken in case of a RTI with HMPV especially because these patient groups are at greater risk for severer disease and no proven treatment and/or vaccination strategies against HMPV are available up till now [42,103,134,139].

Till now a lot of experience on treatment of HMPV has been gained in individual cases and small case series [120,122,140–142]. The combination of ribavirin with IVIG seems to be very promising, although this combination is expensive and has disadvantages. Several other treatment regimes have been investigated and proven to be effective *in vitro* and in animal studies. Both immunoglobulins (like mAb 338 and Fab DS7) and synthetic fusion inhibitors showed to be efficient against HMPV. The recently discovered approach of *RNA interference* (RNAi) could be the technique of the future. However, up till now, no treatment proven to be effective in large clinical trials is available and treatment of HMPV infection is mainly supportive.

Since HMPV is an important cause of morbidity and mortality in frail patients, a vaccine is desirable and several *in vitro* and animal studies investigating the development of an HMPV vaccine have been performed. The development of a vaccine against HMPV is hampered by the fact that natural infection with HMPV does not elicits complete immunity and that studies in which is vaccinated with inactivated HMPV show an enlarged immune reaction with even lethal outcome. However, other studies showed promising results, although no vaccine is available up till now.

12. Conclusion

HMPV is an important pathogen causing viral RTI. People at risk are the elderly, the immunocompromised patients and patients with cardiac or pulmonary diseases. While HMPV infections are mild and self-limiting in the majority of adults, clinical course can be complicated in these risk groups and associated morbidity and mortality are considerable.

13. Key Issues

- HMPV is an important pathogen causing viral RTI in adults.
- The elderly, immunocompromised patients and patients with cardiac or pulmonary diseases are at risk for severe infection.
- Distinguishing HMPV clinically from other respiratory viruses is difficult. Diagnosis relies mainly on RT-PCR.
- Although a lot of research has been performed last years, treatment of HMPV infection is mainly supportive and no vaccine is available up till now.
- In case of severe infections, treatment with ribavirin and IVIG might be considered.

References

1. Freymuth, F.; Vabret, A.; Gouarin, S.; Petitjean, J.; Charbonneau, P.; Lehoux, P.; Galateau-Salle, F.; Tremolieres, F.; Carette, M.F.; Mayaud, C.; *et al.* Epidemiology and diagnosis of respiratory syncitial virus in adults. *Rev. Mal. Respir.* **2004**, *21*, 35–42.

2. Osterhaus, A.; Fouchier, R. Human metapneumovirus in the community. *Lancet* **2003**, *361*, 890–891.

3. Falsey, A.R.; Erdman, D.; Anderson, L.J.; Walsh, E.E. Human metapneumovirus infections in young and elderly adults. *J. Infect. Dis.* **2003**, *187*, 785–790.

4. Van den Hoogen, B.G.; de Jong, J.C.; Groen, J.; Kuiken, T.; de Groot, R.; Fouchier, R.A.; Osterhaus, A.D. A newly discovered human pneumovirus isolated from young children with respiratory tract disease. *Nat. Med.* **2001**, *7*, 719–724.

5. Stockton, J.; Stephenson, I.; Fleming, D.; Zambon, M. Human metapneumovirus as a cause of community-acquired respiratory illness. *Emerg. Infect. Dis.* **2002**, *8*, 897–901.

6. Boivin, G.; Abed, Y.; Pelletier, G.; Ruel, L.; Moisan, D.; Cote, S.; Peret, T.C.; Erdman, D.D.; Anderson, L.J. Virological features and clinical manifestations associated with human metapneumovirus: A new paramyxovirus responsible for acute respiratory-tract infections in all age groups. *J. Infect. Dis.* **2002**, *186*, 1330–1334.

7. Peret, T.C.; Boivin, G.; Li, Y.; Couillard, M.; Humphrey, C.; Osterhaus, A.D.; Erdman, D.D.; Anderson, L.J. Characterization of human metapneumoviruses isolated from patients in North America. *J. Infect. Dis.* **2002**, *185*, 1660–1663.

8. Widmer, K.; Zhu, Y.; Williams, J.V.; Griffin, M.R.; Edwards, K.M.; Talbot, H.K. Rates of hospitalizations for respiratory syncytial virus, human metapneumovirus, and influenza virus in older adults. *J. Infect. Dis.* **2012**, *206*, 56–62.

9. Walsh, E.E.; Peterson, D.R.; Falsey, A.R. Human metapneumovirus infections in adults: Another piece of the puzzle. *Ann. Intern. Med.* **2008**, *168*, 2489–2496.

10. Biacchesi, S.; Skiadopoulos, M.H.; Boivin, G.; Hanson, C.T.; Murphy, B.R.; Collins, P.L.; Buchholz, U.J. Genetic diversity between human metapneumovirus subgroups. *Virology* **2003**, *315*, 1–9.

11. Agapov, E.; Sumino, K.C.; Gaudreault-Keener, M.; Storch, G.A.; Holtzman, M.J. Genetic variability of human metapneumovirus infection: Evidence of a shift in viral genotype without a change in illness. *J. Infect. Dis.* **2006**, *193*, 396–403.

12. van den Hoogen, B.G.; Herfst, S.; Sprong, L.; Cane, P.A.; Forleo-Neto, E.; de Swart, R.L.; Osterhaus, A.D.; Fouchier, R.A. Antigenic and genetic variability of human metapneumoviruses. *Emerg. Infect. Dis.* **2004**, *10*, 658–666.

13. Mackay, I.M.; Bialasiewicz, S.; Jacob, K.C.; McQueen, E.; Arden, K.E.; Nissen, M.D.; Sloots, T.P. Genetic diversity of human metapneumovirus over 4 consecutive years in Australia. *J. Infect. Dis.* **2006**, *193*, 1630–1633.

14. Skiadopoulos, M.H.; Biacchesi, S.; Buchholz, U.J.; Riggs, J.M.; Surman, S.R.; Amaro-Carambot, E.; McAuliffe, J.M.; Elkins, W.R.; St Claire, M.; Collins, P.L.; *et al.* The two major human metapneumovirus genetic lineages are highly related antigenically, and the fusion (F) protein is a major contributor to this antigenic relatedness. *J. Virol.* **2004**, *78*, 6927–6937.

15. Huck, B.; Scharf, G.; Neumann-Haefelin, D.; Puppe, W.; Weigl, J.; Falcone, V. Novel human metapneumovirus sublineage. *Emerg. Infect. Dis.* **2006**, *12*, 147–150.

16. Schildgen, V.; van den Hoogen, B.; Fouchier, R.; Tripp, R.A.; Alvarez, R.; Manoha, C.; Williams, J.; Schildgen, O. Human metapneumovirus: Lessons learned over the first decade. *Clin. Microbiol. Rev.* **2011**, *24*, 734–754.

17. Hamelin, M.E.; Yim, K.; Kuhn, K.H.; Cragin, R.P.; Boukhvalova, M.; Blanco, J.C.; Prince, G.A.; Boivin, G. Pathogenesis of human metapneumovirus lung infection in BALB/c mice and cotton rats. *J. Virol.* **2005**, *79*, 8894–8903.

18. Hamelin, M.E.; Prince, G.A.; Gomez, A.M.; Kinkead, R.; Boivin, G. Human metapneumovirus infection induces long-term pulmonary inflammation associated with airway obstruction and hyperresponsiveness in mice. *J. Infect. Dis.* **2006**, *193*, 1634–1642.

19. Darniot, M.; Pitoiset, C.; Petrella, T.; Aho, S.; Pothier, P.; Manoha, C. Age-associated aggravation of clinical disease after primary metapneumovirus infection of BALB/c mice. *J. Virol.* **2009**, *83*, 3323–3332.

20. Ditt, V.; Lusebrink, J.; Tillmann, R.L.; Schildgen, V.; Schildgen, O. Respiratory infections by HMPV and RSV are clinically indistinguishable but induce different host response in aged individuals. *PLoS One* **2011**, *6*, e16314.

21. Lusebrink, J.; Wiese, C.; Thiel, A.; Tillmann, R.L.; Ditt, V.; Muller, A.; Schildgen, O.; Schildgen, V. High seroprevalence of neutralizing capacity against human metapneumovirus in all age groups studied in Bonn, Germany. *Clin. Vaccine Immunol.* **2010**, *17*, 481–484.

22. Sastre, P.; Ruiz, T.; Schildgen, O.; Schildgen, V.; Vela, C.; Rueda, P. Seroprevalence of human respiratory syncytial virus and human metapneumovirus in healthy population analyzed by recombinant fusion protein-based enzyme linked immunosorbent assay. *Virol. J.* **2012**, *9*, 130-422X-9-130.

23. Falsey, A.R.; Hennessey, P.A.; Formica, M.A.; Criddle, M.M.; Biear, J.M.; Walsh, E.E. Humoral immunity to human metapneumovirus infection in adults. *Vaccine* **2010**, *28*, 1477–1480.

24. Van den Hoogen, B.G.; van Doornum, G.J.; Fockens, J.C.; Cornelissen, J.J.; Beyer, W.E.; de Groot, R.; Osterhaus, A.D.; Fouchier, R.A. Prevalence and clinical symptoms of human metapneumovirus infection in hospitalized patients. *J. Infect. Dis.* **2003**, *188*, 1571–1577.

25. Williams, J.V.; Wang, C.K.; Yang, C.F.; Tollefson, S.J.; House, F.S.; Heck, J.M.; Chu, M.; Brown, J.B.; Lintao, L.D.; Quinto, J.D.; *et al.* The role of human metapneumovirus in upper respiratory tract infections in children: A 20-year experience. *J. Infect. Dis.* **2006**, *193*, 387–395.

26. Esper, F.; Martinello, R.A.; Boucher, D.; Weibel, C.; Ferguson, D.; Landry, M.L.; Kahn, J.S. A 1-year experience with human metapneumovirus in children aged <5 years. *J. Infect. Dis.* **2004**, *189*, 1388–1396.

27. Williams, J.V.; Harris, P.A.; Tollefson, S.J.; Halburnt-Rush, L.L.; Pingsterhaus, J.M.; Edwards, K.M.; Wright, P.F.; Crowe, J.E., Jr. Human metapneumovirus and lower respiratory tract disease in otherwise healthy infants and children. *N. Engl. J. Med.* **2004**, *350*, 443–450.

28. Williams, J.V.; Edwards, K.M.; Weinberg, G.A.; Griffin, M.R.; Hall, C.B.; Zhu, Y.; Szilagyi, P.G.; Wang, C.K.; Yang, C.F.; Silva, D.; *et al.* Population-based incidence of human metapneumovirus infection among hospitalized children. *J. Infect. Dis.* **2010**, *201*, 1890–1898.

29. Boivin, G.; De Serres, G.; Cote, S.; Gilca, R.; Abed, Y.; Rochette, L.; Bergeron, M.G.; Dery, P. Human metapneumovirus infections in hospitalized children. *Emerg. Infect. Dis.* **2003**, *9*, 634–640.

30. Mullins, J.A.; Erdman, D.D.; Weinberg, G.A.; Edwards, K.; Hall, C.B.; Walker, F.J.; Iwane, M.; Anderson, L.J. Human metapneumovirus infection among children hospitalized with acute respiratory illness. *Emerg. Infect. Dis.* **2004**, *10*, 700–705.

31. Van den Hoogen, B.G.; Osterhaus, D.M.; Fouchier, R.A. Clinical impact and diagnosis of human metapneumovirus infection. *J. Pediatr. Infect. Dis.* **2004**, *23*, S25–S32.

32. Crowe, J.E., Jr. Human metapneumovirus as a major cause of human respiratory tract disease. *J. Pediatr. Infect. Dis.* **2004**, *23*, S215–S221.

33. Debiaggi, M.; Canducci, F.; Ceresola, E.R.; Clementi, M. The role of infections and coinfections with newly identified and emerging respiratory viruses in children. *Virol. J.* **2012**, *9*, 247.

34. Hustedt, J.W.; Vazquez, M. The changing face of pediatric respiratory tract infections: How human metapneumovirus and human bocavirus fit into the overall etiology of respiratory tract infections in young children. *Yale J. Biol. Med.* **2010**, *83*, 193–200.

35. Papenburg, J.; Boivin, G. The distinguishing features of human metapneumovirus and respiratory syncytial virus. *Rev. Med. Virol.* **2010**, *20*, 245–260.

36. Papenburg, J.; Hamelin, M.E.; Ouhoummane, N.; Carbonneau, J.; Ouakki, M.; Raymond, F.; Robitaille, L.; Corbeil, J.; Caouette, G.; Frenette, L.; *et al.* Comparison of risk factors for human metapneumovirus and respiratory syncytial virus disease severity in young children. *J. Infect. Dis.* **2012**, *206*, 178–189.

37. Pavlin, J.A.; Hickey, A.C.; Ulbrandt, N.; Chan, Y.P.; Endy, T.P.; Boukhvalova, M.S.; Chunsuttiwat, S.; Nisalak, A.; Libraty, D.H.; Green, S.; *et al.* Human metapneumovirus reinfection among children in thailand determined by elisa using purified soluble fusion protein. *J. Infect. Dis.* **2008**, *198*, 836–842.

38. Van den Hoogen, B.G.; Herfst, S.; de Graaf, M.; Sprong, L.; van Lavieren, R.; van Amerongen, G.; Yuksel, S.; Fouchier, R.A.; Osterhaus, A.D.; de Swart, R.L. Experimental infection of macaques with human metapneumovirus induces transient protective immunity. *J. Gen. Virol.* **2007**, *88*, 1251–1259.

39. Falsey, A.R. Respiratory syncytial virus infection in elderly and high-risk adults. *Exp. Lung Res.* **2005**, *31*, 77.

40. Matsuzaki, Y.; Itagaki, T.; Ikeda, T.; Aoki, Y.; Abiko, C.; Mizuta, K. Human metapneumovirus infection among family members. *Epidemiol. Infect.* **2012**, 1–6.

41. Tu, C.C.; Chen, L.K.; Lee, Y.S.; Ko, C.F.; Chen, C.M.; Yang, H.H.; Lee, J.J. An outbreak of human metapneumovirus infection in hospitalized psychiatric adult patients in Taiwan. *Scand. J. Infect. Dis.* **2009**, *41*, 363–367.

42. Kim, S.; Sung, H.; Im, H.J.; Hong, S.J.; Kim, M.N. Molecular epidemiological investigation of a nosocomial outbreak of human metapneumovirus infection in a pediatric hemato-oncology patient population. *J. Clin. Microbiol.* **2009**, *47*, 1221–1224.

43. Te Wierik, M.J.; Nguyen, D.T.; Beersma, M.F.; Thijsen, S.F.; Heemstra, K.A. An outbreak of severe respiratory tract infection caused by human metapneumovirus in a residential care facility for elderly in Utrecht, the Netherlands, January to March 2010. *Euro. Surveill.* **2012**, *17*, 20132.

44. Peiris, J.S.; Tang, W.H.; Chan, K.H.; Khong, P.L.; Guan, Y.; Lau, Y.L.; Chiu, S.S. Children with respiratory disease associated with metapneumovirus in Hong Kong. *Emerg. Infect. Dis.* **2003**, *9*, 628–633.

45. Bruno, R.; Marsico, S.; Minini, C.; Apostoli, P.; Fiorentini, S.; Caruso, A. Human metapneumovirus infection in a cohort of young asymptomatic subjects. *New Microbiol.* **2009**, *32*, 297–301.

46. Falsey, A.R.; Criddle, M.C.; Walsh, E.E. Detection of respiratory syncytial virus and human metapneumovirus by reverse transcription polymerase chain reaction in adults with and without respiratory illness. *J. Clin. Virol.* **2006**, *35*, 46–50.

47. Hall, W.B.; Kidd, J.M.; Campbell-Bright, S.; Miller, M.; Aris, R.M. Clinical manifestations and impact of human metapneumovirus in healthy adults: A retrospective analysis of 28 patients over 2 years. *Am. J. Respir. Crit. Care Med.* **2011**, *183*, 4927.

48. Li, I.W.; To, K.K.; Tang, B.S.; Chan, K.H.; Hui, C.K.; Cheng, V.C.; Yuen, K.Y. Human metapneumovirus infection in an immunocompetent adult presenting as mononucleosis-like illness. *J. Infect.* **2008**, *56*, 389–392.

49. Falsey, A.R.; Erdman, D.; Anderson, L.J.; Walsh, E.E. Human metapneumovirus infections in young and elderly adults. *J. Infect. Dis.* **2003**, *187*, 785–790.

50. Johnstone, J.; Majumdar, S.R.; Fox, J.D.; Marrie, T.J. Human metapneumovirus pneumonia in adults: Results of a prospective study. *Clin. Infect. Dis.* **2008**, *46*, 571–574.

51. Van den Hoogen, B.G. Respiratory tract infection due to human metapneumovirus among elderly patients. *Clin. Infect. Dis.* **2007**, *44*, 1159–1160.

52. Tu, C.C.; Chen, L.K.; Lee, Y.S.; Ko, C.F.; Chen, C.M.; Yang, H.H.; Lee, J.J. An outbreak of human metapneumovirus infection in hospitalized psychiatric adult patients in Taiwan. *Scand. J. Infect. Dis.* **2009**, *41*, 363–367.

53. O'Gorman, C.; McHenry, E.; Coyle, P.V. Human metapneumovirus in adults: A short case series. *Euro. J. Clin. Micorbiol. Infect. Dis.* **2006**, *25*, 190–192.

54. Boivin, G.; de Serres, G.; Hamelin, M.E.; Cote, S.; Argouin, M.; Tremblay, G.; Maranda-Aubut, R.; Sauvageau, C.; Ouakki, M.; Boulianne, N.; *et al.* An outbreak of severe respiratory tract infection due to human metapneumovirus in a long-term care facility. *Clin. Infect. Dis.* **2007**, *44*, 1152–1158.

55. Pelletier, G.; Dery, P.; Abed, Y.; Boivin, G. Respiratory tract reinfections by the new human metapneumovirus in an immunocompromised child. *Emerg. Infect. Dis.* **2002**, *8*, 976–978.

56. Syha, R.; Beck, R.; Hetzel, J.; Ketelsen, D.; Grosse, U.; Springer, F.; Horger, M. Humane metapneumovirus (HMPV) associated pulmonary infections in immunocompromised adults-initial ct findings, disease course and comparison to respiratory-syncytial-virus (RSV) induced pulmonary infections. *Eur. J. Radiol.* **2012**, *81*, 4173–4178.

57. Franquet, T.; Rodriguez, S.; Martino, R.; Salinas, T.; Gimenez, A.; Hidalgo, A. Human metapneumovirus infection in hematopoietic stem cell transplant recipients: High-resolution computed tomography findings. *J. Comput. Assist. Tomo.* **2005**, *29*, 223–227.

58. Kamboj, M.; Gerbin, M.; Huang, C.K.; Brennan, C.; Stiles, J.; Balashov, S.; Park, S.; Kiehn, T.E.; Perlin, D.S.; Pamer, E.G.; *et al.* Clinical characterization of human metapneumovirus infection among patients with cancer. *J. Infect.* **2008**, *57*, 464–471.

59. Hamelin, M.E.; Boivin, G. Development and validation of an enzyme-linked immunosorbent assay for human metapneumovirus serology based on a recombinant viral protein. *Clin. Diagn. Lab. Immunol.* **2005**, *12*, 249–253.

60. Cheng, M.F.; Chen, B.C.; Kao, C.L.; Kao, C.H.; Hsieh, K.S.; Liu, Y.C. Human metapneumovirus as a causative agent of lower respiratory tract infection in four patients: The first report of human metapneumovirus infection confirmed by rna sequences in Taiwan. *Scand. J. Infect. Dis.* **2006**, *38*, 392–396.

61. Chiu, C.Y.; Alizadeh, A.A.; Rouskin, S.; Merker, J.D.; Yeh, E.; Yagi, S.; Schnurr, D.; Patterson, B.K.; Ganem, D.; DeRisi, J.L. Diagnosis of a critical respiratory illness caused by human metapneumovirus by use of a pan-virus microarray. *J. Clin. Microbiol.* **2007**, *45*, 2340–2343.

62. Sookoian, S.; Castano, G.; Flichman, D.; Cello, J. Effects of ribavirin on cytokine production of recall antigens and phytohemaglutinin-stimulated peripheral blood mononuclear cells. (Inhibitory effects of ribavirin on cytokine production). *Ann. Hepatol.* **2004**, *3*, 104–107.

63. Graci, J.D.; Cameron, C.E. Mechanisms of action of ribavirin against distinct viruses. *Rev. Med. Virol.* **2006**, *16*, 37–48.

64. Wyde, P.R.; Chetty, S.N.; Jewell, A.M.; Boivin, G.; Piedra, P.A. Comparison of the inhibition of human metapneumovirus and respiratory syncytial virus by ribavirin and immune serum globulin *in vitro*. *Antivir. Res.* **2003**, *60*, 51–59.

65. Hamelin, M.E.; Prince, G.A.; Boivin, G. Effect of ribavirin and glucocorticoid treatment in a mouse model of human metapneumovirus infection. *Antimicrob. Agents Chemother.* **2006**, *50*, 774–777.

66. Shachor-Meyouhas, Y.; Ben-Barak, A.; Kassis, I. Treatment with oral ribavirin and ivig of severe human metapneumovirus pneumonia (HMPV) in immune compromised child. *Pediatr. Blood Cancer* **2011**, *57*, 350–351.

67. Egli, A.; Bucher, C.; Dumoulin, A.; Stern, M.; Buser, A.; Bubendorf, L.; Gregor, M.; Servida, P.; Sommer, G.; Bremerich, J.; *et al.* Human metapneumovirus infection after allogeneic hematopoietic stem cell transplantation. *Infection* **2012**, *40*, 677–684.

68. Kroll, J.L.; Weinberg, A. Human metapneumovirus. *Semin. Respir. Crit. Care Med.* **2011**, *32*, 447–453.

69. Shahda, S.; Carlos, W.G.; Kiel, P.J.; Khan, B.A.; Hage, C.A. The human metapneumovirus: A case series and review of the literature. *Transpl. Infect. Dis.* **2011**, *13*, 324–328.

70. American Academy of Pediatrics Committee on Infectious Diseases and Committee on Fetus and Newborn. Revised indications for the use of palivizumab and respiratory syncytial virus immune globulin intravenous for the prevention of respiratory syncytial virus infections. *Pediatrics* **2003**, *112*, 1442–1446.

71. Ulbrandt, N.D.; Ji, H.; Patel, N.K.; Barnes, A.S.; Wilson, S.; Kiener, P.A.; Suzich, J.; McCarthy, M.P. Identification of antibody neutralization epitopes on the fusion protein of human metapneumovirus. *J. Gen. Virol.* **2008**, *89*, 3113–3118.

72. Feltes, T.F.; Cabalka, A.K.; Meissner, H.C.; Piazza, F.M.; Carlin, D.A.; Top, F.H., Jr.; Connor, E.M.; Sondheimer, H.M.; Cardiac Synagis Study Group. Palivizumab prophylaxis reduces hospitalization due to respiratory syncytial virus in young children with hemodynamically significant congenital heart disease. *J. Pediatr.* **2003**, *143*, 532–540.

73. The IMpact-RSV Study Group. Palivizumab, a humanized respiratory syncytial virus monoclonal antibody, reduces hospitalization from respiratory syncytial virus infection in high-risk infants. *Pediatrics* **1998**, *102*, 531–537.

74. Carbonell-Estrany, X.; Simoes, E.A.; Dagan, R.; Hall, C.B.; Harris, B.; Hultquist, M.; Connor, E.M.; Losonsky, G.A.; Motavizumab Study Group. Motavizumab for prophylaxis of respiratory syncytial virus in high-risk children: A noninferiority trial. *Pediatrics* **2010**, *125*, e35–e51.

75. Ulbrandt, N.D.; Ji, H.; Patel, N.K.; Riggs, J.M.; Brewah, Y.A.; Ready, S.; Donacki, N.E.; Folliot, K.; Barnes, A.S.; Senthil, K.; *et al.* Isolation and characterization of monoclonal antibodies which neutralize human metapneumovirus *in vitro* and *in vivo*. *J. Virol.* **2006**, *80*, 7799–7806.

76. Hamelin, M.E.; Couture, C.; Sackett, M.; Kiener, P.; Suzich, J.; Ulbrandt, N.; Boivin, G. The prophylactic administration of a monoclonal antibody against human metapneumovirus attenuates viral disease and airways hyperresponsiveness in mice. *Antivir. Ther.* **2008**, *13*, 39–46.

77. Hamelin, M.E.; Gagnon, C.; Prince, G.A.; Kiener, P.; Suzich, J.; Ulbrandt, N.; Boivin, G. Prophylactic and therapeutic benefits of a monoclonal antibody against the fusion protein of human metapneumovirus in a mouse model. *Antivir. Res.* **2010**, *88*, 31–37.

78. Williams, J.V.; Chen, Z.; Cseke, G.; Wright, D.W.; Keefer, C.J.; Tollefson, S.J.; Hessell, A.; Podsiad, A.; Shepherd, B.E.; Sanna, P.P.; *et al.* A recombinant human monoclonal antibody to human metapneumovirus fusion protein that neutralizes virus *in vitro* and is effective therapeutically *in vivo*. *J. Virol.* **2007**, *81*, 8315–8324.

79. Wyde, P.R.; Moylett, E.H.; Chetty, S.N.; Jewell, A.; Bowlin, T.L.; Piedra, P.A. Comparison of the inhibition of human metapneumovirus and respiratory syncytial virus by NMSO3 in tissue culture assays. *Antivir. Res.* **2004**, *63*, 51–59.

80. Hamelin, M.E.; Prince, G.A.; Boivin, G. Effect of ribavirin and glucocorticoid treatment in a mouse model of human metapneumovirus infection. *Antimicrob. Agents Chemother.* **2006**, *50*, 774–777.

81. Kilham, L.; Ferm, V.H. Congenital anomalies induced in hamster embryos with ribavirin. *Science* **1977**, *195*, 413–414.

82. Wyde, P.R.; Chetty, S.N.; Jewell, A.M.; Boivin, G.; Piedra, P.A. Comparison of the inhibition of human metapneumovirus and respiratory syncytial virus by ribavirin and immune serum globulin *in vitro*. *Antivir. Res.* **2003**, *60*, 51–59.

83. Deffrasnes, C.; Hamelin, M.E.; Prince, G.A.; Boivin, G. Identification and evaluation of a highly effective fusion inhibitor for human metapneumovirus. *Antimicrob. Agents Chemother.* **2008**, *52*, 279–287.

84. Miller, S.A.; Tollefson, S.; Crowe, J.E., Jr.; Williams, J.V.; Wright, D.W. Examination of a fusogenic hexameric core from human metapneumovirus and identification of a potent synthetic peptide inhibitor from the heptad repeat 1 region. *J. Virol.* **2007**, *81*, 141–149.

85. Sah, D.W. Therapeutic potential of rna interference for neurological disorders. *Life Sciences* **2006**, *79*, 1773–1780.

86. Alvarez, R.; Elbashir, S.; Borland, T.; Toudjarska, I.; Hadwiger, P.; John, M.; Roehl, I.; Morskaya, S.S.; Martinello, R.; Kahn, J.; *et al.* RNA interference-mediated silencing of the respiratory syncytial virus nucleocapsid defines a potent antiviral strategy. *Antimicrob. Agents Chemother.* **2009**, *53*, 3952–3962.

87. DeVincenzo, J.; Lambkin-Williams, R.; Wilkinson, T.; Cehelsky, J.; Nochur, S.; Walsh, E.; Meyers, R.; Gollob, J.; Vaishnaw, A. A randomized, double-blind, placebo-controlled study of an rnai-based therapy directed against respiratory syncytial virus. *Proc. Natl. Acad. Sci. USA* **2010**, *107*, 8800–8805.

88. Deffrasnes, C.; Cavanagh, M.H.; Goyette, N.; Cui, K.; Ge, Q.; Seth, S.; Templin, M.V.; Quay, S.C.; Johnson, P.H.; Boivin, G. Inhibition of human metapneumovirus replication by small interfering RNA. *Antivir. Ther.* **2008**, *13*, 821–832.

89. Preston, F.M.; Straub, C.P.; Ramirez, R.; Mahalingam, S.; Spann, K.M. SiRNA against the g gene of human metapneumovirus. *Virol. J.* **2012**, *9*, 105-422X-9-105.

90. Wyde, P.R.; Moylett, E.H.; Chetty, S.N.; Jewell, A.; Bowlin, T.L.; Piedra, P.A. Comparison of the inhibition of human metapneumovirus and respiratory syncytial virus by NMSO3 in tissue culture assays. *Antivir. Res.* **2004**, *63*, 51–59.

91. Herfst, S.; Fouchier, R.A. Vaccination approaches to combat human metapneumovirus lower respiratory tract infections. *J. Clin. Virol.* **2008**, *41*, 49–52.

92. Tang, R.S.; Mahmood, K.; Macphail, M.; Guzzetta, J.M.; Haller, A.A.; Liu, H.; Kaur, J.; Lawlor, H.A.; Stillman, E.A.; Schickli, J.H.; *et al.* A host-range restricted parainfluenza virus type 3 (PIV3) expressing the human metapneumovirus (hMPV) fusion protein elicits protective immunity in african green monkeys. *Vaccine* **2005**, *23*, 1657–1667.

93. Skiadopoulos, M.H.; Biacchesi, S.; Buchholz, U.J.; Riggs, J.M.; Surman, S.R.; Amaro-Carambot, E.; McAuliffe, J.M.; Elkins, W.R.; St Claire, M.; Collins, P.L.; *et al.* The two major human metapneumovirus genetic lineages are highly related antigenically, and the fusion (F) protein is a major contributor to this antigenic relatedness. *J. Virol.* **2004**, *78*, 6927–6937.

94. Herfst, S.; Fouchier, R.A. Vaccination approaches to combat human metapneumovirus lower respiratory tract infections. *J. Clin. Virol.* **2008**, *41*, 49–52.

95. Herfst, S.; de Graaf, M.; Schrauwen, E.J.; Ulbrandt, N.D.; Barnes, A.S.; Senthil, K.; Osterhaus, A.D.; Fouchier, R.A.; van den Hoogen, B.G. Immunization of syrian golden hamsters with f subunit vaccine of human metapneumovirus induces protection against challenge with homologous or heterologous strains. *J. Gen. Virol.* **2007**, *88*, 2702–2709.

96. Cseke, G.; Wright, D.W.; Tollefson, S.J.; Johnson, J.E.; Crowe, J.E., Jr.; Williams, J.V. Human metapneumovirus fusion protein vaccines that are immunogenic and protective in cotton rats. *J. Virol.* **2007**, *81*, 698–707.

97. Mok, H.; Tollefson, S.J.; Podsiad, A.B.; Shepherd, B.E.; Polosukhin, V.V.; Johnston, R.E.; Williams, J.V.; Crowe, J.E., Jr. An alphavirus replicon-based human metapneumovirus vaccine is immunogenic and protective in mice and cotton rats. *J. Virol.* **2008**, *82*, 11410–11418.

98. Ryder, A.B.; Tollefson, S.J.; Podsiad, A.B.; Johnson, J.E.; Williams, J.V. Soluble recombinant human metapneumovirus g protein is immunogenic but not protective. *Vaccine* **2010**, *28*, 4145–4152.

99. Yim, K.C.; Cragin, R.P.; Boukhvalova, M.S.; Blanco, J.C.; Hamlin, M.E.; Boivin, G.; Porter, D.D.; Prince, G.A. Human metapneumovirus: Enhanced pulmonary disease in cotton rats immunized with formalin-inactivated virus vaccine and challenged. *Vaccine* **2007**, *25*, 5034–5040.

100. Hamelin, M.E.; Couture, C.; Sackett, M.K.; Boivin, G. Enhanced lung disease and th2 response following human metapneumovirus infection in mice immunized with the inactivated virus. *J. Gen. Virol.* **2007**, *88*, 3391–3400.

101. De Swart, R.L.; van den Hoogen, B.G.; Kuiken, T.; Herfst, S.; van Amerongen, G.; Yuksel, S.; Sprong, L.; Osterhaus, A.D. Immunization of macaques with formalin-inactivated human metapneumovirus induces hypersensitivity to hMPV infection. *Vaccine* **2007**, *25*, 8518–8528.

102. Buchholz, U.J.; Nagashima, K.; Murphy, B.R.; Collins, P.L. Live vaccines for human metapneumovirus designed by reverse genetics. *Expet. Rev. Vaccine.* **2006**, *5*, 695–706.

103. Boivin, G.; De Serres, G.; Hamelin, M.E.; Cote, S.; Argouin, M.; Tremblay, G.; Maranda-Aubut, R.; Sauvageau, C.; Ouakki, M.; Boulianne, N.; *et al.* An outbreak of severe respiratory tract infection due to human metapneumovirus in a long-term care facility. *Clin. Infect. Dis.* **2007**, *44*, 1152–1158.

104. Osbourn, M.; McPhie, K.A.; Ratnamohan, V.M.; Dwyer, D.E.; Durrheim, D.N. Outbreak of human metapneumovirus infection in a residential aged care facility. *Comm. Dis. Intell.* **2009**, *33*, 38–40.

105. Louie, J.K.; Schnurr, D.P.; Pan, C.Y.; Kiang, D.; Carter, C.; Tougaw, S.; Ventura, J.; Norman, A.; Belmusto, V.; Rosenberg, J.; *et al.* A summer outbreak of human metapneumovirus infection in a long-term-care facility. *J. Infect. Dis.* **2007**, *196*, 705–708.

106. http://www.wip.nl.

107. Siegel, J.D.; Rhinehart, E.; Jackson, M.; Chiarello, L.; Health Care Infection Control Practices Advisory Committee. 2007 guideline for isolation precautions: Preventing transmission of infectious agents in health care settings. *Am. J. Infect. Control* **2007**, *35*, S65–S164.

108. Duncan, C.B.; Walsh, E.E.; Peterson, D.R.; Lee, F.E.; Falsey, A.R. Risk factors for respiratory failure associated with respiratory syncytial virus infection in adults. *J. Infect. Dis.* **2009**, *200*, 1242–1246.

109. Beckham, J.D.; Cadena, A.; Lin, J.; Piedra, P.A.; Glezen, W.P.; Greenberg, S.B.; Atmar, R.L. Respiratory viral infections in patients with chronic, obstructive pulmonary disease. *J. Infect.* **2005**, *50*, 322–330.

110. Walsh, E.E.; Falsey, A.R.; Hennessey, P.A. Respiratory syncytial and other virus infections in persons with chronic cardiopulmonary disease. *Am. J. Respir. Crit. Care Med.* **1999**, *160*, 791–795.

111. Johnstone, J.; Majumdar, S.R.; Fox, J.D.; Marrie, T.J. Viral Infection in Adults Hospitalized with Community-Acquired Pneumonia: Prevalence, Pathogens, and Presentation. *Chest* **2008**, *134*, 1141–1148.

112. Hamelin, M.E.; Boivin, G. Human metapneumovirus: A ubiquitous and long-standing respiratory pathogen. *J. Pediatr. Infect. Dis.* **2005**, *24*, S203–S207.

113. Martinello, R.A.; Esper, F.; Weibel, C.; Ferguson, D.; Landry, M.L.; Kahn, J.S. Human metapneumovirus and exacerbations of chronic obstructive pulmonary disease. *J. Infect.* **2006**, *53*, 248–254.

114. Williams, J.V.; Crowe, J.E., Jr.; Enriquez, R.; Minton, P.; Peebles, R.S., Jr; Hamilton, R.G.; Higgins, S.; Griffin, M.; Hartert, T.V. Human metapneumovirus infection plays an etiologic role in acute asthma exacerbations requiring hospitalization in adults. *J. Infect. Dis.* **2005**, *192*, 1149–1153.

115. Williams, J.V.; Crowe, J.E.,Jr; Enriquez, R.; Minton, P.; Peebles, R.S.,Jr; Hamilton, R.G.; Higgins, S.; Griffin, M.; Hartert, T.V. Human metapneumovirus infection plays an etiologic role in acute asthma exacerbations requiring hospitalization in adults. *J. Infect. Dis.* **2005**, *192*, 1149–1153.

116. Haas, L.E.; de Rijk, N.X.; Thijsen, S.F. Human metapneumovirus infections on the ICU: A report of three cases. *Ann. Intensive Care* **2012**, *2*, 30.

117. Miller, R.A. The aging immune system: Primer and prospectus. *Science* **1996**, *273*, 70–74.

118. Honda, H.; Iwahashi, J.; Kashiwagi, T.; Imamura, Y.; Hamada, N.; Anraku, T.; Ueda, S.; Kanda, T.; Takahashi, T.; Morimoto, S. Outbreak of human metapneumovirus infection in elderly inpatients in Japan. *J. Am. Geriatr. Soc.* **2006**, *54*, 177–180.

119. Liao, R.S.; Appelgate, D.M.; Pelz, R.K. An outbreak of severe respiratory tract infection due to human metapneumovirus in a long-term care facility for the elderly in Oregon. *J. Clin. Virol.* **2012**, *53*, 171–173.

120. Raza, K.; Ismailjee, S.B.; Crespo, M.; Studer, S.M.; Sanghavi, S.; Paterson, D.L.; Kwak, E.J.; Rinaldo, C.R., Jr.; Pilewski, J.M.; McCurry, K.R.; *et al.* Successful outcome of human metapneumovirus (hMPV) pneumonia in a lung transplant recipient treated with intravenous ribavirin. *J. Heart Lung Transplant.* **2007**, *26*, 862–864.

121. Huck, B.; Egger, M.; Bertz, H.; Peyerl-Hoffman, G.; Kern, W.V.; Neumann-Haefelin, D.; Falcone, V. Human metapneumovirus infection in a hematopoietic stem cell transplant recipient with relapsed multiple myeloma and rapidly progressing lung cancer. *J. Clin. Microbiol.* **2006**, *44*, 2300–2303.

122. Kamble, R.T.; Bollard, C.; Demmler, G.; LaSala, P.R.; Carrum, G. Human metapneumovirus infection in a hematopoietic transplant recipient. *Bone Marrow Transplant.* **2007**, *40*, 699–700.

123. Muller, A.; Kupfer, B.; Vehreschild, J.; Cornely, O.; Kaiser, R.; Seifert, H.; Viazov, S.; Tillmann, R.L.; Franzen, C.; Simon, A.; *et al.* Fatal pneumonia associated with human metapneumovirus (HMPV) in a patient with myeloid leukemia and adenocarcinoma in the lung. *Eur. J. Med. Res.* **2007**, *12*, 183–184.

124. Kamboj, M.; Gerbin, M.; Huang, C.K.; Brennan, C.; Stiles, J.; Balashov, S.; Park, S.; Kiehn, T.E.; Perlin, D.S.; Pamer, E.G.; *et al.* Clinical Characterization of Human Metapneumovirus Infection among Patients with Cancer. *J. Infect.* **2008**, *57*, 464–471.

125. Williams, J.V.; Martino, R.; Rabella, N.; Otegui, M.; Parody, R.; Heck, J.M.; Crowe, J.E., Jr. A prospective study comparing human metapneumovirus with other respiratory viruses in adults with hematologic malignancies and respiratory tract infections. *J. Infect. Dis.* **2005**, *192*, 1061–1065.

126. Martino, R.; Porras, R.P.; Rabella, N.; Williams, J.V.; Ramila, E.; Margall, N.; Labeaga, R.; Crowe, J.E., Jr.; Coll, P.; Sierra, J. Prospective study of the incidence, clinical features, and outcome of symptomatic upper and lower respiratory tract infections by respiratory viruses in adult recipients of hematopoietic stem cell transplants for hematologic malignancies. *Biol. Blood Marrow Transplant.* **2005**, *11*, 781–796.

127. Peck, A.J.; Englund, J.A.; Kuypers, J.; Guthrie, K.A.; Corey, L.; Morrow, R.; Hackman, R.C.; Cent, A.; Boeckh, M. Respiratory virus infection among hematopoietic cell transplant recipients: Evidence for asymptomatic parainfluenza virus infection. *Blood* **2007**, *110*, 1681–1688.

128. Debiaggi, M.; Canducci, F.; Sampaolo, M.; Marinozzi, M.C.; Parea, M.; Terulla, C.; Colombo, A.A.; Alessandrino, E.P.; Bragotti, L.Z.; Arghittu, M.; *et al.* Persistent symptomless human metapneumovirus infection in hematopoietic stem cell transplant recipients. *J. Infect. Dis.* **2006**, *194*, 474–478.

129. Sumino, K.C.; Agapov, E.; Pierce, R.A.; Trulock, E.P.; Pfeifer, J.D.; Ritter, J.H.; Gaudreault-Keener, M.; Storch, G.A.; Holtzman, M.J. Detection of severe human metapneumovirus infection by real-time polymerase chain reaction and histopathological assessment. *J. Infect. Dis.* **2005**, *192*, 1052–1060.

130. Debur, M.C.; Vidal, L.R.; Stroparo, E.; Nogueira, M.B.; Almeida, S.M.; Takahashi, G.A.; Rotta, I.; Pereira, L.A.; Silveira, C.S.; Delfraro, A.; *et al.* Impact of human metapneumovirus infection on in and outpatients for the years 2006–2008 in Southern Brazil. *Memorias do Instituto Oswaldo Cruz* **2010**, *105*, 1010–1018.

131. Englund, J.A.; Boeckh, M.; Kuypers, J.; Nichols, W.G.; Hackman, R.C.; Morrow, R.A.; Fredricks, D.N.; Corey, L. Brief communication: Fatal human metapneumovirus infection in stem-cell transplant recipients. *Ann. Intern. Med.* **2006**, *144*, 344–349.

132. Cane, P.A.; van den Hoogen, B.G.; Chakrabarti, S.; Fegan, C.D.; Osterhaus, A.D. Human metapneumovirus in a haematopoietic stem cell transplant recipient with fatal lower respiratory tract disease. *Bone Marrow Transplant.* **2003**, *31*, 309–310.

133. Weinberg, A.; Lyu, D.M.; Li, S.; Marquesen, J.; Zamora, M.R. Incidence and morbidity of human metapneumovirus and other community-acquired respiratory viruses in lung transplant recipients. *Transpl. Infect. Dis.* **2010**, *12*, 330–335.

134. Larcher, C.; Geltner, C.; Fischer, H.; Nachbaur, D.; Muller, L.C.; Huemer, H.P. Human metapneumovirus infection in lung transplant recipients: Clinical presentation and epidemiology. *J. Heart Lung Transplant.* **2005**, *24*, 1891–1901.

135. Kumar, D.; Erdman, D.; Keshavjee, S.; Peret, T.; Tellier, R.; Hadjiliadis, D.; Johnson, G.; Ayers, M.; Siegal, D.; Humar, A. Clinical impact of community-acquired respiratory viruses on bronchiolitis obliterans after lung transplant. *Am. J. Transplant.* **2005**, *5*, 2031–2036.

136. Sharples, L.D.; McNeil, K.; Stewart, S.; Wallwork, J. Risk factors for bronchiolitis obliterans: A systematic review of recent publications. *J. Heart Lung Transplant.* **2002**, *21*, 271–281.

137. Kukavica-Ibrulj, I.; Hamelin, M.E.; Prince, G.A.; Gagnon, C.; Bergeron, Y.; Bergeron, M.G.; Boivin, G. Infection with human metapneumovirus predisposes mice to severe pneumococcal pneumonia. *J. Virol.* **2009**, *83*, 1341–1349.

138. Ludewick, H.P.; Aerts, L.; Hamelin, M.E.; Boivin, G. Long-term impairment of streptococcus pneumoniae lung clearance is observed after initial infection with influenza a virus but not human metapneumovirus in mice. *J. Gen. Virol.* **2011**, *92*, 1662–1665.

139. Louie, J.K.; Schnurr, D.P.; Pan, C.Y.; Kiang, D.; Carter, C.; Tougaw, S.; Ventura, J.; Norman, A.; Belmusto, V.; Rosenberg, J.; *et al.* A summer outbreak of human metapneumovirus infection in a long-term-care facility. *J. Infect. Dis.* **2007**, *196*, 705–708.

140. Bonney, D.; Razali, H.; Turner, A.; Will, A. Successful treatment of human metapneumovirus pneumonia using combination therapy with intravenous ribavirin and immune globulin. *Br. J. Haematol.* **2009**, *145*, 667–669.

141. Safdar, A. Immune modulatory activity of ribavirin for serious human metapneumovirus disease: Early i.v. therapy may improve outcomes in immunosuppressed SCT recipients. *Bone Marrow Transplant.* **2008**, *41*, 707–708.

142. Shachor-Meyouhas, Y.; Ben-Barak, A.; Kassis, I. Treatment with oral ribavirin and IVIG of severe human metapneumovirus pneumonia (HMPV) in immune compromised child. *Pediatr. Blood Canc.* **2011**, *57*, 350–351.

12

Respiratory Syncytial Virus Persistence in Macrophages Alters the Profile of Cellular Gene Expression

Evelyn Rivera-Toledo * and Beatríz Gómez

Department of Microbiology and Parasitology, Faculty of Medicine,
Universidad Nacional Autónoma de México, Circuito exterior s/n, Ciudad Universitaria,
México D.F., C.P. 04510, Mexico; E-Mail: begomez@servidor.unam.mx

*   Author to whom correspondence should be addressed; E-Mail: evelynmicro@gmail.com

Abstract: Viruses can persistently infect differentiated cells through regulation of expression of both their own genes and those of the host cell, thereby evading detection by the host's immune system and achieving residence in a non-lytic state. Models *in vitro* with cell lines are useful tools in understanding the mechanisms associated with the establishment of viral persistence. In particular, a model to study respiratory syncytial virus (RSV) persistence in a murine macrophage-like cell line has been established. Compared to non-infected macrophages, macrophages persistently infected with RSV show altered expression both of genes coding for cytokines and trans-membrane proteins associated with antigen uptake and of genes related to cell survival. The biological changes associated with altered gene expression in macrophages as a consequence of persistent RSV infection are summarized.

Keywords: Respiratory syncytial virus; viral persistence; macrophages; P388D1; altered gene expression

1. The Virus: Characteristics, Pathogenesis, and Epidemiology

Respiratory syncytial virus (RSV; family Paramyxoviridae, genus Pneumovirus) is a highly infectious agent—more so than other respiratory viruses—and worldwide is the principal cause of serious lower-respiratory tract illness in infants and young children [1]. Structurally, RSV is an enveloped and pleomorphic virus, with a single-stranded, negative-sense RNA genome encoding 11 proteins [1,2]. Epidemiological studies of RSV indicate that this pathogen is frequently isolated from children with bronchiolitis [3,4] and is the most frequent cause of hospitalization of infants in industrialized countries [5]. Risk factors, such as premature birth, congenital heart disease, and immune deficiencies, predispose children <6 months of age to severe respiratory disease, thus increasing the frequency of RSV-related hospitalizations by as much as 56% [6–8]. Most infants experience RSV infection during the first year of life and there exists an association between early severe RSV infection and recurrent wheezing or asthma in later childhood [9–11]. RSV is also an important cause of morbidity and mortality in the elderly and in immunocompromised patients [12,13]. In the elderly, RSV is the second leading cause of viral death, with an annual incidence up to 5% [14]. The World Health Organization (WHO) reports 64 million cases and 160,000 deaths each year due to RSV—more than that caused by any other respiratory virus [15]. Seasonal RSV outbreaks occur each year throughout the world during the winter months: in the northern hemisphere, the annual epidemics normally start in November, peak in January and February and end in May; in the southern hemisphere, the epidemic season runs from May through September [16,17].

Prospective studies of cohorts of patients with chronic obstructive pulmonary disease (COPD) have revealed, through reverse-transcription polymerase chain reaction (RT-PCR), that RSV is the virus most frequently detected in nasopharyngeal aspirates during stable COPD and exacerbated episodes [18,19]. The effects of the sequelae of severe RSV disease may be explained, in part, by viral persistence, with the RSV infection causing an alteration of the airway structure and/or inducing an aberrant immune response [9,10,19]. Continuous stimulation of the immune system by persistent viral infections may cause chroniflammation or alter the expression of immunoregulatory molecules [20–22]; such outcomes may explain the clinical manifestations that persist long after acute viral infection. Infected epithelial cells and macrophages secrete cytokines, chemokines, and other factors that attract lymphocytes and other cells to the site of infection, thus resulting in airway inflammation [23,24].

2. RSV Persistence

Although RSV persistence in humans has not been demonstrated, some observations indicate that this may be the case: (1) the presence of RSV antigen in bone biopsies and in osteoclasts cultured from patients with Paget disease was detected by using immunohistological assays [25]; (2) RSV was isolated repeatedly from the nasopharynx of apparently healthy children [26]; (3) RSV nucleoprotein mRNA was detected in archival postmortem lung tissue from infants, who had died during the summer, without apparent clinical disease having been reported [27]; and (4) RSV genome has been detected in human naïve primary bone marrow stromal cells from adults (6/8) and children (3/3) [28].

Persistent RSV infection has been established *in vivo* in mouse and guinea pig models [29–31]. In studies using BALB/c mice, persistent RSV infection has been followed through kinetic studies, revealing that infectious virus can be isolated from bronchioalveolar fluid or lymph nodes only during the first 14 days post-infection, whereas in lung homogenates, viral genomic RNA and mRNA can still be detected after 100 days, even though signs of acute infection have disappeared [30]. In guinea pigs, after resolution of acute bronchiolitis and at 60 days post-infection, viral genomic RNA and RSV proteins, along with polymorphonuclear cell infiltrates, can be detected in lungs by RT-PCR and immunohistochemistry [29]. Although, in these models *in vivo*, the cell type that RSV is able to persistently infect has not been determined, studies *in vitro* indicate that RSV can establish persistent infection in epithelial cells, macrophages and dendritic cells [32–36].

The predominant cell type recovered from bronchioalveolar lavages from children with acute severe lower-respiratory tract symptoms is the alveolar macrophage; these macrophages express RSV antigens along with pro-inflammatory cytokines [37]. Also, experiments with calves acutely infected with bovine respiratory syncytial virus (BRSV), a virus closely related to RSV, indicate that upper and lower airway epithelial cells and alveolar macrophages are target cells for the virus, as they became productively infected [38]. In addition, experiments with isolated human alveolar macrophages have shown that this cell type can support prolonged RSV replication (up to 25 days post-infection) without an apparent effect on cell viability, suggesting that macrophages may be an important reservoir for RSV *in vivo* [39].

Succeeding in a persistent infection depends on the ability of the virus to regulate not only its own genes but also the host genes in order to avoid killing the host cell. This is achieved by an alternative viral strategy of replication and the ability to evade the immunologic surveillance system of the host. In this way, the continuous replication of a virus in a differentiated cell can alter the normal functions of said cell without destroying it; this in turn disturbs the homeostasis of the host, thus producing disease [40].

Given that macrophages are important target cells for RSV and that, once infected, they can support a persistent viral infection, this brief review is focused on alterations in the biological functions of a murine macrophage-like cell line persistently infected with RSV.

3. Establishment and Characteristics of a Persistently RSV-Infected Macrophage-Like Culture

A model to study the RSV persistence in macrophages was established by using the murine macrophage-like cell line, P388D1, which was derived from serial passages in mice of an original methylcholanthrene-induced lymphoid neoplasm in a DBA/2 mouse [41]. When this cell line was infected at a multiplicity of infection (m.o.i.) of 1.0 with the prototype RSV Long strain (wild-type RSV), both a low frequency of syncytia and a high percentage of cell death during the first 48 h post infection were observed. Nevertheless, after 72 h, the number of macrophages started to increase and the surviving cells were propagated. In the first few passages, 40%–60% of the cells presented viral antigen on their cell membrane; after cloning the cells by limited dilution and reinfecting the clones at an m.o.i. of 1.0, subsequent passages were stabilized, with a constant viral expression in 90%–95% of the cells being achieved [33]. Currently, after more than 85 passages, this line of macrophages persistently infected with RSV (MφP) continues to express the viral genome: mRNA of the N viral gene is detected by RT-PCR and viral proteins are expressed on the cell membrane, as demonstrated by immunofluorescence [42].

One of the effects of persistent virus infection in immortalized cells is alteration of the viral genome, thus producing viral variants adapted for a prolonged period of replication without killing the host cell [40]. Similarly, the RSV in MφP shows genotypic changes, at least in the viral membrane fusion protein (F), compared to the wild-type RSV [43]. The genotypic change in persistent RSV was associated with a decreased fusogenic activity and was manifested by reduced size and frequency of syncytia, as well as with low extracellular viral titer in Vero cells, an RSV-permissive cell line [43]. When the deduced amino acid sequences of the F protein from the persistent and wild-type RSV were compared, changes in nine amino acids were observed, three of which are adjacent to the cleavage domain and the fusion peptide. The particular changes in the region of the cleavage domain suggest that the processing of the F0 precursor by cellular proteases may not be efficient, thus reducing its membrane fusion capacity. This hypothesis is supported by experiments in which the number of syncytia was augmented approximately five-fold when Vero cells infected with persistent RSV were cultured either in the presence of trypsin or in a low pH environment—conditions that have been shown to improve activation of viral fusogenic proteins [44–46]. However, it seems that the efficiency of F0 processing from persistent RSV is cell-line dependent, because when lung carcinoma cells H358 were used as target cells for the same persistent virus, neither the enzymatic nor acidic treatment improved the fusogenic activity; in fact, the fusogenic activity was similar to that obtained without treatment, indicating that the intracellular protease activation of the persistent RSV F protein is less efficient in Vero cells than in H358 cells [43].

4. Persistent RSV Infection Alters Macrophage Gene Expression and Biological Activities

Macrophages, important cells of the innate immune system, act as a first-line of defense against invading pathogens and help to initiate T-cell responses by processing and presenting antigens. The non-specific defense function of macrophages depends mainly on their ability to take up particulate material by phagocytosis [47]. Phagocytosis can be mediated either directly by receptors on the macrophages recognizing foreign structures of particles or indirectly by receptors that recognize self-ligands (e.g., when a foreign particle is opsonized by complement or by antibodies) [48,49].

Specific phagocytosis mediated by Fcγ receptors (FcγR) of IgG-opsonized sheep red blood cells is three- to six-fold enhanced in MφP, compared to mock infected macrophages (MφN); this relevant change is likely a consequence of an increased level of expression of FcγRII and FcγRIII in the MφP [50]. Arrevillaga et al. [42] showed that non-opsonized phagocytosis is also altered in MφP. In that work, MφP show a decreased efficiency in phagocytizing non-typeable Haemophilus influenzae (NTHi), a pathogen associated with exacerbations of COPD, with bacterial adhesion and ingestion being 1.7- and 11-fold less, respectively, than the values obtained with MφN [42]. This diminished uptake of bacteria by MφP is linked to a reduced expression (~50%) of both the ICAM-1 mRNA and ICAM-1 protein on the cell membrane, the latter serving as a ligand to bind bacteria. Although ICAM-1 is not the only ligand for NTHi, the negative transcriptional regulation of this molecule, as a consequence of the persistent RSV infection, could contribute to inefficient bacterial clearance by macrophages.

Dendritic cells, macrophages, and B lymphocytes are "professional" antigen-presenting cells (APCs). Although dendritic cells and their subsets are the most potent stimulators of T lymphocytes, the relevance of particular APCs can be determined according to their abundance in a particular tissue [51]. Alveolar macrophages comprise 95% of the cells of the lung lavage with the remaining portion consisting mostly of leukocytes, thus indicating that macrophages may be important in establishing an early non-specific defense and by functioning as presenting cells to initiate the adaptive immune response in the lung [52]. A study by Guerrero-Plata et al. [53], which focused on determining whether MφP preserve their ability to present antigens, showed that persistent infection with RSV increases expression levels of alleles K and D of the MHC class-I molecules to levels similar to those obtained at 24-h post-acute infection. The augmented MHC-I expression in MφP correlates with an efficient processing and presentation of RSV antigens to RSV-specific CD8 T cells, as determined by cytotoxicity assays. Also, MφP maintain the ability to process and present other viral antigens, such as a peptide derived from the influenza virus nucleoprotein (NP147-155). In addition, the profiles of cytokine expression in supernatants of MφP and MφN cultures indicate that the cytokines IL-1β and IL-6 are statistically significantly augmented in the MφP, suggesting that persistent RSV infection keeps macrophages in a permanently activated state [50]. Acute RSV infection of lung epithelial cells and granulocytes induced prolonged survival of infected cells by increasing the expression of anti-apoptotic molecules of the Bcl-2 family [54,55]. MφP, under normal culture conditions, display similar viability as MφN [56]. However, treatment of these macrophage cultures with staurosporine—an inhibitor of protein kinases, which induces cellular apoptosis in the original P388D1 cell line [57]—induces cell death of almost all MφN after 24 h, whereas more than 75% of MφP are refractory [56]. MφP resistance to apoptosis is associated with reduced expression of the protein pro-caspase 9, although its mRNA levels are normal or even higher than in MφN, suggesting that persistent infection regulates caspase 9 expression at a post-transcriptional level. Furthermore, chronic RSV infection of MφP up-regulates mRNA and the protein products of anti-apoptotic genes such as Bcl-2, Bcl-x, and XIAP, indicating that abrogation of the intrinsic pathway of apoptosis is a mechanism crucial for the establishment and maintenance of viral persistence [56]. Figure 1 summarizes changes in virus and MφP as a consequence of persistent infection.

Figure 1. Changes in respiratory syncytial virus (RSV) and macrophages by persistent infection. RSV persistence in macrophages leads to genotypic changes, at least in the viral membrane fusion protein F and in the profile of cellular gene expression. Arrows indicate increase or decrease in biological activities or molecule expression.

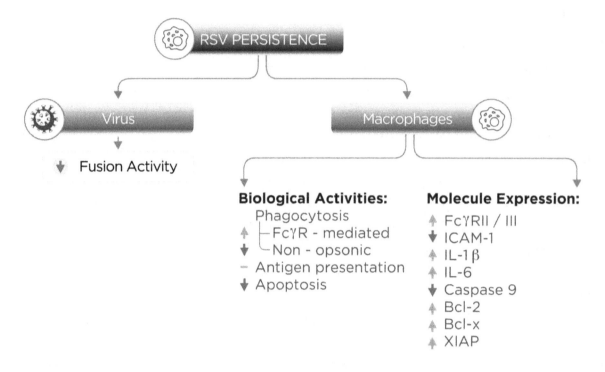

5. Relevance of RSV Persistence in Macrophages and Epithelial Cells

Understanding the virus-cell interactions during acute and persistent RSV infections is fundamental for the development of strategies to inhibit viral infection and to eliminate viral reservoirs. Models *in vitro* and *in vivo* have been useful tools in advancing comprehension both of the mechanisms by which RSV establishes persistence and of the pathology associated with chronic infection. Models *in vitro* with macrophages and epithelial cell lines have been particularly useful in determining, at the molecular level, alterations produced in the host cell by long-term RSV infection [32,42,53,56]. To date, in addition to MφP, the only other cell model of persistent infection by RSV, in which changes in cellular gene expression have been studied, are persistently RSV-infected HEp-2 epithelial cells. Martínez *et al.* [32] reported that, as determined by microarray analysis, several genes with diverse functional categories were either up- or down-regulated in persistently RSV-infected HEp-2 cells. In particular, it was observed that some of the genes that were up-regulated were those involved in cell survival, such as those encoding for the anti-apoptotic molecules TRAF-1 and BIRC3, and that some of the genes that were down-regulated were pro-apoptotic genes, such as tnf-α, bcl2l11, and caspase 9. In contrast to that in MφP, persistent RSV infection in HEp-2 cells regulates caspase 9 expression at the translational level. The study also showed that, although the chemokines CCL3 and RANTES are up-regulated during acute and persistent RSV infection, the levels of these chemokines in persistently infected HEp-2 cells are up to two-fold greater than those in acutely infected HEp-2 cells. It has also been reported that, in a model of RSV persistence in human epithelial cells A549, the level of the cytokine IL-8, evaluated by ELISA in supernatants, is up to 2.6-fold greater than that in mock-infected cells [34]. Thus, when taken together, the findings (1) that RSV can establish persistent infection in macrophages and epithelial cell *in vitro*; (2) that alterations in gene expression lead to survival of persistently infected cells; and (3) that persistently infected cells produce excessive level of cytokines and chemokines that are associated with chronic inflammation lend strong support to the hypothesis that RSV persistence in patients may be a cause of chronic respiratory diseases. It is still to be determined whether altered expression of membrane molecules related to antigen uptake by macrophages occurs in models *in vivo* and, if so, whether such altered expression is relevant to pathogenesis.

6. Conclusion

RSV can productively infect macrophages *in vivo* and *in vitro* and can establish persistent infection in macrophage-like cells *in vitro*. The consequence of persistent RSV infection in macrophages is the altered expression of genes coding for pro-inflammatory cytokines, for trans-membrane proteins related to antigen uptake, and for those proteins related to cell survival. The evidence suggests that macrophages may be one of the cell populations that can serve as viral reservoirs for RSV *in vivo*. Understanding how RSV manipulates host cells during persistent infection may provide important insights into new approaches for rational drug design and vaccines.

Acknowledgments

The authors thank Enrique Graue Wiechers for his support, Andi Espinoza-Sánchez for his help in figure preparation and Veronica Yakoleff for revision of the original English version, editing of the manuscript, and helpful comments.

References

1. Cane, P.A. Molecular epidemiology of respiratory syncytial virus. *Rev. Med. Virol.* **2007**, *11*, 103–116.

2. Collins, P.L.; Graham, B.S. Viral and host factors in human respiratory syncytial virus pathogenesis. *J. Virol.* **2008**, *82*, 2040–2055.

3. Ogra, P.L. Respiratory syncytial virus: The virus, the disease and the immune response. *Paediatr. Respir. Rev.* **2004**, *5*, 119–126.

4. Hall, C.B.; Weinberg, G.A.; Iwane, M.K.; Blumkin, A.K.; Edwards, K.M.; Staat, M.A.; Auinger, P.; Griffin, M.R.; Poehling, K.A.; Erdman, D.; *et al.* The burden of respiratory syncytial virus infection in young children. *N. Engl. J. Med.* **2009**, *360*, 588–598.

5. Law, B.J.; Carbonell-Estrany, X.; Simoes, E.A. An update on respiratory syncytial virus epidemiology: A developed country perspective. *Respir. Med.* **2002**, *96*, 1–7.

6. Hervás, D.; Reina, J.; Yañez, A.; del Valle, J.M.; Figuerola, J.; Hervás, J.A. Epidemiology of hospitalization for acute bronchiolitis in children: Differences between RSV and non-RSV bronchiolitis. *Eur. J. Clin. Microbiol. Infect. Dis.* **2012**, *31*, 1975–1981.

7. Langley, G.F.; Anderson, L.J. Epidemiology and prevention of respiratory syncytial virus infections among infants and young children. *Pediatr. Infect. Dis. J.* **2011**, *30*, 510–517.

8. Welliver, R.C. Review of epidemiology and clinical risk factors for severe respiratory syncytial virus (RSV) infection. *J. Pediatr.* **2003**, *143*, 112–117.

9. Mejías, A.; Chávez-Bueno, S.; Ramilo, O. Respiratory syncytial virus pneumonia: Mechanisms of inflammation and prolonged airway hyperresponsiveness. *Curr. Opin. Infect. Dis.* **2005**, *18*, 199–204.

10. Sigurs, N.; Gustafsson, P.M.; Bjarnason, R.; Lundberg, F.; Schmidt, S.; Sigurbergsson, F.; Kjellman, B. Severe respiratory syncytial virus bronchiolitis in infancy and asthma and allergy at age 13. *Am. J. Respir. Crit. Care Med.* **2005**, *171*, 137–141.

11. Staat, M.A. Respiratory syncytial virus infections in children. *Semin. Respir. Infect.* **2002**, *17*, 15–20.

12. Dowell, S.F.; Anderson, L.J.; Gary, H.E., Jr.; Erdman, D.D.; Plouffe, J.F.; File, T.M., Jr.; Marston, B.J.; Breiman, R.F. Respiratory syncytial virus is an important cause of community-acquired lower respiratory infection among hospitalized adults. *J. Infect. Dis.* **1996**, *174*, 456–462.

13. Falsey, A.R.; Hennessey, P.A.; Formica, M.A.; Cox, C.; Walsh, E.E. Respiratory syncytial virus infection in elderly and high-risk adults. *N. Engl. J. Med.* **2005**, *352*, 1749–1759.

14. Falsey, A.R.; Walsh, E.E. Respiratory syncytial virus infection in adults. *Clin. Microbiol. Rev.* **2000**, *13*, 371–384.

15. World Health Organization. Initiative for Vaccine Research: Respiratory Syncytial Virus. Available online: http://www.who.int/vaccine_research/diseases/ari/en/index3.html (accessed on 22 August 2012).

16. Bhatt, J.M.; Everard, M.L. Do environmental pollutants influence the onset of respiratory syncytial virus epidemics or disease severity? *Paediatr. Respir. Rev.* **2004**, *5*, 333–338.

17. Collins, P.L.; Melero, J.A. Progress in understanding and controlling respiratory syncytial virus: Still crazy after all these years. *Virus Res.* **2011**, *162*, 80–99.

18. Seemungal, T.; Harper-Owen, R.; Bhowmik, A.; Moric, I.; Sanderson, G.; Message, S.; Maccallum, P.; Meade, T.W.; Jeffries, D.J.; Johnston, S.L.; *et al.* Respiratory viruses, symptoms, and inflammatory markers in acute exacerbations and stable chronic obstructive pulmonary disease. *Am. J. Respir. Crit. Care Med.* **2001**, *164*, 1618–1623.

19. Sikkel, M.B.; Quint, J.K.; Mallia, P.; Wedzicha, J.A.; Johnston, S.L. Respiratory syncytial virus persistence in chronic obstructive pulmonary disease. *Pediatr. Infect. Dis. J.* **2008**, *27*, 63–70.

20. Kim, E.Y.; Battaile, J.T.; Patel, A.C.; You, Y.; Agapov, E.; Grayson, M.H.; Benoit, L.A.; Byers, D.E.; Alevy, Y.; Tucker, J.; *et al.* Persistent activation of an innate immune response translates respiratory viral infection into chronic lung disease. *Nat. Med.* **2008**, *14*, 633–640.

21. Di Rosa, F.; Barnaba, V. Persisting viruses and chronic inflammation: Understanding their relation to autoimmunity. *Immunol. Rev.* **1998**, *164*, 17–27.

22. Wald, O.; Weiss, I.D.; Galun, E.; Peled, A. Chemokines in hepatitis C virus infection: Pathogenesis, prognosis and therapeutics. *Cytokine* **2007**, *39*, 50–62.

23. Culley, F.J.; Pennycook, A.M.; Tregoning, J.S.; Hussell, T.; Openshaw, P.J. Differential chemokine expression following respiratory virus infection reflects Th1- or Th2-biased immunopathology. *J. Virol.* **2006**, *80*, 4521–4527.

24. Krishnan, S.; Halonen, M.; Welliver, R.C. Innate immune responses in respiratory syncytial virus infections. *Viral Immunol.* **2004**, *17*, 220–233.

25. Mills, B.G.; Singer, F.R.; Weiner, L.P.; Holst, P.A. Immunohistological demonstration of respiratory syncytial virus antigens in Paget disease of bone. *Proc. Natl. Acad. Sci. USA* **1981**, *78*, 1209–1213.

26. Isaia G.; Teodosiu, O.; Popescu, G.; Athanasiu, P.; Sternberg, I.; Dumitriu, Z. Persistence of viruses in the nasopharynx of apparently healthy children aged 0–5 years. Results of investigations performed in 1982–83. *Virologie* **1985**, *36*, 175–179.

27. Cubie, H.A.; Duncan, L.A.; Marshall, L.A.; Smith, N.M. Detection of respiratory syncytial virus nucleic acid in archival postmortem tissue from infants. *Pediatr. Pathol. Lab. Med.* **1997**, *17*, 927–938.

28. Rezaee, F.; Gibson, L.F.; Piktel, D.; Othumpangat, S.; Piedimonte, G. Respiratory syncytial virus infection in human bone marrow stromal cells. *Am. J. Respir. Cell Mol. Biol.* **2011**, *45*, 277–286.

29. Hegele, R.G.; Hayashi, S.; Bramley, A.M.; Hogg, J.C. Persistence of respiratory syncytial virus genome and protein after acute bronchiolitis in guinea pigs. *Chest* **1994**, *105*, 1848–1854.

30. Schwarze, J.; O'Donnell, D.R.; Rohwedder, A.; Openshaw, P.J. Latency and persistence of respiratory syncytial virus despite T cell immunity. *Am. J. Respir. Crit. Care Med.* **2004**, *169*, 801–805.

31. Sutton, T.C.; Tayyari, F.; Khan, M.A.; Manson, H.E.; Hegele, R.G. T helper 1 background protects against airway hyperresponsiveness and inflammation in guinea pigs with persistent respiratory syncytial virus infection. *Pediatr. Res.* **2007**, *61*, 525–529.

32. Martínez, I.; Lombardía, L.; Herranz, C.; García-Barreno, B.; Domínguez, O.; Melero, J.A. Cultures of HEp-2 cells persistently infected by human respiratory syncytial virus differ in chemokine expression and resistance to apoptosis as compared to lytic infections of the same cell type. *Virology* **2009**, *388*, 31–41.

33. Sarmiento, R.E.; Tirado, R.; Gómez, B. Characteristics of a respiratory syncytial virus persistently infected macrophage-like culture. *Virus Res.* **2002**, *84*, 45–58.

34. Tirado, R.; Ortega, A.; Sarmiento, R.E.; Gómez, B. Interleukin-8 mRNA synthesis and protein secretion are continuously up-regulated by respiratory syncytial virus persistently infected cells. *Cell Immunol.* **2005**, *233*, 61–71.

35. Valdovinos, M.R.; Gómez, B. Establishment of respiratory syncytial virus persistence in cell lines: Association with defective interfering particles. *Intervirology* **2003**, *46*, 190–198.

36. Hobson, L.; Everard, M.L. Persistent of respiratory syncytial virus in human dendritic cells and influence of nitric oxide. *Clin. Exp. Immunol.* **2008**, *151*, 359–366.

37. Midulla, F.; Villani, A.; Panuska, J.R.; Dab, I.; Kolls, J.K.; Merolla, R.; Ronchetti, R. Respiratory syncytial virus lung infection in infants: Immunoregulatory role of infected alveolar macrophages. *J. Infect. Dis.* **1993**, *168*, 1515–1519.

38. Castleman, W.L.; Lay, J.C.; Dubovi, E.J.; Slauson, D.O. Experimental bovine respiratory syncytial virus infection in conventional calves: Light microscopic lesions, microbiology, and studies on lavaged lung cells. *Am. J. Vet. Res.* **1985**, *46*, 547–553.

39. Panuska, J.R.; Cirino, N.M.; Midulla, F.; Despot, J.E.; McFadden, E.R., Jr.; Huang, Y.T. Productive infection of isolated human alveolar macrophages by respiratory syncytial virus. *J. Clin. Investig.* **1990**, *86*, 113–119.

40. Oldstone, M.B. Viral persistence: Parameters, mechanisms and future predictions. *Virology* **2006**, *344*, 111–118.

41. Koren, H.S.; Handwerger, B.S.; Wunderlich, J.R. Identification of macrophage-like characteristics in a cultured murine tumor line. *J. Immunol.* **1975**, *114*, 894–897.

42. Arrevillaga, G.; Gaona, J.; Sánchez, C.; Rosales, V.; Gómez, B. Respiratory syncytial virus persistence in macrophages downregulates intercellular adhesion molecule-1 expression and reduces adhesion of non-typeable haemophilus influenzae. *Intervirology* **2012**, *55*, 442–450.

43. Sarmiento, R.E.; Arias, C.F.; Méndez, E.; Gómez, B. Characterization of a persistent respiratory syncytial virus showing a low-fusogenic activity associated to an impaired F protein. *Virus Res.* **2009**, *139*, 39–47.

44. Matsuyama, S.; Delos, S.E.; White, J.M. Sequential roles of receptor binding and low pH in forming prehairpin and hairpin conformations of a retroviral envelope glycoprotein. *J. Virol.* **2004**, *78*, 8201–8209.

45. Skehel, J.J.; Wiley, D.C. Receptor binding and membrane fusion in virus entry: The influenza hemagglutinin. *Annu. Rev. Biochem.* **2000**, *69*, 531–569.

46. Thoennes, S.; Li, Z.N.; Lee, B.J.; Langley, W.A.; Skehel, J.J.; Russell, R.J.; Steinhauer, D.A. Analysis of residues near the fusion peptide in the influenza hemagglutinin structure for roles in triggering membrane fusion. *Virology* **2008**, *370*, 403–414.

47. Hume, D.A. The mononuclear phagocyte system. *Curr. Opin. Immunol.* **2006**, *18*, 49–53.

48. Swanson, J.A.; Hoppe, A.D. The coordination of signaling during Fc receptor-mediated phagocytosis. *J. Leukoc. Biol.* **2004**, *76*, 1093–1103.

49. Van Lookeren Campagne, M.; Wiesmann, C.; Brown, E.J. Macrophage complement receptors and pathogen clearance. *Cell. Microbiol.* **2007**, *9*, 2095–2102.

50. Guerrero-Plata, A.; Ortega, E.; Gomez, B. Persistence of respiratory syncytial virus in macrophages alters phagocytosis and pro-inflammatory cytokine production. *Viral Immunol.* **2001**, *14*, 19–30.

51. Liu, K.; Nussenzweig, M.C. Origin and development of dendritic cells. *Immunol. Rev.* **2010**, *234*, 45–54.

52. Guth, A.M.; Janssen, W.J.; Bosio, C.M.; Crouch, E.C.; Henson, P.M.; Dow, S.W. Lung environment determines unique phenotype of alveolar macrophages. *Am. J. Physiol. Lung Cell. Mol. Physiol.* **2009**, *296*, 936–946.

53. Guerrero-Plata, A.; Ortega, E.; Ortíz-Navarrete, V.; Gómez, B. Antigen presentation by a macrophage-like cell line persistently infected with respiratory syncytial virus. *Virus Res.* **2004**, *99*, 95–100.

54. Lindemans, C.A.; Coffer, P.J.; Schellens, I.M.; de Graaff, P.M.; Kimpen, J.L.; Koenderman, L. Respiratory syncytial virus inhibits granulocyte apoptosis through a phosphatidylinositol 3-kinase and NF-kappaB-dependent mechanism. *J. Immunol.* **2006**, *176*, 5529–5537.

55. Monick, M.M.; Cameron, K.; Staber, J.; Powers, L.S.; Yarovinsky, T.O.; Koland, J.G.; Hunninghake, G.W. Activation of the epidermal growth factor receptor by respiratory syncytial virus results in increased inflammation and delayed apoptosis. *J. Biol. Chem.* **2005**, *280*, 2147–2158.

56. Nakamura-López, Y.; Villegas-Sepúlveda, N.; Sarmiento-Silva, R.E.; Gómez, B. Intrinsic apoptotic pathway is subverted in mouse macrophages persistently infected by RSV. *Virus Res.* **2011**, *158*, 98–107.

57. Nakamura-López, Y.; Sarmiento-Silva, R.E.; Moran-Andrade, J.; Gómez-García, B. Staurosporine-induced apoptosis in P388D1 macrophages involves both extrinsic and intrinsic pathways. *Cell Biol. Int.* **2009**, *33*, 1026–1031.

13

Th17 Lymphocytes in Respiratory Syncytial Virus Infection

Jonas Bystrom [1,*], Nasra Al-Adhoubi [2], Mohammed Al-Bogami [1], Ali S. Jawad [2] and Rizgar A. Mageed [1]

[1] Bone and Joint Research Unit, William Harvey Research Institute,
   Queen Mary University of London, London EC1M 6BQ, UK;
   E-Mails: m.al-bogami@qmul.ac.uk (M.A.-B.); r.a.mageed@qmul.ac.uk (R.A.M.)

[2] Department of Rheumatology, The Royal London Hospital, Mile End, Barts and The London,
   Queen Mary University of London, London EC1M 6BQ, UK;
   E-Mails: nasrak2004@yahoo.com (N.A.-A.); alismjawad1@hotmail.com (A.S.J.)

* Author to whom correspondence should be addressed; E-Mail: j.bystrom@qmul.ac.uk

---

Abstract: Infection by respiratory syncytial virus (RSV) affects approximately 33 million infants annually worldwide and is a major cause of hospitalizations. Helper T lymphocytes (Th) play a central role in the immune response during such infections. However, Th lymphocytes that produce interleukin 17 (IL-17), known as Th17 lymphocytes, in addition to been protective can also cause pathology that accompany this type of infection. The protective effects of Th17 is associated with better prognosis in most infected individuals but heightened Th17 responses cause inflammation and pathology in others. Studies employing animal models have shown that activated Th17 lymphocytes recruit neutrophils and facilitate tertiary lymphoid structure development in infected lungs. However, IL-17 also inhibits the ability of $CD8^+$ lymphocytes to clear viral particles and acts synergistically with the innate immune system to exacerbate inflammation. Furthermore, IL-17 enhances IL-13 production which, in turn, promotes the activation of Th2 lymphocytes and excessive mucus production. Studies of animal models have also shown that a lack of, or inadequate, responses by the Th1 subset of T lymphocytes enhances Th17-mediated responses and that this is detrimental during RSV co-infection in experimental asthma. The available evidence, therefore, indicates that Th17 can play contradictory roles during RSV infections. The factors that determine the shift in the balance between beneficial and adverse Th17 mediated effects during RSV infection remains to be determined.

Keywords: RSV; pneumovirus; mucus; interleukin 17; interleukin 23; interleukin 13; Th17

---

1. Th17 Lymphocytes and IL-17 and the Immune System—Basic biology

Th17 lymphocytes play a central role in host defences against a range of extracellular pathogens including bacteria, viruses and fungi [1–3]. This subset of helper T lymphocytes differs from the other subsets, Th1, Th2 and regulatory T lymphocytes (T-reg lymphocytes) both in their requirements for differentiation and expansion factors and in their targets pathogens. In addition, excess Th17 lymphocyte numbers have been associated with inflammatory autoimmune diseases [4–6]. In contrast to Th1 and Th2 lymphocytes which predominantly produce interferon gamma (IFNγ) and IL-4/IL-5/IL13, Th17 lymphocytes produce IL-17A, IL-17F, IL-21 and IL-22. IL-17A and IL-17F are members of IL-17 family of cytokines which includes six members; IL-17A-F. All members of this family are involved in inflammatory responses; however, only IL-17A, F and E (IL-25) are produced by haematopoietic cells. IL-17A and IL-17F show 50% homology and both bind IL-17 receptor (IL-17R) which is a complex of IL-17RA and IL-17RC. IL-17A binds with higher affinity to the IL-17RA/C and induces stronger intracellular signalling than IL-17F. Both IL-17A and F are active as dimers; homodimers and heterodimers [7]. The studies reviewed in this article are mainly about IL-17A and this cytokine will thereafter be referred to as IL-17.

IL-17 acts on stromal cells to promote the production chemokines such as CXCL1, IL-8, CCL20 (MIP-3α) and IL-6 which then promote neutrophil recruitment to sites of infection (see Table 1) [8]. IL-17 itself is a weak inducer of these cytokines/chemokines but acts by stabilizing mRNA transcripts induced by other cytokines [9]. IL-17 also down-regulates micro-RNA 23b (miR-23b), which negatively regulates inflammatory responses [10]. Furthermore, IL-17 induces mucus production in the respiratory tract and increases the expression of polymeric Ig receptors that facilitate the release of IgA and IgM antibodies into the respiratory tract [11]. Of the other cytokines produced by Th17 lymphocytes, IL-21 promotes Th17 proliferation and antibody production by B lymphocytes [12]. Paradoxically, however, Il-21 also antagonizes some IL-17-mediated responses during RSV infection [13]. IL-22, in contrast, promotes mucosal homeostasis and induces the production of antibacterial peptides [14].

The production of low-levels of IL-17 by resident Th17 lymphocytes is necessary for maintaining immunological homeostasis in the gut. This occurs under the influence of IL-1β and transforming growth factor beta (TGFβ) that are produced by gut epithelial cells [15]. During inflammation, IL-6 and prostaglandin E_2 (PGE_2) are produced and these induce IL-23 receptor expression which is necessary for the differentiation of naive $CD4^+$ T lymphocytes to Th17 lymphocytes [16,17]. The differentiation of Th17 cells involves an intricate network of cytokines and transcription factors predominant among which is the retinoic orphan receptor gamma t (RORγt) and retinoic acid receptor alpha (RARα) [18]. Interestingly, recent studies have revealed that low level CD3/TCR engagement, as compared with high level receptor engagement, preferentially promotes human Th17 differentiations and the effect is mediated through activating the NFAT-1 transcription factor [19,20]. Hypoxia also promotes Th17 differentiation through the hypoxia-inducible factor alpha (HIF-1α) transcription factor which binds to the promoter of RORγt in naïve T lymphocytes [21,22]. The production of IL-23, in contrast, is associated with the expansion of Th17 lymphocytes in pathogenic settings such as in autoimmune disease [23]. In this respect, IL-23 production by DCs during RSV infection has been suggested to be responsible for Th17 propagation and exacerbated inflammation associated with the infection [24,25].

2. Th17 Lymphocytes in the Respiratory Tract

Th17 lymphocytes are present in the respiratory tract and there is evidence that they play a key role in responses to fungal infections. These cells, however, also contribute to inflammatory disorders that afflict the respiratory tract, such as asthma and chronic obstructive pulmonary disease (COPD). Increased production of the Th17-related cytokines, such as IL-17A, IL-22 and IL-23 in COPD patients reflects the involvement of Th17 lymphocytes in initiating and driving the disease process [26,27]. In addition, excess IL-17 production has been reported in animal models and human patients has been associated with neutrophil dominated asthma and with cortisone-resistant severe airway and hyper-reactivity (AHR) [28,29]. Although both IL-17A and IL-17F have been shown to play a role in asthma, studies of gene knockout mice have suggested that IL-17F may in fact ameliorate the disease process [30]. Th17 lymphocytes have also been implicated in effector mechanisms triggered in response to RSV and other types of respiratory viral infections [31,32].

3. IL-17 and Th17 Lymphocytes in Human RSV Infection

3.1. The Immune Response at the Onset of RSV Infection

Worldwide, infants are affected by lower respiratory tract infections caused by RSV. Although many such infections have a mild course, in certain infants the infection leads to bronchiolitis needing hospitalization and respiratory support in an intensive care unit [31,34,35]. Inhaled RSV particles bind glucose amino glycans on respiratory epithelial cells through their glycoproteins, major attachment protein G and fusion protein F. The particles then fuse with the cells and initiate their propagation and spreading [36,37]. There is evidence that cells other than epithelial cells, including macrophages and dendritic cells (DCs), are also infected by the virus [38,39]. Infected epithelial cells initially respond either by releasing acute phase proteins or promoting their production, such as causing complement component C3 activation and the release of its pro-anaphylactic factor C3a [40]. The subsequent response to the infection is of innate immune-type resulting in the influx of neutrophils which become the dominant cells during the first four days of infection [41,42].

Figure 1. IL-17 mediated responses in the respiratory tract during RSV infections. RSV virus particles infect ciliated epithelial cells in the lower respiratory tract. C3a and other mediators of inflammation are then released from epithelial cells in response to the infection and this, in turn, induces IL-17 production (dark blue colour). During the early phase of the response to RSV infection, IL-17 is produced by CD11b[+] innate immune cells. Subsequently, the production of IL-17 is predominantly by CD4[+] Th17 lymphocytes. The production of IL-17 initiates a number of effects in the respiratory tract. Thus, IL-17 induces mild inflammation and exacerbates inflammatory responses triggered by other signals and cytokines. In this scenario, single stranded RNA in RSV particles bind to TLR3 and synergize with IL-17 to induce IL-6 (orange colour) and IL-8 (blue colour) by fibroblasts (Fc). The binding of double stranded RNA to TLR7, however, is inhibitory to IL-17-mediated responses and, instead, promotes Th1-mediated responses. IL-17 co-operates with IL-1β and TNFα to induce the release of chemokines that mediate neutrophil recruitment. Furthermore, IL-17 induces mucus production from epithelial cells. IL-17 also binds receptors on CD8[+] T lymphocytes and inhibits their ability to reduce viral load. Cytokines produced by Th1 and Th2 lymphocytes, IFNγ and IL-13, in contrast, inhibit IL-17 production [25,33].

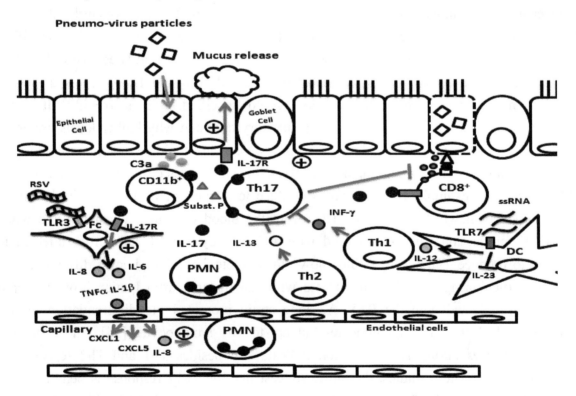

Figure: IL-17 responses in the respiratory tract during RSV infections.

3.2. The Adaptive Immune Response to RSV Infection

RSV infection activates T lymphocytes in lung draining lymph nodes with the help of DCs that migrate from sites of infection. This results in the induction and differentiation of T lymphocytes into viral-specific Th1 and Th2 lymphocytes in detectable numbers in the lung 6–8 days post RSV infection [43,46]. CD8$^+$ T lymphocytes emerge after the initial inflammatory response that follows RSV infection to clear viral particles [42]. Th1 lymphocytes are also induced and these produce pro-inflammatory cytokines, such as IFNγ and TNFα and the combination of the two cellular responses efficiently clears RSV infections in most individuals [44]. However, humans and mice deficient in the transcription factor STAT1, which is activated following IFNγ binding to its receptor, are prone to severe RSV infections [45,46]. In addition to cytotoxic and Th1 lymphocytes, the immune response also includes Th2 lymphocytes which cause key symptomatic features of RSV infections, such as excessive mucus production and wheezing that normally accompany asthma [47]. Measurement of cytokines in the *bronchoalveolar lavage* (*BAL*) of infected infants (1.5–6 months of age) has identified similar levels of Th1- and Th2-type cytokines [48,49]. In animal models of RSV infection, the lack of Th1 effects resulting from IFNγ receptor deletion leads to a dominant Th2 response and worse pathology suggesting that Th1 responses ameliorate Th2-mediated effects during RSV infection in humans [50]. A recent study analysing the cytokine profile in the plasma of RSV infected infants (6 months or younger), however, revealed that infants with a moderate response to the virus had higher plasma levels of IL-17 than infants with a severe response to RSV. In this study IFNγ and TNFα levels were shown to be lower in RSV infected infants than in control infants [51]. Furthermore, IL-17 levels were higher in BAL from paediatric patients (13 months and below) with non-ventilated RSV disease at admission and at discharge compared with BAL from more severe, ventilated cases. IFNγ was undetectable in this study but IL-6 levels were 30 times higher in the ventilated cases [31]. A further study which examined tracheal aspirates reported increased IL-6 and IL-17 levels in severely ill ventilated infants compared with healthy infants (age not specified in this study) [32]. It is currently unknown what the function of IL-17 is in the respiratory tract and why higher levels are associated with better outcome in some but not all infected infants. One clue could be that the immune system of the newly born is immature with an impaired Th1 response [52]. DCs derived from infants' umbilical cord blood have, for example, been shown to produce low levels of IL-12 [53]. Furthermore, DCs from cord blood of newly born, but not DCs from the blood of adults, when infected with RSV induced IL-17 production when co-cultured with T lymphocytes [39]. DCs from infected infants were shown to produce TGFβ, a cytokine known to promote Th17 lymphocyte differentiation [39]. Furthermore, co-culturing adult T lymphocytes with supernatants from human bronchial epithelial cells chronically-infected with the RSV A2 long strain promoted the differentiation of naïve T lymphocytes to Th2 and Th17 lymphocytes but not to Th1 lymphocytes [54]. These studies of T lymphocyte responses during RSV infection indicate that besides Th1 and Th2 responses, Th17 responses also occur. These studies, therefore, suggest that the Th17 response is beneficial in some cases of RSV infection. Th17 responses have, however, also been linked with pathology in the respiratory tract during severe neutrophil dominated asthma. More research is, therefore, needed to unravel the complex consequences of IL-17 production and when this is beneficial, when not and why.

4. The Role of Th17 Lymphocytes in the Patho-Physiology of RSV Infection: Some Insights from *in Vitro* and Animal Model Studies

To better understand the role that Th17 lymphocytes play in the patho-physiology of RSV infection animal models and *in vitro* systems have been studied. Different strains of RSV were used to immunize mice and assess the immune response to RSV infection. In addition, cell lines were used to assess the direct effect viral particles have on immune cells. RSV strains "A2" and "A2 long" were used to immunize mice to define the nature of the response including immune cell infiltration during RSV infection. The RSV strain "line 19", by contrast, was used to study cellular and molecular mechanisms involved in excessive mucus secretion and IL-13 production. Studies using the three strains of RSV revealed that infection induces IL-17 production in mice. However, no studies have been carried out to compare and contrast the responses initiated by the three strains in the same experiment.

4.1. Infection with RSV Induces IL-17 Production which Promotes Neutrophil Influx during the Early Response

Immunization of wild-type mice with RSV strain A2 resulted in complement activation by infected epithelial cells leading to the production of C3a which induced tachykinin and Substance P release. These mediators bound to their receptors on T lymphocytes, neutrophils and monocytes and lead to IL-17A production by CD11b$^+$ myeloid cells during the early phase of the response [55]. In addition, RSV RNA particles trigger innate immune system-mediated inflammatory responses by binding to TLRs. Studies on the interaction between viral particles and cell lines *in vitro* revealed that IL-17 acted synergistically with RSV RNA particles to induce IL-6 and IL-8 production by fibroblasts. Thus, RSV strain A2 RNA induced an innate immune-like response by binding to TLR3 and this response was enhanced by IL-17 [56]. Furthermore, IL-17 produced during the infection increased the influx of neutrophils. The influx of neutrophils was also observed following infection with the RSV strain A line 19. In this setting neutrophils were recruited by IL-8 which was induced by IL-17 [32] (Figure 1).

The impact of RSV infection on the cooperation between the innate system and IL-17/IL-17 producing cells is, however, complex. Thus, in addition to binding TLR3, single stranded RSV RNA particles bind TLR7 on DCs, plasmacytoid DCs, B lymphocytes and macrophages and induce IL-12 production, which promotes Th1-mediated responses (Figure 1). This can impact the balance between Th1 and Th17 responses and the patho-physiological response *in vivo*. For example, infection of TLR7 deficient mice with RSV Strain A line 19 resulted in increased numbers of Th17 lymphocytes due to an increase in IL-23 production by DCs. This response caused more pathology through the consequent increase in IL-13 and mucus production in TLR7 deficient mice compared with wild-type mice [24]. Furthermore, the inflammatory response to the mouse homologue of RSV, pneumo virus of mice (PVM), was diminished when TLR7 was missing [57]. This is somewhat analogous to the situation in newly born infants in whom effector Th17 lymphocytes are recruited when the activation of Th1 responses is inadequate.

4.2. Activation of Th17 and Th2 Cells in Response to RSV Infection

An efficient immune response to RSV infection is dependent on antigen recognition and presentation by DCs in local lymph nodes. Viral antigen presentation by DCs results in the activation and migration of CD4$^+$ and CD8$^+$ lymphocytes to the lung. The process of DC migration is dependent on the chemokine CCR7. Kallal and colleagues noted that CCR7 deficient mice had impaired lymph node formation and, instead, responded by activating T lymphocytes in local ectopic lymphoid structures in response to infection with RSV Strain A, line 19. The T lymphocyte response to RSV infection in these structures was dominated by Th17 lymphocytes. These Th17 lymphocytes promoted pathology by inducing the production of IL-13 and IL-21 which induced excessive mucus production [58]. A similar response was observed in the absence of IFNγ signaling in STAT1-deficient mice. Thus, infection of STAT1-deficient mice with RSV strain A2 resulted in elevated IL-13 and IL-17 levels, production of excess mucus and airway inflammation. Just as was the case in TLR7$^{-/-}$ mice, elevated IL-17 levels in STAT1-deficient mice were due to increased production of IL-23 [25]. In addition, to the inflammatory effects mediated by excess IL-17, it suppressed the ability of CD8$^+$ to kill cells infected with RSV [59]. This latter study revealed that Th17-derived IL-17 bound to IL-17RA on CD8$^+$ T lymphocytes and impaired their ability to reduce viral load and reduce the number of infected cells in the lung. The role of excess IL-17 in promoting pathology is further supported by the ability of neutralizing anti-IL-17 antibodies to reduce mucus and IL-13 production and increase viral clearance [36] (Table 1 and Figure 1). *In vitro* studies revealed that IL-17 enhanced mucus production by directly upregulating transcription of the mucus gene *MUC5B* in human tracheal and bronchial epithelial cell lines [60,61]. This upregulation of the *MUC5B* gene was shown to be dependent on ERK signalling and the activation NF-κB [60,61]

A number of studies in which mice were infected with RSV particles have shown that the mice simultaneously produced IL-17 and IL-13 suggesting that the Th17 response is concomitant with the Th2 response [25,32,54,58]. The molecular mechanisms that underpin the co-production of IL-13 and IL-17 were further explored in STAT1-deficient mice. Newcomb *et al.* observed that IL-13 produced during infection of mice with RSV Strain A2 was capable, perhaps paradoxically, of suppressing IL-17 production [73]. Using double STAT1- and IL-13-deficient mice for immunization experiments, these investigators observed higher levels of IL-17 production than in mice deficient in STAT1 alone. Increased IL-17 production in STAT1/IL-13-deficient mice was explained by the fact that IL-10 production, which is induced by IL-13, reduces IL-17 production by Th17 lymphocytes. In addition, Th17 lymphocytes have been reported to express IL-13 receptor alpha (IL-13Rα, also known as IL-13RA) suggesting that these cells could be directly modulated by IL-13 [62]. As IL-17 has been shown to increase mucus production through enhancing IL-13 production, these findings may suggest that IL-13 can also negatively regulate Th17 lymphocytes through a negative feedback mechanism [33].

4.3. IL-17 Causes RSV-Mediated Exacerbation of Asthma

IL-13 and mucus production are not only associated with IL-17 production but a feature of virally-exacerbated asthma. In addition, a number of studies have indicated that IL-17 is involved in severe asthma [28,29]. Therefore, the involvement of IL-17 has been explored in animal models of RSV infection concomitant with experimental asthma. For example, infection of mice with RSV Strain A2 subsequent to immunization with ovalbumin (OVA) induced experimental asthma and increased the production of mucus-associated proteins, Muc5ac and Gob-5 [63]. Mice injected with OVA, or with RSV alone, also upregulated the expression of genes encoding the mucus-associated proteins but gene expression persisted for longer periods in the OVA and RSV-immunized mice compared with those immunized with either OVA or RSV alone. Importantly, the increase in mucus production was associated with increased levels of IL-17 in the lungs [63]. Another study in which investigators used cockroach allergen (CRA) with RSV Strain A line 19 to induce asthma in mice provided further evidence for Th17 lymphocytes involvement in experimental asthma. Thus, stimulated T lymphocytes from lymph nodes of RSV/CRA-immunized mice produced IL-17 while mice immunized with CRA alone did not. Furthermore, administration of anti-IL17 antibody intraperitoneally suppressed the expression of Muc5ac and Gob5 in the lung, and IL-13 production in lymph nodes but increased the number of $CD8^+$ lymphocytes [32]. These observations are further evidence for a role for IL-17 in viral exacerbation of asthma.

Table 1. Responses and products released by the cells present in the respiratory tract when stimulated with IL-17.

Cell type	Response	*In vitro/in vivo*	Reference
CD8+ lymphocyte	Reduced RSV clearance	*in vivo*	[32]
Epithelial cells	IL-6, IL-8, PGE_2	*in vitro*	[64]
	MUC5B, MUC5AC	*in vitro*	[60,61]
	CCL20	*in vitro*	[65]
	beta defensin 2	*in vitro*	[66]
	IL-19 **	*in vitro*	[67]
Endothelial cells	IL-6, IL-8, PGE_2		
Lung microvascular endothelial cells	CXCL1 (GROα), CXCL5, and IL-8 *	*in vitro*	[68]
Fibroblasts	IL-6, IL-8, PGE_2	*in vitro*	[64] [69] *
Smooth muscle	AHR (OVA induced asthma)	*in vivo*	[70]
	Contraction	*in vitro*	

* IL-17 potentiates the response by IL-1 beta and TNFα. ** IL-17 potentiates the response by IL-13.

5. Summary

Th17 lymphocytes are important contributors to both protective immune responses and the pathology associated with RSV infection. The involvement of Th17 cells in the patho-physiology that accompanies RSV infections is of great topical interest. Measurements of IL-17 levels in plasma and BAL fluids from RSV-infected infants have indicated that the cytokine can be beneficial. These studies have also suggested that Th17 responses during RSV infections are independent of Th1 and Th2 responses and that they are, in some infants, supersede an immature/inadequate Th1 immune response in the newly born [39]. Studies of IL-17 in animal models and *in vitro* culture systems have revealed that the lack of INFγ-mediated response enhances Th17 response. Such a response is driven by IL-23 which is produced in preference to IL-12 [24,25]. *In vitro* systems and animal models have showed that IL-17 *per se*, or together with RSV RNA particles, can induce inflammatory cytokine and chemokine responses that promote the influx of neutrophils to sites of infection [32]. As have been shown in other models of inflammation, IL-17 can also orchestrate the development of tertiary lymphoid tissues in the lung [58,71,72]. These structures are termed inducible bronchus-associated lymphoid tissues and are similar to structures found in RA patients with pulmonary complications (an autoimmune disease associated with IL-17) [73]. In addition to enhancing the inflammatory response that accompanies RSV infections, IL-17 has also been shown to suppress the ability of CD8+ lymphocytes to kill virally-infected cells and reduce the viral load [32]. Furthermore, both *in vitro* and animal model studies have confirmed that IL-17 enhances mucus production by acting directly on epithelial cells. This mucus production was also shown to be accompanied by IL-13 production which acts synergistically with IL-17 to enhance mucus production. However, high levels of IL-13 were also reported to inhibit IL-17 production. The induction of IL-17 production by RSV infection exacerbates asthma through enhancing mucus production. It is intriguing that IL-17F was not upregulated concomitant with IL-17A in one model of RSV infection [32]. Further studies to determine if IL-17F has a distinct role in RSV infection are warranted. The involvement of other Th17 cytokines, such as IL-21 and IL-22 in RSV patho-physiology also remains to be determined.

Taken together, studies of infected individuals and animal models have revealed that IL-17 can have both beneficial and pathogenic effects during RSV infection. In animal models, just as in cases of patients with asthma, IL-17 induces pathology by enhancing neutrophil influx, mucus and IL-13 production. However, the beneficial effects of IL-17 continue to be debated. It is intriguing to note that although Th17 lymphocytes have evolved together with the rest of the adaptive immune system, the emergence of the IL-17 family of cytokines predates chordates [74]. Th17 lymphocytes differentiate in response to inflammatory cytokines, preferably with low level of TCR engagement and their expansion is favoured by low oxygen levels [21,22]. The cells might, therefore, emerge as a weak alternative to the more efficient antiviral response mediated by a missing, or immature/inadequate Th1 lymphocyte response. Under such circumstances, Th17 lymphocytes may provide a response that straddles adaptive and innate immune responses resulting in mucus release, neutrophil influx and augmentation of local tertiary lymphoid structures.

Acknowledgments

Studies of the role of IL-17 in arthritis carried out in our laboratory are generously supported by a research grant from Pfizer.

References

1. Milner, J.D.; Brenchley, J.M.; Laurence, A.; Freeman, A.F.; Hill, B.J.; Elias, K.M.; Kanno, Y.; Spalding, C.; Elloumi, H.Z.; Paulson, M.L.; *et al.* Impaired T(H)17 cell differentiation in subjects with autosomal dominant hyper–IgE syndrome. *Nature* **2008**, *452*, 773–776.

2. Chen, Z.; O'Shea, J.J. Th17 cells: A new fate for differentiating helper T cells. *Immunol. Res.* **2008**, *41*, 87–102.

3. Sutton, C.; Brereton, C.; Keogh, B.; Mills, K.H.G.; Lavelle, E.C. A crucial role for interleukin (IL)–1 in the induction of IL–17–producing T cells that mediate autoimmune encephalomyelitis. *J. Exp. Med.* **2006**, *203*, 1685–1691.

4. Toussirot, E. The IL23/Th17 pathway as a therapeutic target in chronic inflammatory diseases. *Inflamm. Allergy Drug Targets* **2012**, *11*, 159–168.

5. Leonardi, C.; Matheson, R.; Zachariae, C.; Cameron, G.; Li, L.; Edson-Heredia, E.; Braun, D.; Banerjee, S. Anti–interleukin–17 monoclonal antibody ixekizumab in chronic plaque psoriasis. *N. Engl. J. Med.* **2012**, *366*, 1190–1199.

6. Papp, K.A.; Leonardi, C.; Menter, A.; Ortonne, J.-P.; Krueger, J.G.; Kricorian, G.; Aras, G.; Li, J.; Russell, C.B.; Thompson, E.H.Z.; *et al.* Brodalumab, an anti–interleukin–17–receptor antibody for psoriasis. *N. Engl. J. Med.* **2012**, *366*, 1181–1189.

7. Gaffen, S.L. Recent advances in the IL–17 cytokine family. *Curr. Opin. Immunol.* **2011**, *23*, 613–619.

8. Khader, S.A.; Gaffen, S.L.; Kolls, J.K. Th17 cells at the crossroads of innate and adaptive immunity against infectious diseases at the mucosa. *Mucosal Immunol.* **2009**, *2*, 403–411.

9. Hartupee, J.; Liu, C.; Novotny, M.; Li, X.; Hamilton, T. IL–17 enhances chemokine gene expression through mRNA stabilization. *J. Immunol.* **2007**, *179*, 4135–4141.

10. Zhu, S.; Pan, W.; Song, X.; Liu, Y.; Shao, X.; Tang, Y.; Liang, D.; He, D.; Wang, H.; Liu, W.; *et al.* The microRNA miR–23b suppresses IL–17–associated autoimmune inflammation by targeting TAB2, TAB3 and IKK–alpha. *Nat. Med.* **2012**, *18*, 1077–1086.

11. Jaffar, Z.; Ferrini, M.E.; Herritt, L.A.; Roberts, K. Cutting edge: Lung mucosal Th17–mediated responses induce polymeric Ig receptor expression by the airway epithelium and elevate secretory IgA levels. *J. Immunol.* **2009**, *182*, 4507–4511.

12. Mitsdoerffera, M.; Leea, Y.; Jägera, A.; Kimb, H.-J.; Kornc, T.; Koolsd, J.K.; Cantorb, H.; Bettellie, E.; Kuchrooa, V.K. Proinflammatory T helper type 17 cells are effective B–cell helpers. *Proc. Natl. Acad. Sci. USA* **2010**, *107*, 14292–14297.

13. Dodd, J.S.; Clark, D.; Muir, R.; Korpis, C.; Openshaw P.J. Endogenous IL–21 regulates pathogenic mucosal CD4 T–cell responses during enhanced RSV disease in mice. *Mucosal Immunol.* **2013**, *6*, 704–717.

14. Zheng, Y.; Valdez, P.A.; Danilenko, D.M.; Hu, Y.; Sa, S.M.; Gong, Q.; Abbas, A.R.; Modrusan, Z.; Ghilardi, N.; de Sauvage, F.J.; *et al.* Interleukin–22 mediates early host defense against attaching and effacing bacterial pathogens. *Nat. Med.* **2008**, *14*, 282–289.

15. Shaw, M.H.; Kamada, N.; Kim, Y.G.; Núñez, G. Microbiota–induced IL–1beta, but not IL–6, is critical for the development of steady–state TH17 cells in the intestine. *J. Exp. Med.* **2012**, *209*, 251–258.

16. Zhou, L.; Ivanov, I.I.; Spolski, R.; Min, R.; Shenderov, K.; Egawa, T.; Levy, D.E.; Leonard, W.J.; Littman, D.R. IL–6 programs T(H)–17 cell differentiation by promoting sequential engagement of the IL–21 and IL–23 pathways. *Nat. Immunol.* **2007**, *8*, 967–974.

17. Boniface, K.; Bak-Jensen, K.S.; Li, Y.; Blumenschein, W.M.; McGeachy, M.J.; McClanahan, T.K.; McKenzie, B.S.; Kastelein, R.A.; Cua, D.J.; de Waal Malefyt, R. Prostaglandin E2 regulates Th17 cell differentiation and function through cyclic AMP and EP2/EP4 receptor signaling. *J. Exp. Med.* **2009**, *206*,535–548.

18. Ivanov, I.I.; McKenzie, B.S.; Zhou, L.; Tadokoro, C.E.; Lepelley, A.; Lafaille, J.J.; Cua, D.J.; Littman, D.R. The orphan nuclear receptor RORgammat directs the differentiation program of proinflammatory IL–17+ T helper cells. *Cell* **2006**, *126*, 1121–1133.

19. Purvis, H.A.; Stoop, J.N.; Mann, J.; Woods, S.; Kozijn, A.E.; Hambleton, S.; Robinson, J.H.; Isaacs, J.D.; Anderson, A.E.; Hilkens, C.M. Low–strength T–cell activation promotes Th17 responses. *Blood* **2010**, *116*, 4829–4837.

20. Liu, X.K.; Lin, X.; Gaffen, S.L. Crucial role for nuclear factor of activated T cells in T cell receptor–mediated regulation of human interleukin–17. *J. Biol. Chem.* **2004**, *279*, 52762–52771.

21. Dang, E.V.; Barbi, J.; Yang, H.Y.; Jinasena, D.; Yu, H.; Zheng, Y.; Bordman, Z.; Fu, J.; Kim, Y.; Yen, H.R.; *et al.* Control of T(H)17/T(reg) balance by hypoxia–inducible factor 1. *Cell* **2011**, *146*, 772–784.

22. Ikejiri, A.; Nagai, S.; Goda, N.; Kurebayashi, Y.; Osada-Oka, M.; Takubo, K.; Suda, T.; Koyasu, S. Dynamic regulation of Th17 differentiation by oxygen concentrations. *Int. Immunol.* **2012**, *24*, 137–146.

23. Hirota, K.; Duarte, J.H.; Veldhoen, M.; Hornsby, E.; Li, Y.; Cua, D.J.; Ahlfors, H.; Wilhelm, C.; Tolaini, M.; Menzel, U.; *et al.* Fate mapping of IL–17–producing T cells in inflammatory responses. *Nat. Immunol.* **2011**, *12*, 255–263.

24. Lukacs, N.W.; Smit, J.J.; Mukherjee, S.; Morris, S.B.; Nunez, G.; Lindell, D.M. Respiratory virus–induced TLR7 activation controls IL–17–associated increased mucus via IL–23 regulation. *J. Immunol.* **2010**, *185*, 2231–2239.

25. Hashimoto, K.; Durbin, J.E.; Zhou, W.; Collins, R.D.; Ho, S.B.; Kolls, J.K.; Dubin, P.J.; Sheller, J.R.; Goleniewska, K.; O'Neal, J.F.; *et al.* Respiratory syncytial virus infection in the absence of STAT 1 results in airway dysfunction, airway mucus, and augmented IL–17 levels. *J. Allergy Clin. Immunol.* **2005**, *116*, 550–557.

26. Di Stefano, A.; Caramori, G.; Gnemmi, I.; Contoli, M.; Vicari, C.; Capelli, A.; Magno, F.; D'Anna, S.E.; Zanini, A.; Brun, P.; *et al.* T helper type 17–related cytokine expression is increased in the bronchial mucosa of stable chronic obstructive pulmonary disease patients. *Clin. Exp. Immunol.* **2009**, *157*, 316–324.

27. Vargas-Rojas, M.I.; Ramírez-Venegas, A.; Limón-Camacho, L.; Ochoa, L.; Hernández-Zenteno, R.; Sansores, R.H. Increase of Th17 cells in peripheral blood of patients with chronic obstructive pulmonary disease. *Respir. Med.* **2011**, *105*, 1648–1654.

28. Wilson, R.H.; Whitehead, G.S.; Nakano, H.; Free, M.E.; Kolls, J.K.; Cook, D.N. Allergic sensitization through the airway primes Th17–dependent neutrophilia and airway hyperresponsiveness. *Am. J. Respir. Crit. Care Med.* **2009**, *180*, 720–730.

29. Zhao, Y.; Yang, J.; Gao, Y.D.; Guo, W. Th17 immunity in patients with allergic asthma. *Int. Arch. Allergy Immunol.* **2010**, *151*, 297–307.

30. Yang, X.O.; Chang, S.H.; Park, H.; Nurieva, R.; Shah, B.; Acero, L.; Wang, Y.H.; Schluns, K.S.; Broaddus, R.R.; Zhu, Z.; *et al.* Regulation of inflammatory responses by IL–17F. *J. Exp. Med.* **2008**, *205*, 1063–1075.

31. Faber, T.E.; Groen, H.; Welfing, M.; Jansen, K.J.; Bont, L.J. Specific increase in local IL–17 production during recovery from primary RSV bronchiolitis. *J. Med. Virol.* **2012**, *84*, 1084–1088.

32. Mukherjee, S.; Lindell, D.M.; Berlin, A.A.; Morris, S.B.; Shanley, T.P.; Hershenson, M.B.; Lukacs, N.W. IL–17–induced pulmonary pathogenesis during respiratory viral infection and exacerbation of allergic disease. *Am. J. Pathol.* **2011**, *179*, 248–258.

33. Newcomb, D.C.; Boswell, M.G.; Huckabee, M.M.; Goleniewska, K.; Dulek, D.E.; Reiss, S.; Lukacs, N.W.; Kolls, J.K.; Peebles, R.S, Jr. IL–13 regulates Th17 secretion of IL–17A in an IL–10–dependent manner. *J. Immunol.* **2012**, *188*, 1027–1035.

34. Polack, F.P.; Irusta, P.M.; Hoffman, S.J.; Schiatti, M.P.; Melendi, G.A.; Delgado, M.F.; Laham, F.R.; Thumar, B.; Hendry, R.M.; Melero, J.A.; *et al.* The cysteine–rich region of respiratory syncytial virus attachment protein inhibits innate immunity elicited by the virus and endotoxin. *Proc. Natl. Acad. Sci. USA* **2005**, *102*, 8996–9001.

35. Hall, C.B.; Weinberg, G.A.; Iwane, M.K.; Blumkin A.K.; Edwards, K.M.; Staat, M.A.; Auinger, P.; Griffin, M.R.; Poehling, K.A.; Erdma, D.; *et al.* The burden of respiratory syncytial virus infection in young children. *N. Engl. J. Med.* **2009**, *360*, 588–598.

36. Zhang, L.; Peeples, M.E.; Boucher, R.C.; Collins, P.L.; Pickles, R.J. Respiratory syncytial virus infection of human airway epithelial cells is polarized, specific to ciliated cells, and without obvious cytopathology. *J. Virol.* **2002**, *76*, 5654–5666.

37. Habibi, M.S.; Openshaw, P.J. Benefit and harm from immunity to respiratory syncytial virus: Implications for treatment. *Curr. Opin. Infect. Dis.* **2012**, *25*, 687–694.

38. Panuska, J.R.; Cirino, N.M.; Midulla, F.; Despot, J.E.; McFadden, E.R., Jr.; Huang, Y.T. Productive infection of isolated human alveolar macrophages by respiratory syncytial virus. *J. Clin. Investig.* **1990**, *86*, 113–119.

39. Thornburg, N.J.; Shepherd, B.; Crowe, J.E., Jr. Transforming growth factor beta is a major regulator of human neonatal immune responses following respiratory syncytial virus infection. *J. Virol.* **2010**, *84*, 12895–12902.

40. Polack, F.P.; Teng, M.N.; Collins, P.L.; Prince, G.A.; Exner, M.; Regele, H.; Lirman, D.D.; Rabold, R.; Hoffman, S.J.; Karp, C.L.; *et al.* A role for immune complexes in enhanced respiratory syncytial virus disease. *J. Exp. Med.* **2002**, *196*, 859–865.

41. McNamara, P.S.; Ritson, P.; Selby, A.; Hart, C.A.; Smyth, R.L. Bronchoalveolar lavage cellularity in infants with severe respiratory syncytial virus bronchiolitis. *Arch. Dis. Child.* **2003**, *88*, 922–926.

42. Lukens, M.V.; van de Pol, A.C.; Coenjaerts, F.E.; Jansen, N.J.; Kamp, V.M.; Kimpen, J.L.; Rossen, J.W.; Ulfman, L.H.; Tacke, C.E.; Viveen, M.C.; *et al.* A systemic neutrophil response precedes robust CD8(+) T–cell activation during natural respiratory syncytial virus infection in infants. *J. Virol.* **2010**, *84*, 2374–2383.

43. Lukens, M.V.; Kruijsen, D.; Coenjaerts, F.E.; Kimpen, J.L.L.; van Bleek, G.M. Respiratory syncytial virus–induced activation and migration of respiratory dendritic cells and subsequent antigen presentation in the lung–draining lymph node. *J. Virol.* **2009**, *83*, 7235–7243.

44. Graham, B.S.; Bunton, L.A.; Wright, P.F.; Karzon, D.T. Role of T lymphocyte subsets in the pathogenesis of primary infection and rechallenge with respiratory syncytial virus in mice. *J. Clin. Investig.* **1991**, *88*, 1026–1033.

45. Averbuch, D.; Chapgier, A.; Boisson–Dupuis, S.; Casanova, J.L.; Engelhard, D. The clinical spectrum of patients with deficiency of Signal Transducer and Activator of Transcription–1. *Pediatr. Infect. Dis. J.* **2011**, *30*, 352–355.

46. Durbin, J.E.; Johnson, T.R.; Durbin, R.K.; Mertz, S.E.; Morotti, R.A.; Peebles, R.S.; Graham, B.S. The role of IFN in respiratory syncytial virus pathogenesis. *J. Immunol.* **2002**, *168*, 2944–2952.

47. Welliver, R.C.; Wong, D.T.; Sun, M.; Middleton, E., Jr.; Vaughan, R.S.; Ogra, P.L. The development of respiratory syncytial virus–specific IgE and the release of histamine in nasopharyngeal secretions after infection. *N. Engl. J. Med.* **1981**, *305*, 841–846.

48. Mobbs, K.J.; Smyth, R.L.; O'Hea, U.; Ashby, D.; Ritson, P.; Hart, C.A. Cytokines in severe respiratory syncytial virus bronchiolitis. *Pediatr. Pulmonol.* **2002**, *33*, 449–452.

49. Hussell, T.; Spender, L.C.; Georgiou, A.; O'Garra, A.; Openshaw, P.J. Th1 and Th2 cytokine induction in pulmonary T cells during infection with respiratory syncytial virus. *J. Gen. Virol.* **1996**, *77*, 2447–2455.

50. Boelen, A.; Kwakkel, J.; Barends, M.; de Rond, L.; Dormans, J.; Kimman T. Effect of lack of Interleukin–4, Interleukin–12, Interleukin–18, or the Interferon–gamma receptor on virus replication, cytokine response, and lung pathology during respiratory syncytial virus infection in mice. *J. Med. Virol.* **2002**, *66*, 552–560.

51. Larranaga, C.L.; Ampuero, S.L.; Luchsinger, V.F.; Carrión, F.A.; Aguilar, N.V.; Morales, P.R.; Palomino, M.A.; Tapia, L.F.; Avendaño, L.F. Impaired immune response in severe human lower tract respiratory infection by respiratory syncytial virus. *Pediatr. Infect. Dis. J.* **2009**, *28*, 867–873.

52. Tregoning, J.S.; Schwarze, J. Respiratory viral infections in infants: Causes, clinical symptoms, virology, and immunology. *Clin. Microbiol. Rev.* **2010**, *23*, 74–98.

53. Goriely, S.; Vincart, B.; Stordeur, P.; Vekemans, J.; Willems, F.; Goldman, M.; De Wit, D. Deficient IL–12(p35) gene expression by dendritic cells derived from neonatal monocytes. *J. Immunol.* **2001**, *166*, 2141–2146.

54. Qin, L.; Hu, C.P.; Feng, J.T.; Xia, Q. Activation of lymphocytes induced by bronchial epithelial cells with prolonged RSV infection. *PLoS One* **2011**, *6*, e27113.

55. Bera, M.M.; Lu, B.; Martin, T.R.; Cui, S.; Rhein, L.M.; Gerard, C.; Gerard, N.P. Th17 cytokines are critical for respiratory syncytial virus–associated airway hyperreponsiveness through regulation by complement C3a and tachykinins. *J. Immunol.* **2011**, *187*, 4245–4255.

56. Ryzhakov, G.; Lai, C.C.; Blazek, K.; To, K.W.; Hussell, T.; Udalova, I. IL–17 boosts proinflammatory outcome of antiviral response in human cells. *J. Immunol.* **2011**, *187*, 5357–5362.

57. Davidson, S.; Kaiko, G.; Loh, Z.; Lalwani, A.; Zhang, V.; Spann, K.; Foo, S.Y.; Hansbro, N.; Uematsu, S.; Akira, S.; *et al.* Plasmacytoid dendritic cells promote host defense against acute pneumovirus infection via the TLR7–MyD88–dependent signaling pathway. *J. Immunol.* **2011**, *186*, 5938–5948.

58. Kallal, L.E.; Hartigan, A.J.; Hogaboam, C.M.; Schaller, M.A.; Lukacs, N.W. Inefficient lymph node sensitization during respiratory viral infection promotes IL–17–mediated lung pathology. *J. Immunol.* **2010**, *185*, 4137–4147.

59. Cannon, M.J.; Openshaw, P.J.; Askonas, B.A. Cytotoxic T cells clear virus but augment lung pathology in mice infected with respiratory syncytial virus. *J. Exp. Med.* **1988**, *168*, 1163–1168.

60. Chen, Y.; Thai, P.; Zhao, Y.H.; Ho, Y.S.; DeSouza, M.M.; Wu, R. Stimulation of airway mucin gene expression by interleukin (IL)–17 through IL–6 paracrine/autocrine loop. *J. Biol. Chem.* **2003**, *278*, 17036–17043.

61. Fujisawa, T.; Chang, M.M.; Velichko, S.; Thai, P.; Hung, L.Y.; Huang, F.; Phuong, N.; Chen, Y.; Wu, R. NF–kappaB mediates IL–1beta– and IL–17A–induced MUC5B expression in airway epithelial cells. *Am. J. Respir. Cell Mol. Biol.* **2011**, *45*, 246–252.

62. Newcomb, D.C.; Boswell, M.G.; Zhou, W.; Huckabee, M.M.; Goleniewska, K.; Sevin, C.M.; Hershey, G.K.; Kolls, J.K.; Peebles, R.S., Jr. Human TH17 cells express a functional IL–13 receptor and IL–13 attenuates IL–17A production. *J. Allergy Clin. Immunol.* **2011**, *127*, 1006–1013.

63. Hashimoto, K.; Graham, B.S.; Ho, S.B.; Adler, K.B.; Collins, R.D.; Olson, S.J.; Zhou, W.; Suzutani, T.; Jones, P.W.; Goleniewska, K.; *et al.* Respiratory syncytial virus in allergic lung inflammation increases Muc5ac and gob–5. *Am. J. Respir. Crit. Care Med.* **2004**, *170*, 306–312.

64. Fossiez, F.; Djossou, O.; Chomarat, P.; Flores-Romo, L.; Ait-Yahia, S.; Maat, C.; Pin, J.J.; Garrone, P.; Garcia, E.; Saeland, S.; *et al.* T cell interleukin–17 induces stromal cells to produce proinflammatory and hematopoietic cytokines. *J. Exp. Med.* **1996**, *183*, 2593–2603.

65. Kao, C.Y.; Huang, F.; Chen, Y.; Thai, P.; Wachi, S.; Kim, C.; Tam, L.; Wu, R. Up–regulation of CC chemokine ligand 20 expression in human airway epithelium by IL–17 through a JAK–independent but MEK/NF–kappaB–dependent signaling pathway. *J. Immunol.* **2005**, *175*, 6676–6685.

66. Kao, C.Y.; Chen, Y.; Thai, P.; Wachi, S.; Huang, F.; Kim, C.; Harper, R.W.; Wu, R. IL–17 markedly up–regulates beta–defensin–2 expression in human airway epithelium via JAK and NF–kappaB signaling pathways. *J. Immunol.* **2004**, *173*, 3482–3491.

67. Huang, F.; Wachi, S.; Thai, P.; Loukoianov, A.; Tan, K.H.; Forteza, R.M.; Wu, R. Potentiation of IL–19 expression in airway epithelia by IL–17A and IL–4/IL–13: Important implications in asthma. *J. Allergy Clin. Immunol.* **2008**, *121*, 1415–1421.

68. Fujie, H.; Niu, K.; Ohba, M.; Tomioka, Y.; Kitazawa, H.; Nagashima, K.; Ohrui, T.; Numasaki, M. A distinct regulatory role of Th17 cytokines IL–17A and IL–17F in chemokine secretion from lung microvascular endothelial cells. *Inflammation* **2012**, *35*, 1119–1131.

69. Katz, Y.; Nadiv, O.; Beer, Y. Interleukin–17 enhances tumor necrosis factor alpha–induced synthesis of interleukins 1,6, and 8 in skin and synovial fibroblasts: A possible role as a "fine–tuning cytokine" in inflammation processes. *Arthritis Rheum.* **2001**, *44*, 2176–2184.

70. Kudo, M.; Melton, A.C.; Chen, C.; Engler, M.B.; Huang, K.E.; Ren, X.; Wang, Y.; Bernstein, X.; Li, J.T.; Atabai, K.; *et al.* IL–17A produced by alphabeta T cells drives airway hyper–responsiveness in mice and enhances mouse and human airway smooth muscle contraction. *Nat. Med.* **2012**, *18*, 547–554.

71. Peters, A.; Pitcher, L.A.; Sullivan, J.M.; Mitsdoerffer, M.; Acton, S.E.; Franz, B.; Wucherpfennig, K.; Turley, S.; Carroll, M.C.; Sobel, R.A.; *et al.* Th17 cells induce ectopic lymphoid follicles in central nervous system tissue inflammation. *Immunity* **2011**, *35*, 986–996.

72. Rangel–Moreno, J.; Carragher, D.M.; de la Luz Garcia–Hernandez, M.; Hwang, J.Y.; Kusser, K.; Hartson, L.; Kolls, J.K.; Khader, S.A.; Randall, T.D. The development of inducible bronchus–associated lymphoid tissue depends on IL–17. *Nat. Immunol.* **2011**, *12*, 639–646.

73. Rangel–Moreno, J.; Hartson, L.; Navarro, C.; Gaxiola, M.; Selman, M.; Randall, T.D. Inducible bronchus–associated lymphoid tissue (iBALT) in patients with pulmonary complications of rheumatoid arthritis. *J. Clin. Investig.* **2006**, *116*, 3183–3194.

74. Chen, K.; McAleer, J.P.; Lin, Y.; Paterson, D.L.; Zheng, M.; Alcorn, J.F.; Weaver, C.T.; Kolls, J.K. Th17 cells mediate clade–specific, serotype–independent mucosal immunity. *Immunity* **2011**, *35*, 997–1009.

Permissions

The contributors of this book come from diverse backgrounds, making this book a truly international effort. This book will bring forth new frontiers with its revolutionizing research information and detailed analysis of the nascent developments around the world.

We would like to thank all the contributing authors for lending their expertise to make the book truly unique. They have played a crucial role in the development of this book. Without their invaluable contributions this book wouldn't have been possible. They have made vital efforts to compile up to date information on the varied aspects of this subject to make this book a valuable addition to the collection of many professionals and students.

This book was conceptualized with the vision of imparting up-to-date information and advanced data in this field. To ensure the same, a matchless editorial board was set up. Every individual on the board went through rigorous rounds of assessment to prove their worth. After which they invested a large part of their time researching and compiling the most relevant data for our readers.

The editorial board has been involved in producing this book since its inception. They have spent rigorous hours researching and exploring the diverse topics which have resulted in the successful publishing of this book. They have passed on their knowledge of decades through this book. To expedite this challenging task, the publisher supported the team at every step. A small team of assistant editors was also appointed to further simplify the editing procedure and attain best results for the readers.

Apart from the editorial board, the designing team has also invested a significant amount of their time in understanding the subject and creating the most relevant covers. They scrutinized every image to scout for the most suitable representation of the subject and create an appropriate cover for the book.

The publishing team has been an ardent support to the editorial, designing and production team. Their endless efforts to recruit the best for this project, has resulted in the accomplishment of this book. They are a veteran in the field of academics and their pool of knowledge is as vast as their experience in printing. Their expertise and guidance has proved useful at every step. Their uncompromising quality standards have made this book an exceptional effort. Their encouragement from time to time has been an inspiration for everyone.

The publisher and the editorial board hope that this book will prove to be a valuable piece of knowledge for researchers, students, practitioners and scholars across the globe.

List of Contributors

Paulo Vitor Marques Simas, Caroline Measso do Bonfim, Felipe Cavassan Nogueira, Claudia Márcia Aparecida Carareto and Paula Rahal
Universidade Estadual Paulista, Instituto de Biociências, Letras e Ciências Exatas de São José do Rio Preto, SP. Departamento de Biologia - Rua Cristóvão Colombo, 2265, Jardim Nazareth – Cep: 15054-000, Brazil

Deriane Elias Gomes and Fátima Pereira de Souza
Universidade Estadual Paulista, Instituto de Biociências, Letras e Ciências Exatas de São José do Rio Preto, SP. Departamento de Física - Rua Cristóvão Colombo, 2265, Jardim Nazareth – Cep: 15054-000 Brazil

Luiz Gustavo Araujo Gardinassi and Gustavo Rocha Garcia
Universidade de São Paulo, Faculdade de Medicina de Ribeirão Preto, SP. Departamento de Bioquímica e Imunologia – Av. dos Bandeirantes, 3900 Monte Alegre – Cep: 14049-900 Brazil

Antonieta Guerrero-Plata
Department of Pathobiological Sciences, Louisiana State University, Baton Rouge, LA 70803, USA
Center for Experimental Infectious Disease Research, Louisiana State University, Baton Rouge, LA 70803, USA

Elske van den Berg, Job B.M. van Woensel and Reinout A. Bem
Pediatric Intensive Care Unit, Emma Children's Hospital, Academic Medical Center, Meibergdreef 9, Amsterdam 1105 AZ, The Netherlands

Sumana Fathima
Provincial Laboratory for Public Health (ProvLab), 3030 Hospital Dr. NW, Calgary, AB T2N 4W4, Canada

Bonita E. Lee
University of Alberta, Room 3-588B, ECHA, 11405 – 87 Avenue, Edmonton, AB T6G 1C9, Canada

Jennifer May-Hadford
Public Health Agency of Canada, 130 Colonnade Road A.L. 6501H Ottawa, ON K1A 0K9, Canada

Shamir Mukhi
Canadian Network for Public Health Intelligence, Public Health Agency of Canada, 1015 Arlington St, Winnipeg, MB R3E 3R2, Canada

Steven J. Drews
Provincial Laboratory for Public Health (ProvLab), 3030 Hospital Dr. NW, Calgary, AB T2N 4W4, Canada
University of Calgary, 2500 University Drive Northwest, Calgary, AB T2N 1N4, Canada

Rajeev Rudraraju, Bart G. Jones, Robert Sealy and Sherri L. Surman
Department of Infectious Diseases, St. Jude Children's Research Hospital, 262 Danny Thomas Place, Memphis, TN 38105, USA

Julia L. Hurwitz
Department of Infectious Diseases, St. Jude Children's Research Hospital, 262 Danny Thomas Place, Memphis, TN 38105, USA
Department of Microbiology, Immunology and Biochemistry, University of Tennessee Health Science Center, 858 Madison Avenue, Memphis, TN 38163, USA

Sutthiwan Thammawat and Gamaliel Muchondo
Department of Microbiology and Infectious Diseases, Flinders University, Flinders Medical Centre, Bedford Park, SA 5042, Australia

Penelope Adamson, Tania Sadlon and David Gordon
Department of Microbiology and Infectious Diseases, Flinders University, Flinders Medical Centre, Bedford Park, SA 5042, Australia
Department of Microbiology and Infectious Diseases, SA Pathology, Flinders Medical Centre, Bedford Park, SA 5042, Australia

Deepthi Kolli and Xiaoyong Bao
Departments of Pediatrics, University of Texas Medical Branch, Galveston, TX 77550, USA

Antonella Casola
Departments of Pediatrics, University of Texas Medical Branch, Galveston, TX 77550, USA
Microbiology and Immunology, University of Texas Medical Branch, Galveston, TX 77550, USA
Sealy Center for Molecular Medicine, University of Texas Medical Branch, Galveston, TX 77550, USA

Peter Mastrangelo and Richard G. Hegele
Department of Laboratory Medicine and Pathobiology, University of Toronto, Toronto, ON M5S 1A8, Canada

Reagan G. Cox
Department of Pathology, Microbiology and Immunology, Vanderbilt University School of Medicine, 1161 21st Ave. S., Nashville, TN 37232, USA

John V. Williams
Departments of Pediatrics and Pathology, Microbiology, and Immunology, Vanderbilt University School of Medicine, 1161 21st Ave. S., Nashville, TN 37232, USA

Joseph B. Domachowske
Department of Pediatrics, SUNY Upstate Medical University, Syracuse, NY 13210, USA

Kimberly D. Dyer, Katia E. Garcia-Crespo, Stephanie Glineur and Helene F. Rosenberg
Laboratory of Allergic Diseases, National Institute of Allergy and Infectious Diseases, National Institutes of Health, Bethesda, MD 20892, USA

Lenneke E. M. Haas
Department of Intensive Care Medicine, Diakonessenhuis, Utrecht, 3582 KE, The Netherlands

Steven F. T. Thijsen and Karen A. Heemstra
Department of Microbiology, Diakonessenhuis, Utrecht, 3582 KE, The Netherlands

Leontine van Elden
Department of Pulmonary Diseases, Diakonessenhuis, Utrecht, 3582 KE, The Netherlands

Evelyn Rivera-Toledo and Beatríz Gómez
Department of Microbiology and Parasitology, Faculty of Medicine, Universidad Nacional Autónoma de México, Circuito exterior s/n, Ciudad Universitaria, México D.F., C.P. 04510, Mexico

Jonas Bystrom, Mohammed Al-Bogami and Rizgar A. Mageed
Bone and Joint Research Unit, William Harvey Research Institute, Queen Mary University of London, London EC1M 6BQ, UK

Nasra Al-Adhoubi and Ali S. Jawad
Department of Rheumatology, The Royal London Hospital, Mile End, Barts and The London, Queen Mary University of London, London EC1M 6BQ, UK

Index

Printed in the USA
CPSIA information can be obtained
at www.ICGtesting.com
JSHW051359091023
49903JS00006B/208